Imaging Diagnosis in Abdomen

Imaging Diagnosis in Abdomen

Guest Editors

Francescamaria Donati
Piero Boraschi

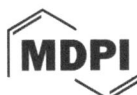

Basel • Beijing • Wuhan • Barcelona • Belgrade • Novi Sad • Cluj • Manchester

Guest Editors

Francescamaria Donati
Department of Radiological
Nuclear and Laboratory
Medicine
Pisa University Hospital
Pisa
Italy

Piero Boraschi
Department of Radiological
Nuclear and Laboratory
Medicine
Pisa University Hospital
Pisa
Italy

Editorial Office
MDPI AG
Grosspeteranlage 5
4052 Basel, Switzerland

This is a reprint of the Special Issue, published open access by the journal *Diagnostics* (ISSN 2075-4418), freely accessible at: www.mdpi.com/journal/diagnostics/special_issues/Abdomen_Imaging.

For citation purposes, cite each article independently as indicated on the article page online and using the guide below:

Lastname, A.A.; Lastname, B.B. Article Title. *Journal Name* **Year**, *Volume Number*, Page Range.

ISBN 978-3-7258-3566-9 (Hbk)
ISBN 978-3-7258-3565-2 (PDF)
https://doi.org/10.3390/books978-3-7258-3565-2

© 2025 by the authors. Articles in this book are Open Access and distributed under the Creative Commons Attribution (CC BY) license. The book as a whole is distributed by MDPI under the terms and conditions of the Creative Commons Attribution-NonCommercial-NoDerivs (CC BY-NC-ND) license (https://creativecommons.org/licenses/by-nc-nd/4.0/).

Contents

Piero Boraschi and Francescamaria Donati
Editorial for the Special Issue "Imaging Diagnosis in the Abdomen"—A Step Forward in Diagnostic Precision
Reprinted from: *Diagnostics* **2025**, *15*, 557, https://doi.org/10.3390/diagnostics15050557 1

Ana P. Borges, Célia Antunes and Filipe Caseiro-Alves
Spectral CT: Current Liver Applications
Reprinted from: *Diagnostics* **2023**, *13*, 1673, https://doi.org/10.3390/diagnostics13101673 3

Gianvito Candita, Sara Rossi, Karolina Cwiklinska, Salvatore Claudio Fanni, Dania Cioni, Riccardo Lencioni and Emanuele Neri
Imaging Diagnosis of Hepatocellular Carcinoma: A State-of-the-Art Review
Reprinted from: *Diagnostics* **2023**, *13*, 625, https://doi.org/10.3390/diagnostics13040625 33

Paolo Niccolò Franco, Chiara Maria Spasiano, Cesare Maino, Elena De Ponti, Maria Ragusi, Teresa Giandola, et al.
Principles and Applications of Dual-Layer Spectral CT in Gastrointestinal Imaging
Reprinted from: *Diagnostics* **2023**, *13*, 1740, https://doi.org/10.3390/diagnostics13101740 50

Sikai Wang, Ping Dai, Guangyan Si, Mengsu Zeng and Mingliang Wang
Multi-Slice CT Features Predict Pathological Risk Classification in Gastric Stromal Tumors Larger Than 2 cm: A Retrospective Study
Reprinted from: *Diagnostics* **2023**, *13*, 3192, https://doi.org/10.3390/diagnostics13203192 63

Inga Zaborienė, Vestina Strakšytė, Povilas Ignatavičius, Giedrius Barauskas, Rūta Dambrauskienė and Kristina Žvinienė
Dynamic Contrast-Enhanced Magnetic Resonance Imaging for Measuring Perfusion in Pancreatic Ductal Adenocarcinoma and Different Tumor Grade: A Preliminary Single Center Study
Reprinted from: *Diagnostics* **2023**, *13*, 521, https://doi.org/10.3390/diagnostics13030521 74

Charikleia Triantopoulou, Sofia Gourtsoyianni, Dimitrios Karakaxas and Spiros Delis
Intraductal Papillary Mucinous Neoplasm of the Pancreas: A Challenging Diagnosis
Reprinted from: *Diagnostics* **2023**, *13*, 2015, https://doi.org/10.3390/diagnostics13122015 86

Ana Veron Sanchez, Nuria Santamaria Guinea, Silvia Cayon Somacarrera, Ilias Bennouna, Martina Pezzullo and Maria Antonietta Bali
Rare Solid Pancreatic Lesions on Cross-Sectional Imaging
Reprinted from: *Diagnostics* **2023**, *13*, 2719, https://doi.org/10.3390/diagnostics13162719 106

Sofia Gourtsoyianni, Michael Laniado, Luis Ros-Mendoza, Giancarlo Mansueto and Giulia A. Zamboni
The Spectrum of Solitary Benign Splenic Lesions—Imaging Clues for a Noninvasive Diagnosis
Reprinted from: *Diagnostics* **2023**, *13*, 2120, https://doi.org/10.3390/diagnostics13122120 148

Ana Veron Sanchez, Ilias Bennouna, Nicolas Coquelet, Jorge Cabo Bolado, Inmaculada Pinilla Fernandez, Luis A. Mullor Delgado, et al.
Unravelling Peritoneal Carcinomatosis Using Cross-Sectional Imaging Modalities
Reprinted from: *Diagnostics* **2023**, *13*, 2253, https://doi.org/10.3390/diagnostics13132253 161

Vincenza Granata, Roberta Fusco, Sergio Venanzio Setola, Igino Simonetti, Carmine Picone, Ester Simeone, et al.
Immunotherapy Assessment: A New Paradigm for Radiologists
Reprinted from: *Diagnostics* **2023**, *13*, 302, https://doi.org/10.3390/diagnostics13020302 . . . . . **200**

Damaris Neculoiu, Lavinia Claudia Neculoiu, Ramona Mihaela Popa and Rosana Mihaela Manea
The Many Hidden Faces of Gallbladder Carcinoma on CT and MRI Imaging—From A to Z
Reprinted from: *Diagnostics* **2024**, *14*, 475, https://doi.org/10.3390/diagnostics14050475 . . . . . **220**

Masumi Nagata, Keisuke Jimbo, Nobuyasu Arai, Kosuke Kashiwagi, Kaori Tokushima, Mitsuyoshi Suzuki, et al.
An Isolated Intestinal Juvenile Polyp Diagnosed by Abdominal Ultrasonography and Resected by Double-Balloon Endoscopy: A Case Report and Literature Review
Reprinted from: *Diagnostics* **2023**, *13*, 494, https://doi.org/10.3390/diagnostics13030494 . . . . . **238**

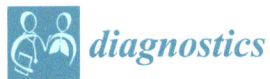 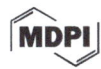

Editorial

Editorial for the Special Issue "Imaging Diagnosis in the Abdomen"—A Step Forward in Diagnostic Precision

Piero Boraschi * and Francescamaria Donati

2nd Unit of Radiology, Department of Radiological Nuclear and Laboratory Medicine, Pisa University Hospital, via Paradisa 2, 56124 Pisa, Italy; f.donati@med.unipi.it
* Correspondence: p.boraschi@gmail.com or p.boraschi@do.med.unipi.it
Tel./Fax: +39-050-996782; +39-3385054954

Abdominal imaging has undergone a significant transformation in recent years, driven by the rapid evolution of diagnostic technologies and their integration into clinical practice. With an expanding range of advanced imaging techniques—such as MRI with hepatobiliary contrast agents [1], diffusion and perfusion imaging [2], contrast-enhanced ultrasound [3], and spectral imaging via dual-energy, multi-energy, and photon-counting CT [4,5]—there has been a revolution in disease detection, staging, and treatment planning. These innovations have greatly enhanced diagnostic accuracy and patient care, particularly in the management of complex abdominal diseases.

Despite these advancements, significant gaps remain in our understanding of certain disease processes and the optimal utilization of emerging imaging modalities. One of the key challenges moving forward is the need for further validation and standardization of newer techniques, such as perfusion imaging and spectral CT, across diverse clinical settings. Additionally, while the potential of advanced imaging in assessing tumor vascularity and predicting prognosis is promising, more research is required to fully leverage these capabilities in personalized treatment planning [6].

The contributions to this Special Issue on *Imaging Diagnosis in the Abdomen* have addressed some of these gaps by presenting the latest advancements in imaging technology and its application in the diagnosis of complex abdominal conditions. For example, studies like Wang et al.'s exploration of multi-slice CT for predicting the pathological risk of gastric stromal tumors [7] and Zaborienė et al.'s use of dynamic contrast-enhanced MRI for assessing pancreatic cancer [8] highlight the ongoing progress in tumor characterization and risk stratification. However, while these studies underscore the promise of advanced imaging techniques, they also point to areas where additional research is needed, particularly in improving the accuracy of tumor grading and enhancing non-invasive diagnostic strategies.

Looking forward, the future of abdominal imaging will likely be shaped by further innovations in artificial intelligence (AI) and machine learning (ML) [9,10]. These technologies have the potential to automate image analysis, improve diagnostic accuracy, and facilitate real-time decision-making. In particular, AI and ML algorithms could play a critical role in integrating multimodal imaging data, enabling clinicians to generate more holistic assessments of disease. Moreover, the increasing role of imaging in monitoring therapeutic responses, particularly in immunotherapy [11,12], will require new frameworks to assess treatment efficacy and tailoring interventions.

While this Special Issue highlights the progress made in abdominal imaging, it also emphasizes the need for continued research to optimize imaging techniques for early disease detection, enhance diagnostic workflows, and improve patient outcomes. Future studies should focus on the development of more refined imaging biomarkers, the greater

Citation: Boraschi, P.; Donati, F. Editorial for the Special Issue "Imaging Diagnosis in the Abdomen"—A Step Forward in Diagnostic Precision. *Diagnostics* 2025, 15, 557. https://doi.org/10.3390/diagnostics15050557

Received: 6 February 2025
Accepted: 13 February 2025
Published: 25 February 2025

Citation: Boraschi, P.; Donati, F. Editorial for the Special Issue "Imaging Diagnosis in the Abdomen"—A Step Forward in Diagnostic Precision. *Diagnostics* 2025, 15, 557. https://doi.org/10.3390/diagnostics15050557

Copyright: © 2025 by the authors. Licensee MDPI, Basel, Switzerland. This article is an open access article distributed under the terms and conditions of the Creative Commons Attribution (CC BY) license (https://creativecommons.org/licenses/by/4.0/).

standardization of imaging protocols, and the potential applications of artificial intelligence in clinical radiology. These efforts will undoubtedly be pivotal in advancing the field and addressing the unmet needs in abdominal imaging.

The research presented in this Special Issue will continue to serve as a valuable resource, laying the foundation for future investigations and shaping the direction of abdominal imaging in the years to come.

Funding: This paper did not receive any specific grant from funding agencies in the public, commercial, or not-for-profit sectors.

Conflicts of Interest: The authors declare no conflicts of interest.

References

1. Seale, M.K.; Catalano, O.A.; Saini, S.; Hahn, P.F.; Sahani, D.V. Hepatobiliary Specific MR Contrast Agents: Role in Imaging the Liver and Biliary Tree. *Radiographics* **2009**, *29*, 1725–1748. [CrossRef] [PubMed]
2. Chandarana, H.; Taouli, B. Diffusion and Perfusion Imaging of the Liver. *Eur. J. Radiol.* **2010**, *76*, 348–358. [CrossRef] [PubMed]
3. D'Onofrio, M.; Crosara, S.; De Robertis, R.; Canestrini, S.; Mucelli, R.P. Contrast-Enhanced Ultrasound of Focal Liver Lesions. *AJR Am. J. Roentgenol.* **2015**, *205*, W56–W66. [CrossRef] [PubMed]
4. Greffier, J.; Villani, N.; Defez, D.; Dabli, D.; Si-Mohamed, S. Spectral CT Imaging: Technical Principles of Dual-Energy CT and Multi-Energy Photon-Counting CT. *Diagn. Interv. Imaging* **2023**, *104*, 167–177. [CrossRef] [PubMed]
5. Onishi, H.; Tsuboyama, T.; Nakamoto, A.; Ota, T.; Fukui, H.; Tatsumi, M.; Honda, T.; Kiso, K.; Matsumoto, S.; Kaketaka, K.; et al. Photon-Counting CT: Technical Features and Clinical Impact on Abdominal Imaging. *Abdom. Radiol.* **2024**, *49*, 4383–4399. [CrossRef] [PubMed]
6. European Society of Radiology (ESR). Medical Imaging in Personalised Medicine: A White Paper of the Research Committee of the European Society of Radiology (ESR). *Insights Imaging* **2015**, *6*, 141–155. [CrossRef] [PubMed]
7. Wang, S.; Dai, P.; Si, G.; Zeng, M.; Wang, M. Multi-Slice CT Features Predict Pathological Risk Classification in Gastric Stromal Tumors Larger Than 2 cm: A Retrospective Study. *Diagnostics* **2023**, *13*, 3192. [CrossRef] [PubMed]
8. Zaborienė, I.; Strakšytė, V.; Ignatavičius, P.; Barauskas, G.; Dambrauskienė, R.; Žvinienė, K. Dynamic Contrast-Enhanced Magnetic Resonance Imaging for Measuring Perfusion in Pancreatic Ductal Adenocarcinoma and Different Tumor Grade: A Preliminary Single Center Study. *Diagnostics* **2023**, *13*, 521. [CrossRef] [PubMed]
9. Syed, A.B.; Zoga, A.C. Artificial Intelligence in Radiology: Current Technology and Future Directions. *Semin. Musculoskelet. Radiol.* **2018**, *22*, 540–545. [CrossRef] [PubMed]
10. Najjar, R. Redefining Radiology: A Review of Artificial Intelligence Integration in Medical Imaging. *Diagnostics* **2023**, *13*, 2760. [CrossRef] [PubMed]
11. Nishino, M.; Hatabu, H.; Hodi, F.S. Imaging of Cancer Immunotherapy: Current Approaches and Future Directions. *Radiology* **2019**, *290*, 9–22. [CrossRef] [PubMed]
12. Dercle, L.; Sun, S.; Seban, R.D.; Mekki, A.; Sun, R.; Tselikas, L.; Hans, S.; Bernard-Tessier, A.; Bouvier, F.M.; Aide, N.; et al. Emerging and Evolving Concepts in Cancer Immunotherapy Imaging. *Radiology* **2023**, *306*, e239003. [CrossRef] [PubMed]

Disclaimer/Publisher's Note: The statements, opinions and data contained in all publications are solely those of the individual author(s) and contributor(s) and not of MDPI and/or the editor(s). MDPI and/or the editor(s) disclaim responsibility for any injury to people or property resulting from any ideas, methods, instructions or products referred to in the content.

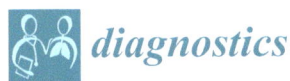

Review

Spectral CT: Current Liver Applications

Ana P. Borges [1,2,3,*], Célia Antunes [1,3] and Filipe Caseiro-Alves [1,2,3]

1. Medical Imaging Department, Coimbra University Hospitals, 3004-561 Coimbra, Portugal
2. Faculty of Medicine, University of Coimbra, 3004-504 Coimbra, Portugal
3. Academic and Clinical Centre of Coimbra, 3000-370 Coimbra, Portugal
* Correspondence: anapsborges0593@gmail.com

Abstract: Using two different energy levels, dual-energy computed tomography (DECT) allows for material differentiation, improves image quality and iodine conspicuity, and allows researchers the opportunity to determine iodine contrast and radiation dose reduction. Several commercialized platforms with different acquisition techniques are constantly being improved. Furthermore, DECT clinical applications and advantages are continually being reported in a wide range of diseases. We aimed to review the current applications of and challenges in using DECT in the treatment of liver diseases. The greater contrast provided by low-energy reconstructed images and the capability of iodine quantification have been mostly valuable for lesion detection and characterization, accurate staging, treatment response assessment, and thrombi characterization. Material decomposition techniques allow for the non-invasive quantification of fat/iron deposition and fibrosis. Reduced image quality with larger body sizes, cross-vendor and scanner variability, and long reconstruction time are among the limitations of DECT. Promising techniques for improving image quality with lower radiation dose include the deep learning imaging reconstruction method and novel spectral photon-counting computed tomography.

Keywords: dual-energy CT; spectral CT; liver disease; pancreatic disease; dual-source CT; fast kVp switching; dual-layer detector CT; split-filter; image quality; photon counting

Citation: Borges, A.P.; Antunes, C.; Caseiro-Alves, F. Spectral CT: Current Liver Applications. *Diagnostics* **2023**, *13*, 1673. https://doi.org/10.3390/diagnostics13101673

Academic Editors: Francescamaria Donati and Piero Boraschi

Received: 26 March 2023
Revised: 2 May 2023
Accepted: 4 May 2023
Published: 9 May 2023

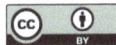

Copyright: © 2023 by the authors. Licensee MDPI, Basel, Switzerland. This article is an open access article distributed under the terms and conditions of the Creative Commons Attribution (CC BY) license (https://creativecommons.org/licenses/by/4.0/).

1. Introduction

Spectral or dual-energy computed tomography (DECT) has improved image contrast resolution by means of acquiring data at two different X-ray tube energy levels, allowing for the differentiation and quantification of tissue elements and materials with different attenuation properties at different energy levels, including those displaying similar attenuation at single-energy computed tomography (SECT), such as calcium and iodine [1,2].

Although DECT was first described in the mid-1970s, its introduction into clinical practice was only possible in 2006 due to technological advances [1,2]. There are different DECT platforms available: dual-source systems, consisting of two independent X-ray tubes operating at different energy levels which are then coupled with two independent detectors mounted orthogonally within the rotating gantry; and systems with a single source. The latter group includes systems with a source capable of rapidly switching between two energy levels, those with spectral separation at the level of a specialized detector composed of two layers with different energy sensitivity, and those with a filter that divides the spectrum into high- and low-energy beams at the source [1–3]. These systems have variable hardware requirements and diagnostic performances, subject to continuous improvement. Recently, photon-counting detector computed tomography (CT) imaging was introduced into clinical practice. This method is capable of counting and measuring the energy of individual photons, enabling improved material decomposition and image quality [4].

The postprocessing of DECT images offers a myriad of opportunities. These include improved contrast-to-noise ratio (CNR) and iodine conspicuity, both of which are capable of ameliorating diagnostic performance and confidence. Additionally, iodine dose reduction is possible, as is a reduction in radiation dose by the creation of virtual non-contrast (VNC) images [1–3]. These and many other advantages of DECT have resulted in the method's widespread use in various clinical applications that keep evolving. In liver imaging, its use is particularly helpful for lesion detection and characterization, accurate staging and treatment response assessment, non-invasive quantification of fat or iron liver deposition and fibrosis, thrombi characterization, and a number of other applications.

The main objective of this article is to review the current applications and challenges of DECT in liver diseases.

2. Materials and Methods

We conducted a comprehensive narrative review of the literature on the most relevant current applications of DECT in liver pathology. We searched MEDLINE and Embase databases for English or Portuguese papers published from January 2010 until December 2022, using the search terms "(((((dual energy) OR (spectral)) AND ((computed tomography) OR (CT))) AND ((liver) OR (hepatic))) AND (((((((((disease) OR (pathology)) OR (diagnosis)) OR (abnormalities)) OR (applications)) OR (advantages)) OR (drawbacks)) OR (limitations)) OR (future)) OR (advances))". Out of 1358 articles, we excluded 1 retracted and 985 duplicates. Out of the remaining 372 papers, those which were most relevant in relation to the search terms were chosen by means of title and abstract analysis, as well as article content when justified.

Representative images were obtained using a single-source twin-beam DECT scanner at 120 kVp (SOMATOM Go.Top, Siemens Healthineers) in the supine position (spiral pitch factor: 0.3; revolution time: 0.33 s; collimation: 38 × 0.6 mm; reconstruction kernel: Qr40; noise reduction iterative reconstruction algorithm: SAFIRE strength 3). Scanning was performed in a dual-energy mode during the late arterial phase or portal venous phase at a fixed delay of 35 and 70 s after the initiation of IV contrast medium injection, respectively. Patients received 150 mL of an intravenous nonionic contrast medium with an iodine concentration of 300 mg I/mL (Iopromide, Ultravist® 300, Bayer AG, Leverkusen, Germany). This was injected into an antecubital fossa vein at a flow rate of 3 mL/s using a power injector (MEDRAD® Salient, Bayer AG, Leverkusen, Germany). The post-processing of the data was performed using Syngo.via® software (Siemens Healthineers, Erlangen, Germany). Figure editing and schematic representations were performed using Microsoft Corporation software (Paint S, Version 7.0.3).

3. Results

3.1. Postprocessing Techniques

The postprocessing of dual-energy data can generate a wide range of useful information by means of material decomposition algorithms, which produce material-selective (decomposition images, mapping atomic number and density) and energy-selective images (reflecting attenuations at a particular photon-energy level). The use of effective atomic number and electron density maps (Figure 1) allow for semiquantitative assessment of materials, providing the calculated concentration of a specified material in units of mass per volume through measurements from a region of interest (ROI). The visual perception of qualitative differences may be improved via color overlay [5]. Different preselected materials (e.g., iodine, fat, calcium) may be quantified, color-coded, or subtracted. For instance, iodine may be superimposed onto grayscale images with a color gradient, generating iodine maps, or it may be subtracted, generating VNC images (Figure 2) [1,6]. The number of "decomposed" materials (usually two or three) depends on each manufacturer's mathematical model and their density values at different energy levels [7].

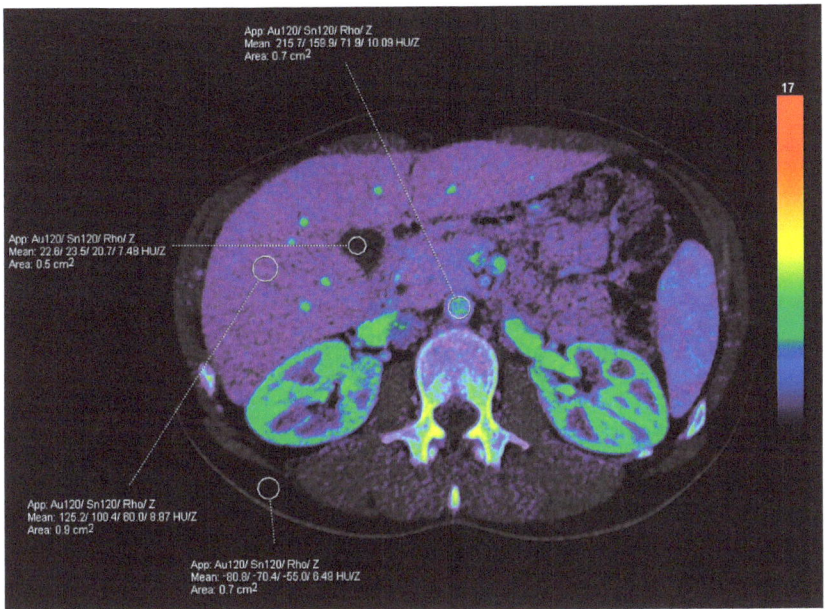

Figure 1. Rho/Z map application. Effective atomic number (Z_{eff}) and electron density (Rho) maps allow for the semiquantitative assessment of materials through measurements drawn within a region of interest (ROI), providing Z_{eff} and HU_{Rho} measurements which can be used to calculate the electron density relative to water (ρe). In the Siemens platform, the electron density values (HU_{Rho}) are converted into the Hounsfield unit scale, in which water has a value of 0 HU and air has a value of −1000 HU. The effective atomic number (Z) is presented in units of 1. The numbers provided in the measured ROI in this figure refer to the attenuation at the Au120 filter/attenuation at Sn120 filter/Rho value/Z value.

Although VNC images have shown reliability in multiple studies and may obviate the need for a true unenhanced acquisition (reducing radiation exposure and scan time), the attenuation values may vary among vendors and with different patient sizes and acquisition phases [2,8,9]. In fact, several studies have shown incomplete iodine subtraction in several abdominal organs, and attenuation differences vary among scanners, software applications, enhancement phase, body tissue, and patient size [10,11]. Additionally, calcifications may appear smaller or be unintentionally subtracted, and pre-existing hyperdense material containing iodine such as lipiodol chemoembolization material may be subtracted and consequently mistaken for contrast enhancement [2,8,12].

Low- and high-energy images may be reconstructed into 120-kilovolt peak (kVp)-like images to simulate the standard SECT scans, but these are less affected by beam-hardening artifacts [1]. Furthermore, the blended energy values may be chosen by the user (Figure 3), balancing the greater conspicuity of differences in contrast to enhancement (at the cost of higher image noise) with low energy values with the opposite effect of high-energy images [7].

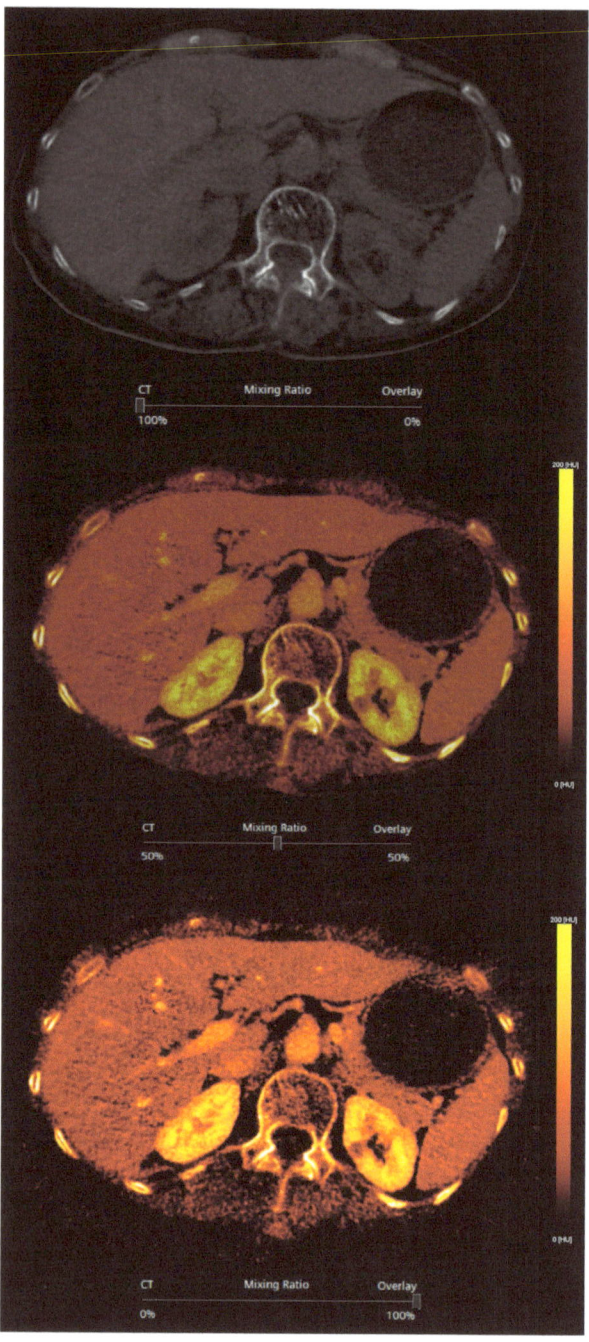

Figure 2. Iodine subtraction and overlay. Iodine may be subtracted, generating virtual non-contrast images (upper image), or superimposed onto grayscale images, generating iodine maps, at a configurable percentage of overlay (50% and 100% in the middle and bottom images, respectively).

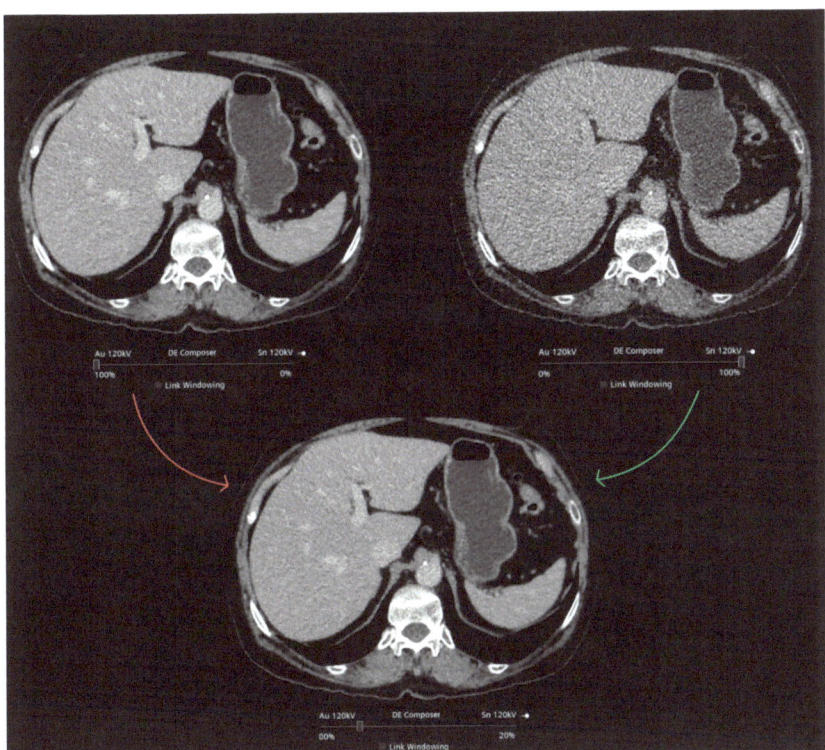

Figure 3. Blended dual-energy image reconstruction. The blended energy values may be chosen by the user, balancing the greater conspicuity of differences in contrast enhancement (at the cost of higher image noise) with low energy values, with the opposite effect of high-energy images. In this example from a TwinBeam DECT scanner (Siemens Healthineers), low- and high-energy beams are derived from a split-filter of gold (Au) and tin (Sn) at the X-ray tube.

Virtual monochromatic images (VMIs) mimic scans obtained at a single energy (Figure 4), described in terms of kiloelectronvolt (keV). Low-keV images improve iodine contrast and lesion conspicuity at the cost of greater noise, whereas high-keV images have less contrast but reduced beam hardening artifacts (Figure 5) and are susceptible to photon-starvation artifacts [6,8]. At 70 keV, these images have shown better objective and subjective image quality compared to conventional polychromatic 120-kVp images at the same radiation dose [13,14].

Spectral attenuation curves (Figure 6) are plots of X-ray beam attenuation measurements across a range of monochromatic energy levels (from 40 to 190 keV). These may be helpful in the characterization of specific materials based on the curve morphology [5].

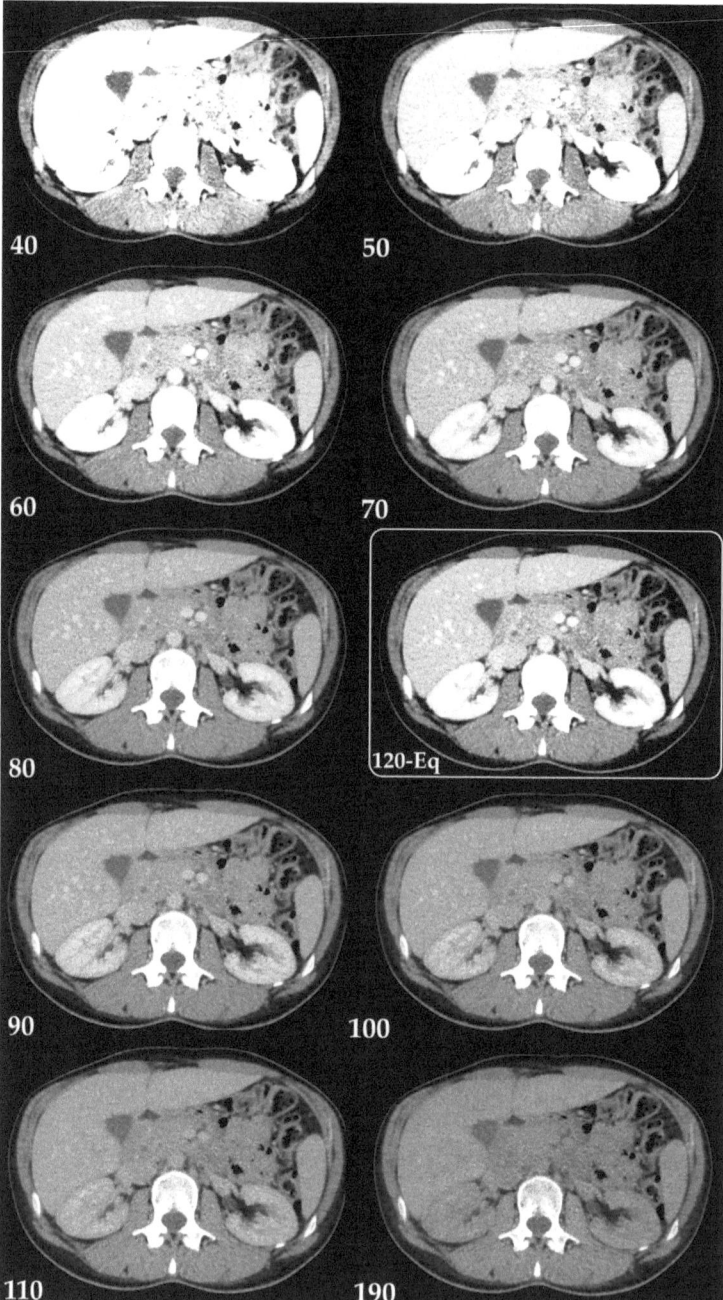

Figure 4. Virtual monochromatic images (Monoenergetic Plus advanced noise-optimized algorithm) from 40 keV to 190 keV in the axial plane (portal venous phase) and mixed 120-kVp-equivalent image (120-Eq). Window settings were kept constant for a more realistic comparability. Note the greater noise with low-keV images and the similarity of the 70 keV VMIs with the blended 120-kVp-equivalent image (120-Eq).

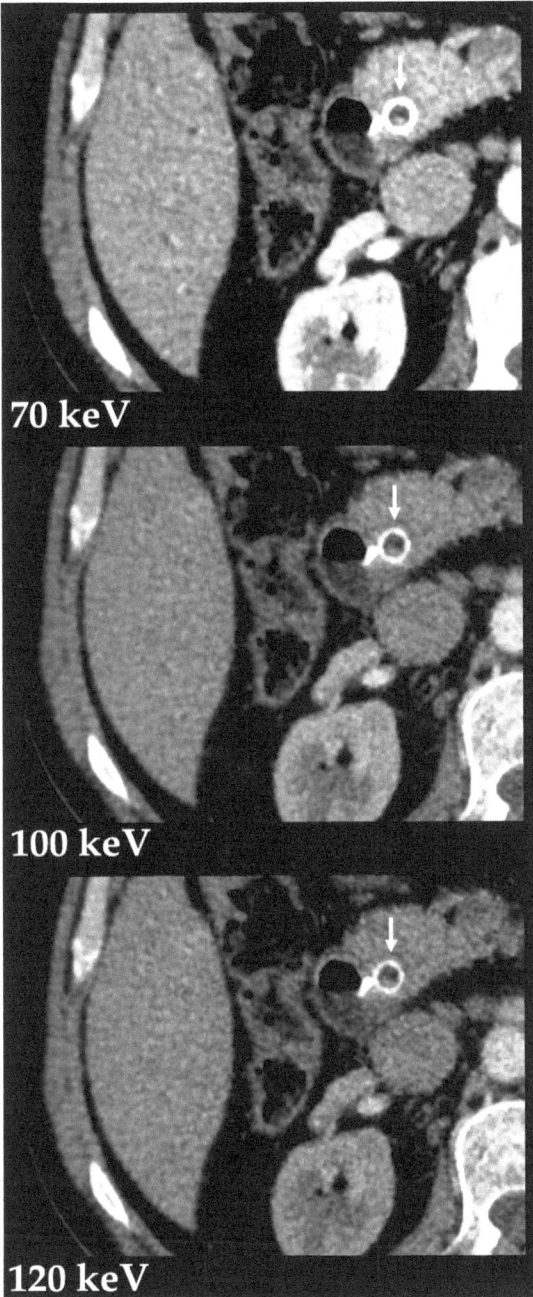

Figure 5. Metal artifact reduction with high-energy VMIs. Virtual monochromatic images (Monoenergetic Plus advanced noise-optimized algorithm) at 70, 100 and 120 keV in the axial plane (portal venous phase) show improved luminal depiction of a metallic biliary stent (arrow) with higher monoenergetic levels due to metal artifact reduction.

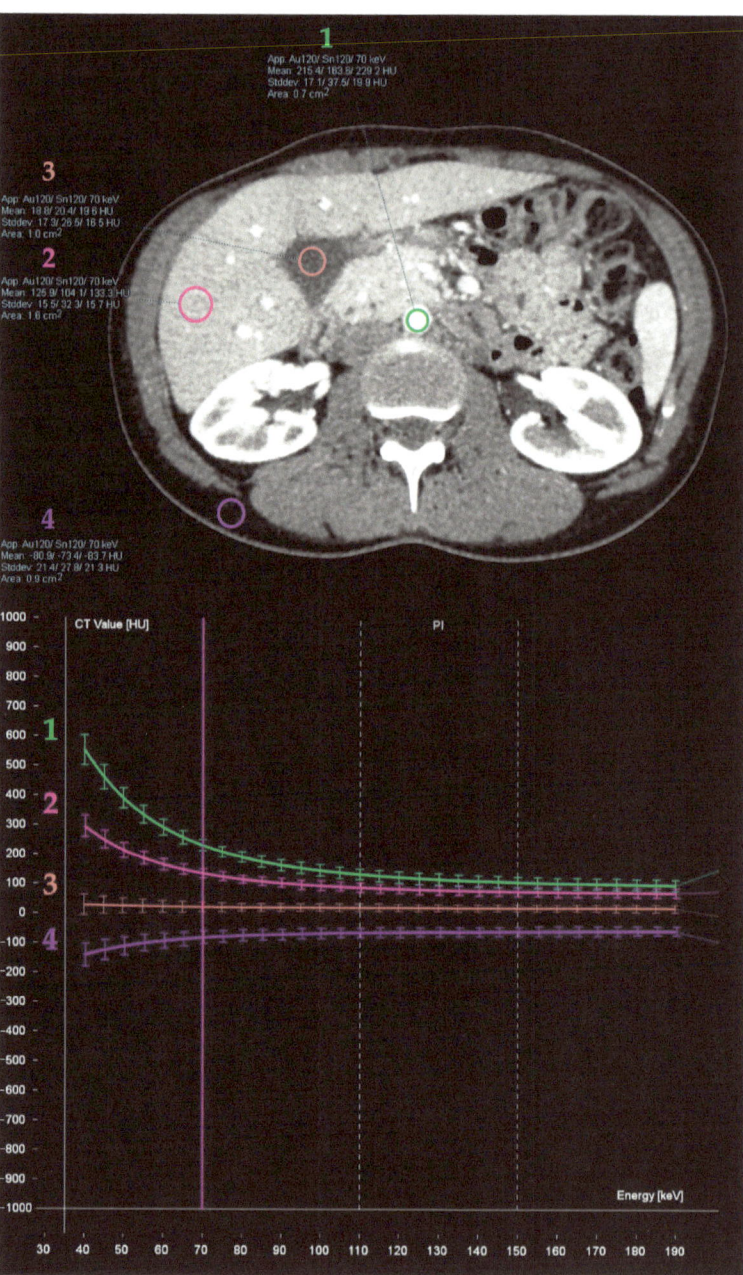

Figure 6. Spectral attenuation curves obtained from iodinated blood in aorta (1), liver parenchyma (2), bile in the gallbladder lumen (3), and abdominal wall fat (4). These are plots of X-ray beam attenuation measurements across a range of monochromatic energy levels, which may be helpful in the characterization of specific materials based on the curve morphology. Note the increasing attenuation of iodine (high atomic number material) at lower energies, as opposed to water materials (stable) and fat (decreasing).

3.2. Liver Diseases

3.2.1. Lesion Detection and Characterization

Hypervascular Lesions

Iodine is better depicted at lower-energy states given its low K-edge of 33.2 keV (material-specific minimum energy above which the attenuation peaks) and predominance of photoelectric interaction [2,15]. Therefore, the use of low tube voltage (80 kVp) can improve the visualization of hypervascular focal liver lesions, with lower radiation dose than exhibited by other methods. However, this comes at the cost of greater image noise [15]. Low-keV VMIs derived from DECT (from 40 to 70 keV) improve the detection of hypervascular liver lesions, including hepatocellular carcinoma (HCC) and hypervascular metastases [2,16,17]. Still, the selection of the optimal monoenergetic level is limited by the nonlinear behavior of noise with lowest-energy keV and by the patient body size [3,18]. These limitations were overcome with the development of an advanced noise-optimized VMIs reconstruction algorithm which combines the greater iodine attenuation at low virtual energies with the lower image noise at higher energies, providing improved diagnostic accuracy for detection of hypervascular lesions (Figures 7 and 8) [19]. Optimal monochromatic image sets have been determined in multiple studies (mostly 40 to 50/55 keV, the latter often preferred due to less image noise) [19–23].

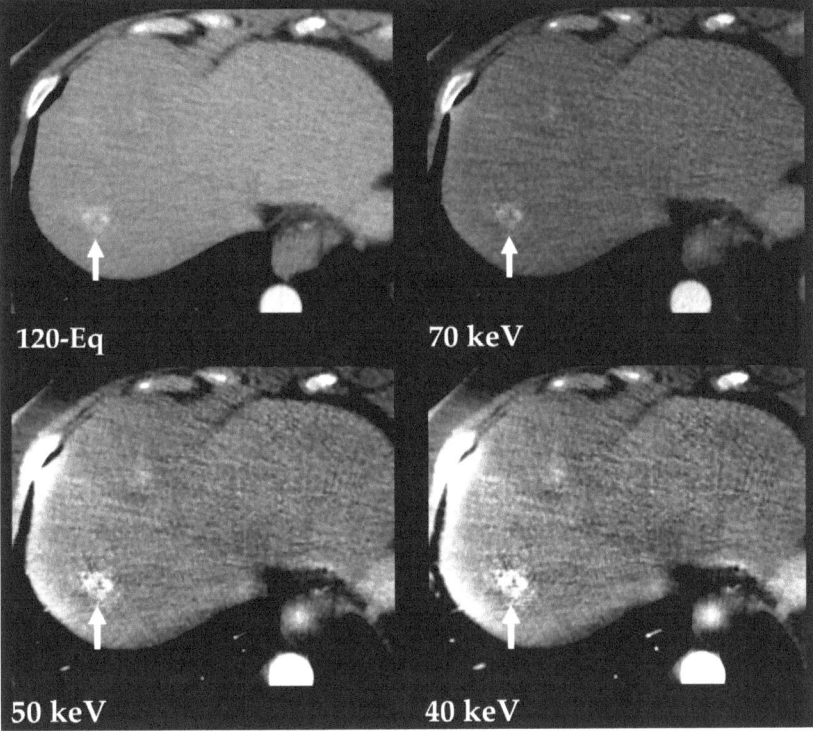

Figure 7. Hypervascular liver metastasis from a pancreatic neuroendocrine tumor, better depicted with low-energy VMIs (70, 50 and 40 keV) obtained from contrast-enhanced DECT in the arterial phase. Postprocessed low-energy VMIs (Monoenergetic Plus advanced noise-optimized algorithm) show the improved conspicuity of the lesion (arrow) compared to the blended 120-kVp-equivalent image (120-Eq) at the cost of increased image noise.

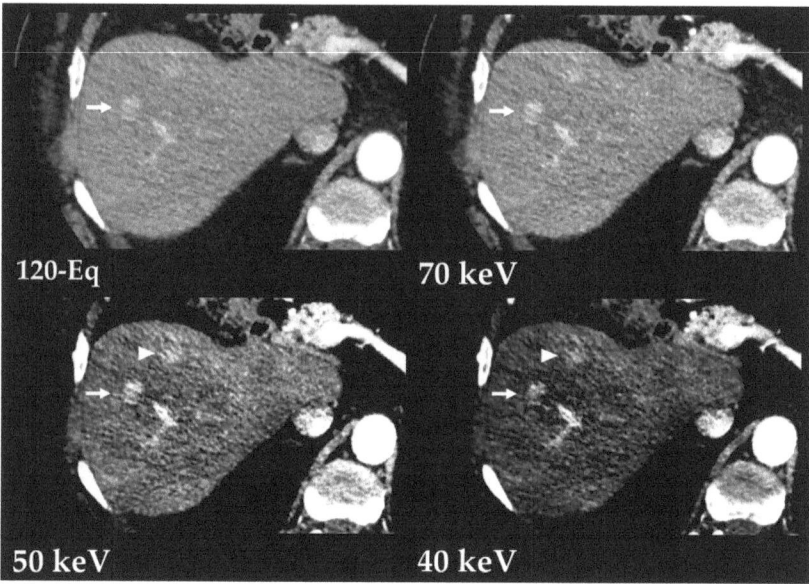

Figure 8. Multifocal hepatocellular carcinoma, better depicted with low-energy VMIs (70, 50 and 40 keV) obtained from contrast-enhanced DECT in the arterial phase. Postprocessed low-energy VMIs (Monoenergetic Plus advanced noise-optimized algorithm) show improved conspicuity of the larger lesion (arrow) compared to the blended 120-kVp-equivalent image (120-Eq) and allow the depiction of a smaller and more subtle lesions at lower keV (arrowhead) at the cost of increased image noise.

Low-energy VMIs also improve the detection of delayed enhancement in tumors with abundant desmoplastic reaction or fibrosis such as cholangiocarcinoma or combined hepatocellular carcinoma–cholangiocarcinoma [24].

Spectral attenuation curves may allow for an accurate discrimination between benign and malignant liver lesions [3,25,26], as well as for the differentiation of primary and metastatic liver neuroendocrine tumors [27].

Early recognition of portal vein and microvascular invasion from HCC is crucial for treatment decisions. Conventional CT only depicts larger vessel invasion, but several DECT parameters can accurately predict microvascular invasion [28]. Iodine quantification correlates with microvessel density and is strongly related with perfusion SECT parameters in HCC, with significantly lower radiation dose [29,30]. Combined with perfusion analysis, DECT predicts microvascular invasion, capsular invasion, and tumor grade, although it does so with a higher radiation dose exposure [31]. Peritumoral and intratumoral volumetric iodine concentration (IC), when used during the arterial phase (Figure 9), are useful for predicting microvascular invasion due to the significantly higher peritumoral normalized iodine concentration (NIC) [32]. Higher values of preoperative NIC in the arterial phase predict early recurrence after resection, meaning it can be a valuable predictive biomarker [33].

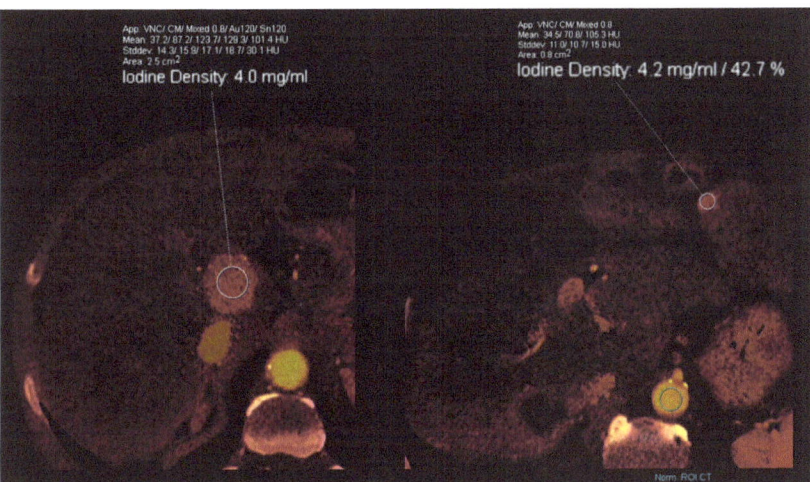

Figure 9. Iodine quantification of hepatocellular carcinomas (HCC). Intratumoral iodine concentration (**left image**) and normalized iodine concentration (**right image**) of HCC in two different patients, measured in the arterial phase. Higher values of preoperative iodine concentrations in the arterial phase predict early recurrence after resection, meaning that they can be valuable predictive biomarkers.

Hypovascular Lesions

The detection of hypovascular liver lesions is also improved with DECT, namely with the use of low kVp data, blending techniques, and monoenergetic imaging [3]. At low-keV images, these lesions show lower attenuation compared to the parenchyma in the portal venous phase (Figure 10) [34]. Optimal reported energy levels for lesion detectability have mostly ranged 40 and 50 keV [35–37], but may also be as high s 70 keV [38,39]. A study also reported highest CNR at 190 keV [40]. The improved definition of margins is useful in assessing the extent of diffuse infiltrative lesions [34].

Iodine maps are helpful in characterizing small hypoattenuating liver lesions, either found incidentally or in patients with a primary malignancy, thus allowing for the distinction between cysts and metastasis based on the absence or presence of iodine within the lesion (Figure 11) [41]. A threshold of 1.2 mg/mL in IC during the portal venous phase (at a fixed delay of 70 s after administration of 150 mL of iopamidol with a concentration of 300 mg I/mL at a flow rate of 3 mL/s) has been found to allow for better differentiation between benign and malignant small hypoattenuating lesions compared to the results obtained from conventional attenuation measurements [42]. In addition, the analysis of the spectral attenuation curve helps to confirm the presence of enhancement in equivocal cases, revealing an exponential increase in attenuation at lower-energy levels, as opposed to pseudoenhancement, which exhibits a flatter curve (Figure 12) [5]. Complex cysts may be also distinguished from simple cysts by means of subtle enhancement depiction [43].

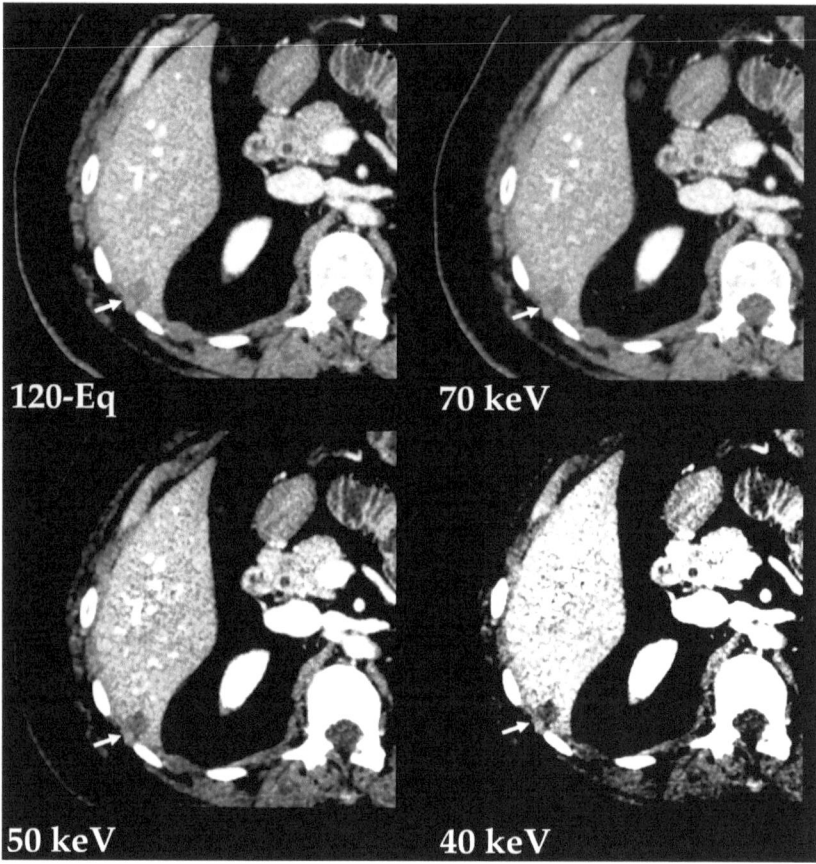

Figure 10. Improved depiction of a hypovascular liver lesion with low-energy VMIs. Contrast-enhanced DECT images in the portal venous phase show a hypovascular liver lesion (arrows). Post-processed low-energy VMIs (Monoenergetic Plus advanced noise-optimized algorithm by Siemens Healthineers) show improved conspicuity of the lesion margins compared to the blended 120-kVp-equivalent image (120-Eq) at the cost of increased image noise.

Liver abscesses can be difficult to differentiate from liver metastasis that develops central necrosis or cystic changes. Quantitative analysis performed by DECT has proven to be helpful as metastasis exhibits higher density, effective atomic number and iodine concentration, and lower fat concentration compared to abscesses. Additionally, the IC in the lesion wall in the venous and delayed phases is significantly higher for abscesses [44]. It is also helpful for differentiating liver abscesses from necrotic HCC [45] or small intrahepatic mass-forming cholangiocarcinomas [46].

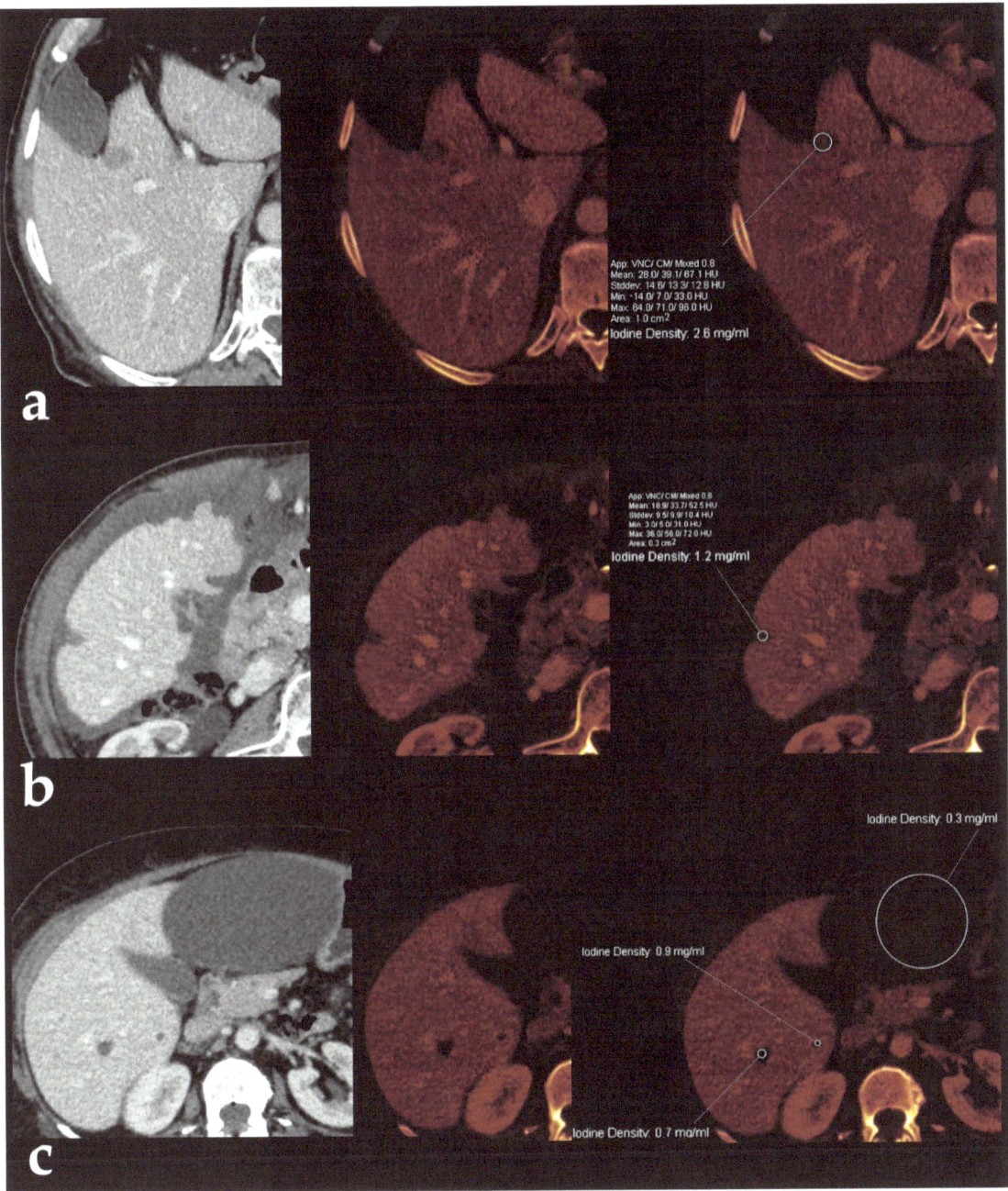

Figure 11. Iodine maps for characterization of hypodense liver lesions. Blended and iodine overlay images from contrast-enhanced DECT images in the portal venous phase in three different patients show small hypodense lesions with iodine densities of 2.6 mg/mL (**a**) and 1.2 mg/mL (**b**) in the cases of liver metastasis from carcinoid tumor and colorectal cancer, respectively, as opposed to simple liver cysts in the bottom images (**c**), which present less than 1 mg/mL of iodine concentration.

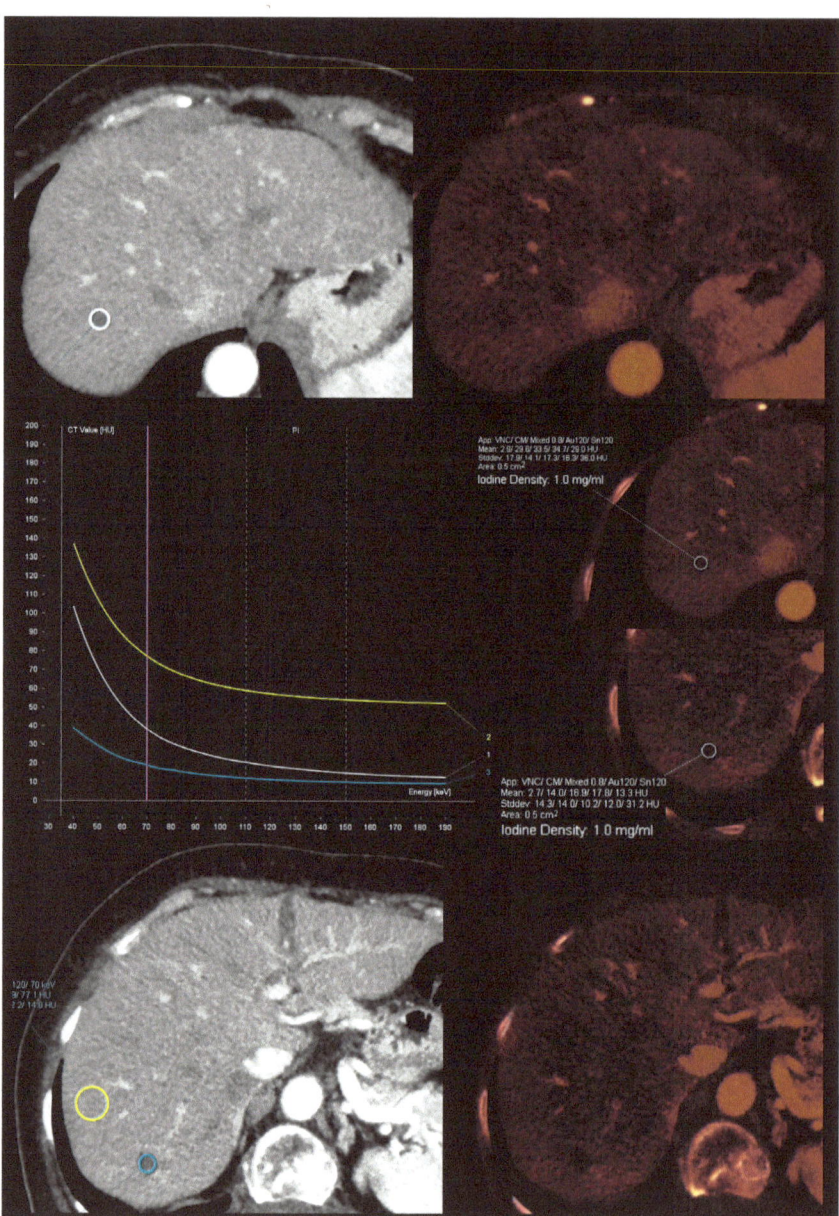

Figure 12. Spectral attenuation curves to confirm the presence of enhancement. Iodine overlay images from contrast-enhanced DECT images in the arterial phase show two small hypodense lesions with iodine density of 1 mg/mL. The superior lesion shows an exponential increase in attenuation at lower energy levels (white curve and circle), as opposed to pseudoenhancement from a cystic lesion, which exhibits a flatter curve (blue curve and circle). The yellow curve and circle correspond to liver parenchyma measurement and is shown for reference.

3.2.2. Treatment Response Evaluation

Sized-based tumor classification systems used to evaluate treatment response, such as version 1.1 of the response evaluation criteria in solid tumors (RECIST 1.1), are limited by variability in lesion target selection or measurement and by the non-consideration of lesion perfusion or composition (lesions with necrosis or myxoid degeneration may remain stable or increase in size despite successful treatment response) [5,6]. This is particularly problematic with emerging immunotherapy agents associated with unconventional response patterns (i.e., pseudo-progression) [6]. Antiangiogenic drugs can also be used to reduce vascularity without changing tumor size. Given its improved capability of vascularity assessment, DECT may serve as a reliable biomarker for tumor viability [5]. The evaluation of HCC angiogenesis with iodine quantification from DECT has shown promising results in animal models [6,47]. Volumetric iodine uptake changes from DECT iodine maps are also valuable for therapy response assessment in advanced HCC patients treated with sorafenib [48].

When evaluating HCC submitted to radiofrequency ablation (RFA), IC allows for accurate differentiation between residual or recurrent HCC, inflammatory reaction zone, and RFA lesions [49]. These parameters have shown the ability to predict the value of HCC progression well within 12 months [50].

In the early assessment after microwave ablation of HCC, 50 keV VMIs provide improved image quality and diagnostic confidence at determining technique efficacy. Additionally, IC is significantly higher in residual tumor compared to the reactive hyperemic rim [51,52].

Transarterial chemoembolization (TACE) is usually performed with a mixture of chemotherapeutic agents and lipiodol, followed by the administration of an embolic agent. Lipiodol deposition within the tumor correlates well with necrosis and predicts tumor recurrence and survival rate. It is not well observed in magnetic resonance imaging (MRI) [53], and its density impairs the detection of enhancing tumor on SECT [54]. Dual-energy CT is capable of lipiodol quantification, allowing more accurate detection of residual or recurrent disease [53–55]. Before TACE, NIC values in the arterial phase closely correlates with the grade of lipiodol accumulation in tumors, meaning it may be a parameter used for the selection of patients who are more likely to benefit from the treatment [56]. After TACE, the arterial phase spectral curve is steeper in the active tumor areas compared to necrotic areas, and the arterial iodine fraction is very good for differentiating tumor active area and adjacent normal hepatic parenchyma (Figures 13 and 14) [57]. Iodine overlay images are capable of discriminating between enhanced viable lesions and iodized oil accumulations [58].

A novel embolic bead has been proposed which would use bismuth as the radiopacifier, distinguishable from iodine on DECT, allowing for the identification of non-targeted delivery or undertreated tumors despite the presence of iodinated contrast agent. Furthermore, iodine-based and bismuth-based beads have the capacity to be loaded with different chemotherapy or immunotherapy drugs, allowing dual drug delivery. In vivo safety studies are still needed [59].

The degree of enhancement uptake after yttrium-90 radioembolization has proven to be a valuable tumor response marker [60]. The volumetric iodine uptake changes in intermediate-advanced HCC can predict response and correlate with overall survival [61].

An excellent correlation has also been demonstrated between DECT parameters and the Choi criteria for treatment response evaluation in liver metastasis from gastrointestinal stromal tumor [62]. This task is particularly difficult due to the presence of treatment-related changes including hemorrhage and calcification, which may have less influence on iodine concentration. A recent study introduced DECT vital iodine tumor burden criteria for posttreatment evaluation in these patients; these outperform RECIST 1.1 and mChoi criteria [63].

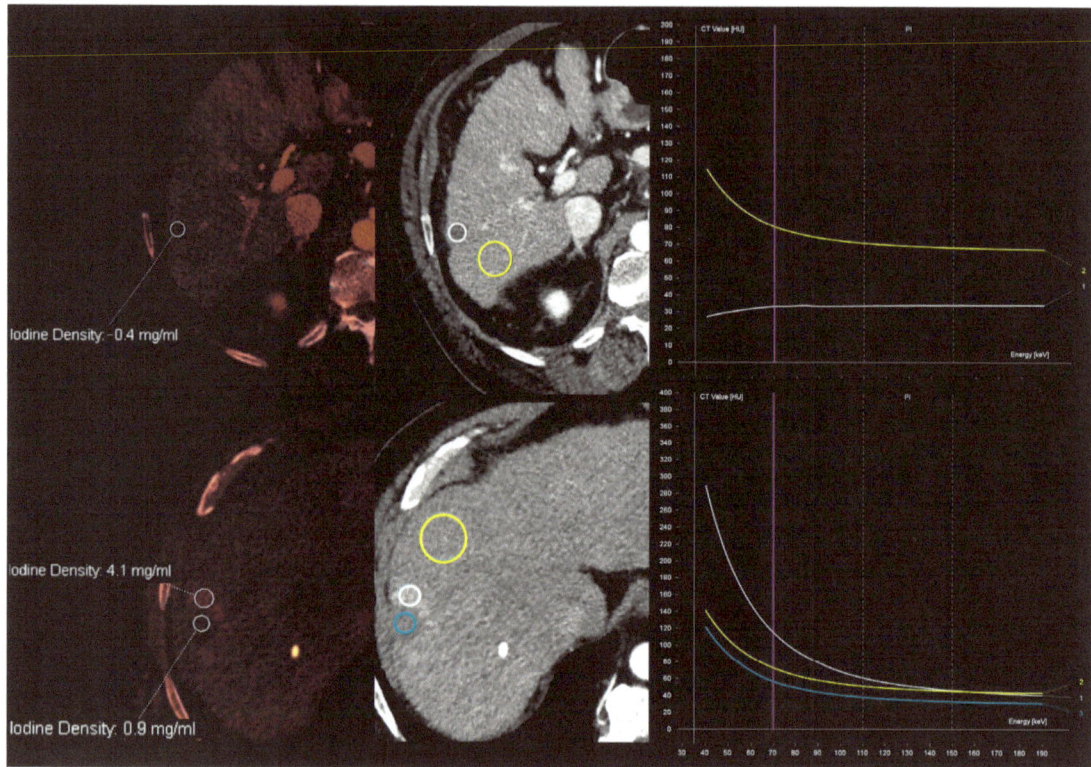

Figure 13. Iodine quantification and spectral attenuation curve analysis obtained from DECT during the arterial phase after transarterial chemoembolization of hepatocellular carcinoma with doxorubicin-eluting microspheres in two different patients. Top images show a hypodense area with iodine density of −0.4 mg/mL and a flat spectral attenuation curve (white curve and circle), consistent with necrotic area. The bottom images show a hypodense area with iodine density of 0.9 mg/mL and a flat spectral attenuation curve (blue curve and circle), with a peripheral thick rim exhibiting iodine density of 4.1 mg/mL and a steep descending spectral attenuation curve (white curve and circle), indicative of active tumor. Yellow curves and circles correspond to liver parenchyma measurements, for reference.

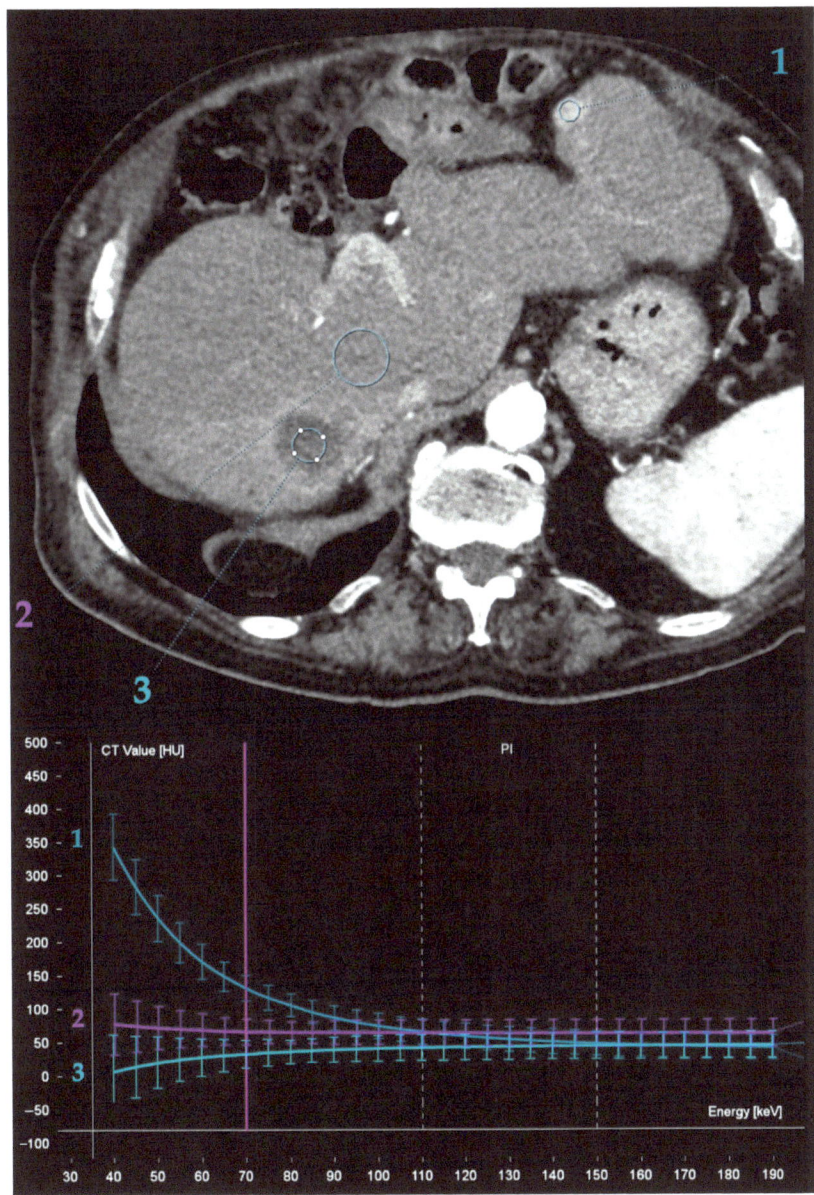

Figure 14. Spectral attenuation curve analysis obtained from DECT during late arterial phase after transarterial chemoembolization (TACE) of hepatocellular carcinoma (HCC) with doxorubicin-eluting microspheres. Recurrent HCC in the left lobe (1) exhibits a steep descending spectral attenuation curve, as opposed to the liver parenchyma (2) and the necrotic area of previous TACE (3).

3.2.3. Diffuse Liver Diseases

Although biopsy is still the reference standard for diagnosing diffuse liver disease, it is invasive and not adequate for monitoring its progression. Regarding non-invasive techniques, MRI is still the most accurate but is contraindicated in some patients [6], expensive and not widely available [64,65].

Fat Deposition

Liver steatosis is associated with metabolic syndrome and non-alcoholic fatty liver disease (NAFLD), which affects 30% of the American and European population [66]. It may progress to steatohepatitis and is currently the main reason for cirrhosis development [6,8]. This occurs in about 20% of patients with NAFLD, making early detection of liver fat and implementation of control measurements essential [6]. Chemotherapy also contributes to the increasing incidence of liver steatosis [67]. It may induce a specific form of steatohepatitis and worsens patient prognosis [68].

Dual-energy CT can provide reliable material composition estimation without the need for unenhanced acquisitions (Figure 15) [6,69,70]. However, it has shown lower performance for fat quantification compared to SECT and has a moderate correlation with MR spectroscopy [66]. Still, a significant correlation has been found between liver fat percentage obtained from a multi-material decomposition algorithm and attenuation measurements. A 10% threshold of liver fat was highly sensitive and specific for predicting the non-contrast CT attenuation indicative of moderate to severe steatosis [65]. Others found a strong correlation between hepatic fat fractions obtained from DECT and those obtained from MRI, without observing significant differences across different scanning phases [71].

For VNC images, a liver attenuation of <40 Hounsfiled units (HU) is highly specific and positively predictive for moderate to severe steatosis using unenhanced SECT criteria, supporting their reliability despite the mild overestimation of liver attenuation compared to true unenhanced images (by 5.4 UH) [72]. A recent study performed using proton density fat fraction MRI as the reference standard found only a moderate correlation between VNC attenuation values and liver fat content with 57–68% sensitivity, but discovered high ($\geq$90%) specificity for diagnosis of steatosis [73]. Others found comparable diagnostic performance of CT parameters measured in VNC and true unenhanced images for diagnosing liver steatosis [74–76]; however, further studies are needed if we are to be able rely on VNC values for the diagnosis of liver steatosis.

On the opposite side, hepatic fat quantification of low-dose unenhanced DECT (volumetric CT dose index of 2.94 mGy) strongly correlates with MRI proton density fat fraction and provides an excellent diagnostic performance for diagnosis of the fatty liver with a cutoff value of $\geq$4.61%. This method could be an option for specific workup of hepatic steatosis [77].

Early studies have also used attenuation differences and curves from low- and high-energy VMIs to grade the severity of fat infiltration. Given its unique property of greater attenuation of high-energy X-rays compared to low-energy X-rays, fat would appear brighter on subtracted images (lower-keV image subtracted from higher-keV image) [67].

Iodine concentration values during the portal venous phase may additionally improve the diagnosis of steatosis in contrast-enhanced CT, being significantly lower in fatty livers compared to healthy liver patients, which is possibly due to a lower interstitial distribution of iodine [78].

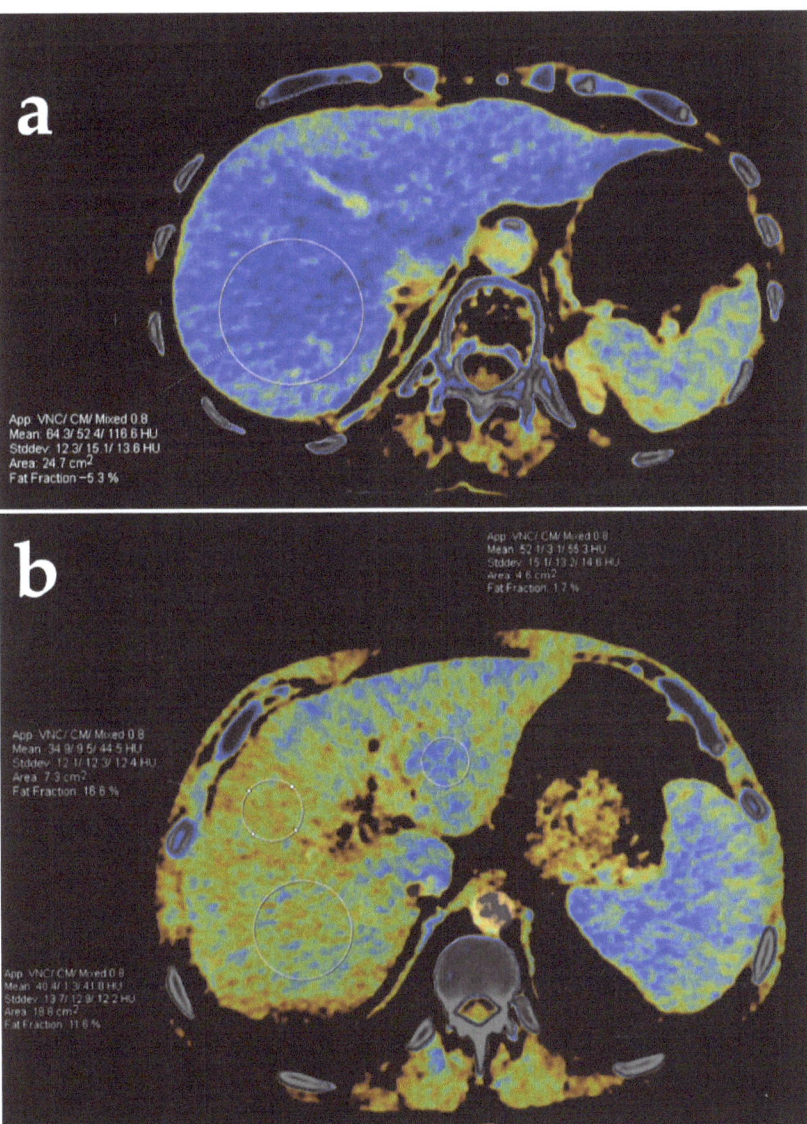

Figure 15. Liver fat quantification using dual-energy CT in two different patients. Fat fraction color-coded maps generated from DECT images in the axial plane show no fat infiltration in the first patient (**a**) and different fat fractions obtained from three regions of interest in another patient (**b**).

Iron Deposition

Iron deposition occurs in chronic liver diseases of multiple causes. This may lead to liver damage and increases the risk of cirrhosis and HCC [6,8,12,79].

The difference between liver attenuation at high- and low-energy acquisitions has shown strong linear correlation with MR R2* relaxometry techniques for estimating iron deposition [6,80]. Virtual iron content determination (3-material decomposition algorithm) has also shown a correlation with serum ferritin levels and displayed sensitivity and specificity comparable to MR R2* relaxometry, but only for clinically relevant liver iron concentration thresholds [6,81]. Despite the good diagnostic accuracy for cases of moderate to severe iron overload, DECT quantification results vary where MRI quantification is limited due to extremely rapid signal decay [8,79], especially for low-grade deposition [8], and a large cohort is still needed for validation to confirm the accuracy and robustness of the method [6,24,82]. Furthermore, maximized spectral separation is important and patient size may impact iron quantification [83].

The opposite effect of fat and iron deposition in CT attenuation limits the assessment of their concurrent accumulation on SECT. Being capable of specific material quantification, DECT may overcome such limitation [8]. However, significant fat deposition may lead to an underestimation of iron accumulation [84]. Being based on a three-tissue decomposition algorithm (iron, soft tissue, and fat), virtual iron content images has the potential to eliminate the effect of fat on iron quantification, but this still requires further investigation [80,85].

Fibrosis

The staging of liver fibrosis is relevant for patient prognosis as early stages may be reversed by treating or controlling the causative factor. The most commonly used imaging tests for diagnosis are MRI and ultrasound elastography. Several CT methods for staging fibrosis have been described but may require specialized software and high radiation dose [8].

The extracellular space expansion induced by the deposition of collagen fibers is strongly correlated with the degree of fibrosis and may be quantified [34]. The hepatic extracellular volume fraction (fECV) on SECT, indicating the absolute contrast enhancement at the equilibrium phase, requires two acquisitions, larger amounts of contrast media, and is prone to misregistration errors. Dual-energy CT allows researchers to perform an accurate quantification of iodine contrast material based only on the equilibrium phase. Multiple studies have shown good results in estimating the degree of fibrosis [64,86]. Both equilibrium phase images at 180 s and 240 s have been used (the latter with slightly greater correlation coefficient) [64]. A 10 min phase has also been proposed, theoretically allowing for greater diffusion of contrast [87]. However, a different study obtained similar results with equilibrium phase images at 180 s and 10 min [88]. Still, existent studies are heterogeneous, with different scanners and protocols, and many rely on liver biopsy specimens, predisposing these methods to staging misclassifications due to heterogeneous fibrosis distribution [64]. Therefore, validation of the use of fECV calculation in DECT for liver fibrosis quantification requires further investigation [8,24].

The hepatic fECV has also been obtained from iodine density maps [89]: liver fibrosis leads to reduced portal flow, with a consequent drop in IC, and the hepatic arterial buffer response increases the IC during the arterial phase (Figure 16) [90]. Several studies have shown good correlation between IC and NIC and histologic fibrosis and cirrhosis, although different scanning phases were used [89–92]. The ratio between IC at arterial and portal venous phases is another promising quantitative parameter [90,93]. Iodine slopes calculated from liver IC at the equilibrium phase, as well as either the arterial or portal venous phase, also correlate positively with the model for end-stage liver disease (MELD) score [94].

A lower iodine washout rate, calculated from portal venous and 3 min delayed phases, has also been reported in patients with clinically significant fibrosis and cirrhosis, providing improved accuracy compared to fECV [95].

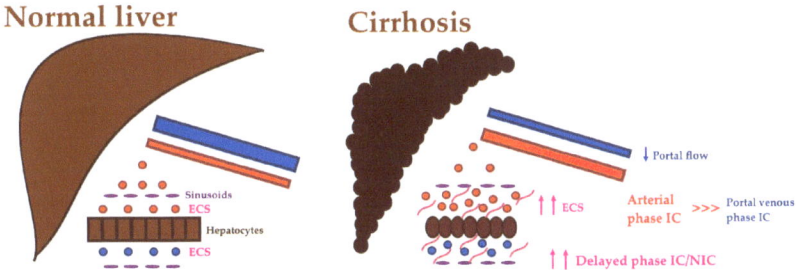

Figure 16. Liver fibrosis staging with dual-energy CT. The extracellular space (ECS) expansion induced by fibrosis may be quantified by measuring iodine concentration (IC), which increases in the delayed phase. Additionally, reduced portal flow with hepatic arterial buffer response in liver fibrosis leads to reduced IC during portal venous phase and increased IC during the arterial phase. NIC—normalized IC.

3.2.4. Trauma

The liver is the second most commonly injured abdominal organ in polytraumatic patients. Important treatment decisions are often performed based on initial CT scans in order to stratify patients who need immediate surgical or angiographic management. Dual-energy CT methods can provide valuable information about the visceral enhancement, vascular injury, and presence of active bleeding. They can accurately differentiate between hemorrhage and calcification and reduce metal-related artifacts that may lead to serious interpretation difficulties [96]. Low-keV images improve the detection of organ lacerations [96,97].

3.2.5. Vascular Applications

The use of low-keV VMIs allowed us to obtain better objective and subjective image quality for the evaluation of hepatic vasculature [98–100]. These allowed for a 25.4% reduction in iodine contrast load [101].

Several factors may impair the quality of liver enhancement, including chronic liver disease, altered hemodynamics, inadequate timing of acquisition, and contrast dose savings in patients with renal dysfunction. Low-energy VMIs showed significant CNR improvement in images obtained with poor intrahepatic contrast enhancement (Figure 17) [102].

Iodine concentration in the portal venous phase is a promising noninvasive measure for accurately assessing portal venous hypertension, showing strong correlation with direct portal venous pressure [103]. Furthermore, it can be used to assess liver blood flow changes after transjugular intrahepatic portosystemic shunt placement based on changes in the quantitative indices of iodine density [104].

Up to 44% of patients with HCC develop malignant portal venous thrombosis (PVT), worsening prognosis and limiting treatment options. Therefore, it is important to distinguish this from bland thrombosis. Thrombus enhancement in the late arterial phase is the most specific sign which suggests a malignant nature. Iodine maps obtained from DECT allow for an accurate noninvasive characterization of PVT, although the optimal scanning phase for thrombus quantification and the optimal iodine threshold are yet to be defined [6,105]. The use of low-keV VMIs (best at 40 keV) significantly improved the diagnostic performance for the detection of PVT compared to other DECT reconstruction algorithms [106].

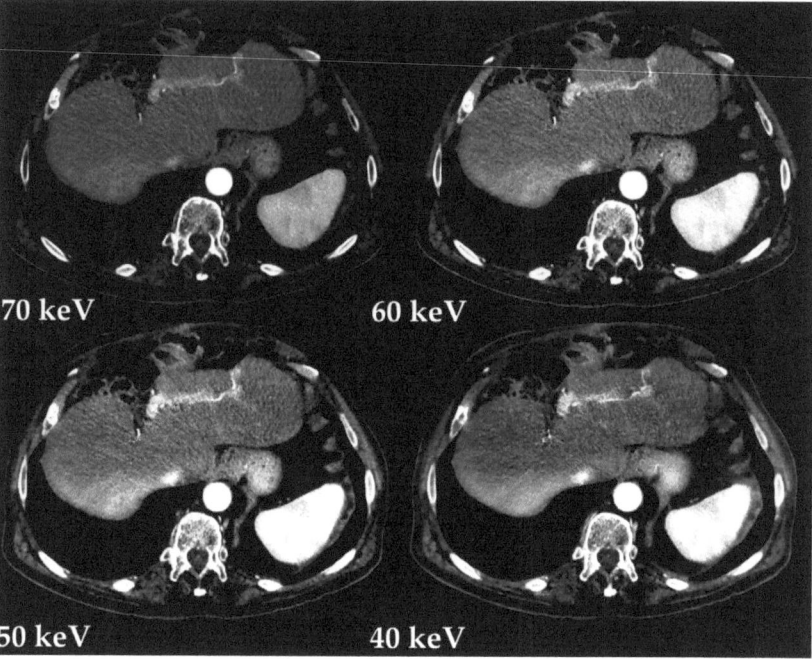

Figure 17. Improved vascular depiction with low-energy VMIs (Monoenergetic Plus advanced noise-optimized algorithm) in a scan with poor intrahepatic contrast enhancement due to the inadequate timing of acquisition.

3.3. Limitations

Current DECT technology is still limited by the significant inter-vendor variability in material-specific decomposition methods, such as in terms of monochromatic data and iodine quantification. Attenuation measurements in VNC images in different organs and scanner settings also need to be compared among those of other vendors. Besides, iodine quantification accuracy is also influenced by other factors related to the patient (e.g., body habitus size) and scanner generation [6].

Dual-energy CT is prone to unique artifacts related with the image post-processing, including subtraction-related artefacts (e.g., inadvertent subtraction of calcifications) [107]. Small lesions are susceptible to volume-averaging originating pseudoenhancement and treated avascular lesions may resemble simple cysts [5].

Workflow limitations related to the increased reconstruction time have been improved with multiple strategies, including the use of lighter workstations or integration of post-processing software in remote workstations [6]. However, large amounts of data require capacious storage systems and demand more interpretation time [73].

Clinical practice decisions, including patient and exam type selection for dual-energy scanning and image reconstruction, have also been limitative. A multi-institutional consensus suggested the use of standardized abdominopelvic CT protocols, recommending DECT in specific scenarios [108].

3.4. Future Perspectives

Radiomics analysis uses advanced mathematical algorithms to extract information from imaging data in order to generate patterns of pathological processes that are beyond visual image interpretation. Although limited, promising results have been published for the potential applications of DECT-based radiomics, including in areas of nodal metastasis prediction in several cancers, the differentiation of solid benign and malignant liver and pancreatic lesions, or the discrimination of normal liver from steatosis and cirrhosis [6,109–111]. However, the limited reproducibility of radiomic features from DECT has been reported [112].

Deep learning imaging reconstruction techniques performed using convolutional neural networks improve CT image quality [8]. These algorithms have demonstrated improved conspicuity of hepatic lesions on DECT [113–115], and the automatic localization and classification of liver lesions [116]. Artificial intelligence is also capable of improving liver segmentation and fat quantification as well as predicting the occurrence of metastatic disease [117,118].

The capability of differentiating between contrast agents with different attenuation properties at low- and high-energy has allowed researchers to perform simultaneous imaging with two contrast agents, providing different vascular phases in a single acquisition [119].

Novel photon-counting detectors convert incident X-rays into individual moving charges that create a current and a signal directly proportional to individual photon energy [6]. Providing more discrete information, photon-counting CT imaging enables K-edge imaging and the differentiation of more than two materials, [4] improving the conspicuity and delineation of tumors. Thinner slices at equivalent radiation doses reduce partial volume averaging. Furthermore, the occurrence common deleterious image artifacts is markedly reduced with the elimination of electronic noise and dose efficiency is improved [120]. An in silico study provided dual-contrast liver imaging with a single-scan after the sequential injection of a gadolinium-based contrast agent (providing arterial enhancement) and an iodine-based contrast agent (providing portal venous enhancement) [121]. This was also validated in rabbits. Future studies are needed to determine the optimal parameters for a clinical protocol [122]. The liposomes or nanoparticles needed to incorporate less biocompatible molecules are under investigation [123].

4. Conclusions

Dual-energy CT has unique capabilities of material differentiation and quantification, provides improved diagnostic performance among many disease processes, allows for the reduction of iodine contrast and radiation dose, among many other advantages over the SECT method. Its value has been proven in many clinical applications, including in the treatment of liver disease. Lesion detection and characterization, accurate staging and treatment response assessment, non-invasive quantification of fat/iron liver deposition and fibrosis, and thrombi characterization are among the most valuable uses of DECT (Table 1). Current limitations include reduced image quality with larger body sizes, cross-vendor and scanner variability, and long reconstruction time. Deep learning imaging reconstruction and the novel spectral photon-counting CT methods are promising techniques for obtaining improved image quality and diagnostic accuracy with lower radiation dose.

Table 1. Summary of current applications of dual-energy CT in liver pathology.

Pathology	Application [Reference Number]
Lesion detection and characterization	- Low-energy VMIs (40–55 keV) improve the detection of hypervascular [2,16,17,19–23] and hypovascular liver lesions [34–37]. - Spectral attenuation curves allow for discrimination between benign and malignant liver lesions [3,25,26]. - Iodine quantification in HCC can predict microvascular invasion [28–32] and early recurrence after resection [33]. - Iodine quantification [41–43] and spectral attenuation curves [5] are helpful in characterizing small hypoattenuating liver lesions. - Quantitative analysis may help to differentiate liver metastasis from abscesses [44], necrotic HCC [45] or small intrahepatic mass-forming cholangiocarcinomas [46].

Table 1. *Cont.*

Pathology	Application [Reference Number]
Treatment response evaluation	- Iodine quantification may be a reliable biomarker for tumor viability in HCC treated with antiangiogenic drugs [5,48], radiofrequency ablation [49], microwave ablation [51,52], TACE [53–55,57,58], and yttrium-90 radioembolization [60]. - Iodine tumor burden criteria for posttreatment evaluation in liver metastasis from GIST outperforms RECIST 1.1 and mChoi criteria [63].
Diffuse liver diseases	- Liver fat percentage obtained from a multi-material decomposition algorithm shows a strong correlation with fat fractions obtained from MRI [71]. - Virtual iron content determination (3-material decomposition algorithm) shows comparable sensitivity and specificity to MR R2* relaxometry, but only for clinically relevant liver iron concentration [6,82]. - The hepatic extracellular volume fraction (fECV) obtained with DECT, either from the absolute contrast enhancement at the equilibrium phase [64,86] or from iodine quantification, shows good correlation with liver fibrosis and cirrhosis [89–92].
Trauma	- Low-keV images improve the detection of liver lacerations [96,97]. - Iodine-selective images are useful for evaluating visceral enhancement, vascular injury, and the presence of active bleeding [96,97].
Vascular applications	- Low-keV VMIs improve the evaluation of hepatic vasculature [98–100,102] and allow for a 25.4% reduction in iodine contrast load [101]. - Iodine concentration is a promising tool for assessing portal venous hypertension [103] and blood flow changes after TIPS placement [104]. - Low-keV VMIs (40 keV) [106] improve the detection of PVT and iodine maps allow for differentiation between malignant and bland PVT [6,105,106].

CT, computed tomography; DECT, dual-energy computed tomography; fECV, extracellular volume fraction; GIST, gastrointestinal stromal tumor; HCC, hepatocellular carcinoma; keV, kiloelectronvolt; MRI, magnetic resonance imaging; PVT, portal venous thrombosis; RECIST, Response Evaluation Criteria in Solid Tumors; TACE, Transarterial chemoembolization; TIPS, transjugular intrahepatic portosystemic shunt; VMIs, virtual monochromatic images.

Author Contributions: Conceptualization, methodology—A.P.B. and F.C.-A.; writing—original draft preparation, A.P.B.; supervision, writing—review and editing, C.A. and F.C.-A. All authors have read and agreed to the published version of the manuscript.

Funding: This research received no external funding.

Institutional Review Board Statement: Not applicable for a review.

Informed Consent Statement: Not applicable.

Data Availability Statement: Not applicable.

Conflicts of Interest: The authors declare no conflict of interest.

Abbreviations

CNR, contrast-to-noise ratio; CT, computed tomography; DECT, dual-energy computed tomography; fECV, extracellular volume fraction; FOV, field of view; GIST, gastrointestinal stromal tumor; HCC, hepatocellular carcinoma; HU, Hounsflied units; IC, iodine concentration; keV, kiloelectronvolt; kVp, kilovolt peak; MELD, Model For End-Stage Liver Disease; MRI, magnetic resonance imaging; NAFLD, non-alcoholic fatty liver disease; NIC, normalized iodine concentration; PVT, portal venous thrombosis; RECIST, Response Evaluation Criteria in Solid Tumors; RFA, radiofrequency ablation; SECT, single-energy computed tomography; TACE, Transarterial chemoembolization; TIPS, transjugular intrahepatic portosystemic shunt; VMIs, virtual monochromatic images; VNC, virtual non-contrast.

References

1. Furlow, B. Dual-energy computed tomography. *Radiol. Technol.* **2015**, *86*, 301ct–321ct. [PubMed]
2. Marin, D.; Boll, D.T.; Mileto, A.; Nelson, R.C. State of the art: Dual-energy CT of the abdomen. *Radiology* **2014**, *271*, 327–342. [CrossRef] [PubMed]

3. Toia, G.V.; Kim, S.; Dighe, M.K.; Mileto, A. Dual-Energy Computed Tomography in Body Imaging. *Semin. Roentgenol.* **2018**, *53*, 132–146. [CrossRef] [PubMed]
4. Nakamura, Y.; Higaki, T.; Kondo, S.; Kawashita, I.; Takahashi, I.; Awai, K. An introduction to photon-counting detector CT (PCD CT) for radiologists. *Jpn. J. Radiol.* **2022**, Epub ahead of print. [CrossRef] [PubMed]
5. Cramer, T.W.; Fletcher, J.G.; Paden, R.G.; Boltz, T.F., 2nd; Stiles, W.L.; Pavlicek, W.; Silva, A.C. A primer on the use of dual-energy CT in the evaluation of commonly encountered neoplasms. *Abdom. Radiol.* **2016**, *41*, 1618–1631. [CrossRef]
6. Toia, G.V.; Mileto, A.; Wang, C.L.; Sahani, D.V. Quantitative dual-energy CT techniques in the abdomen. *Abdom. Radiol.* **2022**, *47*, 3003–3018. [CrossRef]
7. Tamm, E.P.; Le, O.; Liu, X.; Layman, R.R.; Cody, D.D.; Bhosale, P.R. "How to" incorporate dual-energy imaging into a high volume abdominal imaging practice. *Abdom. Radiol.* **2017**, *42*, 688–701. [CrossRef]
8. Kulkarni, N.M.; Fung, A.; Kambadakone, A.R.; Yeh, B.M. Computed Tomography Techniques, Protocols, Advancements, and Future Directions in Liver Diseases. *Magn. Reason. Imaging Clin. N. Am.* **2021**, *29*, 305–320. [CrossRef]
9. Lehti, L.; Söderberg, M.; Höglund, P.; Wassélius, J. Comparing Arterial- and Venous-Phase Acquisition for Optimization of Virtual Noncontrast Images from Dual-Energy Computed Tomography Angiography. *J. Comput. Assist. Tomogr.* **2019**, *43*, 770–774. [CrossRef]
10. Durieux, P.; Gevenois, P.A.; Muylem, A.V.; Howarth, N.; Keyzer, C. Abdominal Attenuation Values on Virtual and True Unenhanced Images Obtained with Third-Generation Dual-Source Dual-Energy CT. *Am. J. Roentgenol.* **2018**, *210*, 1042–1058. [CrossRef]
11. Kim, S.; Kang, B.S.; Kwon, W.J.; Bang, M.; Lim, S.; Park, G.M.; Lee, T.Y. Abdominal Organs Attenuation Values and Abdominal Aortic Calcifications on Virtual and True Noncontrast Images Obtained with Third-Generation Dual-Source Dual-Energy Computed Tomography. *J. Comput. Assist. Tomogr.* **2020**, *44*, 490–500. [CrossRef]
12. Wagner-Bartak, N.A.; Toshav, A.M.; Tamm, E.P.; Le, O.; Agarwal, S.; Ng, C.; Qayyum, A. CT Liver Imaging: What is New? *Curr. Radiol. Rep.* **2015**, *3*, 7. [CrossRef]
13. Yamada, Y.; Jinzaki, M.; Hosokawa, T.; Tanami, Y.; Abe, T.; Kuribayashi, S. Abdominal CT: An intra-individual comparison between virtual monochromatic spectral and polychromatic 120-kVp images obtained during the same examination. *Eur. J. Radiol.* **2014**, *83*, 1715–1722. [CrossRef]
14. Rassouli, N.; Chalian, H.; Rajiah, P.; Dhanantwari, A.; Landeras, L. Assessment of 70-keV virtual monoenergetic spectral images in abdominal CT imaging: A comparison study to conventional polychromatic 120-kVp images. *Abdom. Radiol.* **2017**, *42*, 2579–2586. [CrossRef]
15. Hur, S.; Lee, J.M.; Kim, S.J.; Park, J.H.; Han, J.K.; Choi, B.I. 80-kVp CT using Iterative Reconstruction in Image Space algorithm for the detection of hypervascular hepatocellular carcinoma: Phantom and initial clinical experience. *Korean J. Radiol.* **2012**, *13*, 152–164. [CrossRef]
16. Große Hokamp, N.; Höink, A.J.; Doerner, J.; Jordan, D.W.; Pahn, G.; Persigehl, T.; Maintz, D.; Haneder, S. Assessment of arterially hyper-enhancing liver lesions using virtual monoenergetic images from spectral detector CT: Phantom and patient experience. *Abdom. Radiol.* **2018**, *43*, 2066–2074. [CrossRef]
17. Shuman, W.P.; Green, D.E.; Busey, J.M.; Mitsumori, L.M.; Choi, E.; Koprowicz, K.M.; Kanal, K.M. Dual-energy liver CT: Effect of monochromatic imaging on lesion detection, conspicuity, and contrast-to-noise ratio of hypervascular lesions on late arterial phase. *Am. J. Roentgenol.* **2014**, *203*, 601–606. [CrossRef]
18. Mileto, A.; Nelson, R.C.; Samei, E.; Choudhury, K.R.; Jaffe, T.A.; Wilson, J.M.; Marin, D. Dual-energy MDCT in hypervascular liver tumors: Effect of body size on selection of the optimal monochromatic energy level. *Am. J. Roentgenol.* **2014**, *203*, 1257–1264. [CrossRef]
19. De Cecco, C.N.; Caruso, D.; Schoepf, U.J.; De Santis, D.; Muscogiuri, G.; Albrecht, M.H.; Meinel, F.G.; Wichmann, J.L.; Burchett, P.F.; Varga-Szemes, A.; et al. A noise-optimized virtual monoenergetic reconstruction algorithm improves the diagnostic accuracy of late hepatic arterial phase dual-energy CT for the detection of hypervascular liver lesions. *Eur. Radiol.* **2018**, *28*, 3393–3404. [CrossRef]
20. Marin, D.; Ramirez-Giraldo, J.C.; Gupta, S.; Fu, W.; Stinnett, S.S.; Mileto, A.; Bellini, D.; Patel, B.; Samei, E.; Nelson, R.C. Effect of a Noise-Optimized Second-Generation Monoenergetic Algorithm on Image Noise and Conspicuity of Hypervascular Liver Tumors: An In Vitro and In Vivo Study. *Am. J. Roentgenol.* **2016**, *206*, 1222–1232. [CrossRef]
21. Matsuda, M.; Tsuda, T.; Kido, T.; Tanaka, H.; Nishiyama, H.; Itoh, T.; Nakao, K.; Hirooka, M.; Mochizuki, T. Dual-Energy Computed Tomography in Patients with Small Hepatocellular Carcinoma: Utility of Noise-Reduced Monoenergetic Images for the Evaluation of Washout and Image Quality in the Equilibrium Phase. *J. Comput. Assist. Tomogr.* **2018**, *42*, 937–943. [CrossRef] [PubMed]
22. Voss, B.A.; Khandelwal, A.; Wells, M.L.; Inoue, A.; Venkatesh, S.K.; Lee, Y.S.; Johnson, M.P.; Fletcher, J.G. Impact of dual-energy 50-keV virtual monoenergetic images on radiologist confidence in detection of key imaging findings of small hepatocellular carcinomas using multiphase liver CT. *Acta Radiol.* **2022**, *63*, 1443–1452. [CrossRef] [PubMed]
23. Reimer, R.P.; Große Hokamp, N.; Fehrmann Efferoth, A.; Krauskopf, A.; Zopfs, D.; Kröger, J.R.; Persigehl, T.; Maintz, D.; Bunck, A.C. Virtual monoenergetic images from spectral detector computed tomography facilitate washout assessment in arterially hyper-enhancing liver lesions. *Eur. Radiol.* **2021**, *31*, 3468–3477. [CrossRef] [PubMed]

24. Kim, S.; Shuman, W.P. Clinical Applications of Dual-Energy Computed Tomography in the Liver. *Semin. Roentgenol.* **2016**, *51*, 284–291. [CrossRef]
25. Gordic, S.; Puippe, G.D.; Krauss, B.; Klotz, E.; Desbiolles, L.; Lesurtel, M.; Müllhaupt, B.; Pfammatter, T.; Alkadhi, H. Correlation between Dual-Energy and Perfusion CT in Patients with Hepatocellular Carcinoma. *Radiology* **2016**, *280*, 78–87. [CrossRef]
26. Mulé, S.; Pigneur, F.; Quelever, R.; Tenenhaus, A.; Baranes, L.; Richard, P.; Tacher, V.; Herin, E.; Pasquier, H.; Ronot, M.; et al. Can dual-energy CT replace perfusion CT for the functional evaluation of advanced hepatocellular carcinoma? *Eur. Radiol.* **2018**, *28*, 1977–1985. [CrossRef]
27. Wang, Q.; Shi, G.; Qi, X.; Fan, X.; Wang, L. Quantitative analysis of the dual-energy CT virtual spectral curve for focal liver lesions characterization. *Eur. J. Radiol.* **2014**, *83*, 1759–1764. [CrossRef]
28. Li, J.; Zhao, S.; Ling, Z.; Li, D.; Jia, G.; Zhao, C.; Lin, X.; Dai, Y.; Jiang, H.; Wang, S. Dual-Energy Computed Tomography Imaging in Early-Stage Hepatocellular Carcinoma: A Preliminary Study. *Contrast Media Mol. Imaging.* **2022**, *2022*, 2146343. [CrossRef]
29. Böning, G.; Adelt, S.; Feldhaus, F.; Fehrenbach, U.; Kahn, J.; Hamm, B.; Streitparth, F. Spectral CT in clinical routine imaging of neuroendocrine neoplasms. *Clin. Radiol.* **2021**, *76*, 348–357. [CrossRef]
30. Yang, C.B.; Zhang, S.; Jia, Y.J.; Yu, Y.; Duan, H.F.; Zhang, X.R.; Ma, G.M.; Ren, C.; Yu, N. Dual energy spectral CT imaging for the evaluation of small hepatocellular carcinoma microvascular invasion. *Eur. J. Radiol.* **2017**, *95*, 222–227. [CrossRef]
31. Lewin, M.; Laurent-Bellue, A.; Desterke, C.; Radu, A.; Feghali, J.A.; Farah, J.; Agostini, H.; Nault, J.-C.; Vibert, E.; Guettier, C. Evaluation of perfusion CT and dual-energy CT for predicting microvascular invasion of hepatocellular carcinoma. *Abdom. Radiol.* **2022**, *47*, 2115–2127. [CrossRef]
32. Kim, T.M.; Lee, J.M.; Yoon, J.H.; Joo, I.; Park, S.-J.; Jeon, S.K.; Schmidt, B.; Martin, S. Prediction of microvascular invasion of hepatocellular carcinoma: Value of volumetric iodine quantification using preoperative dual-energy computed tomography. *Cancer Imaging* **2020**, *20*, 60. [CrossRef]
33. Luo, N.; Li, W.; Xie, J.; Fu, D.; Liu, L.; Huang, X.; Su, D.; Jin, G. Preoperative normalized iodine concentration derived from spectral CT is correlated with early recurrence of hepatocellular carcinoma after curative resection. *Eur. Radiol.* **2021**, *31*, 1872–1882. [CrossRef]
34. Tsurusaki, M.; Sofue, K.; Hori, M.; Sasaki, K.; Ishii, K.; Murakami, T.; Kudo, M. Dual-Energy Computed Tomography of the Liver: Uses in Clinical Practices and Applications. *Diagnostics* **2021**, *11*, 161. [CrossRef]
35. Nagayama, Y.; Iyama, A.; Oda, S.; Taguchi, N.; Nakaura, T.; Utsunomiya, D.; Kikuchi, Y.; Yamashita, Y. Dual-layer dual-energy computed tomography for the assessment of hypovascular hepatic metastases: Impact of closing k-edge on image quality and lesion detectability. *Eur. Radiol.* **2019**, *29*, 2837–2847. [CrossRef]
36. Caruso, D.; De Cecco, C.N.; Schoepf, U.J.; Schaefer, A.R.; Leland, P.W.; Johnson, D.; Laghi, A.; Hardie, A.D. Can dual-energy computed tomography improve visualization of hypoenhancing liver lesions in portal venous phase? Assessment of advanced image-based virtual monoenergetic images. *Clin. Imaging* **2017**, *41*, 118–124. [CrossRef]
37. Lenga, L.; Czwikla, R.; Wichmann, J.L.; Leithner, D.; Albrecht, M.H.; Booz, C.; Arendt, C.T.; Yel, I.; D'Angelo, T.; Vogl, T.J.; et al. Dual-energy CT in patients with colorectal cancer: Improved assessment of hypoattenuating liver metastases using noise-optimized virtual monoenergetic imaging. *Eur. J. Radiol.* **2018**, *106*, 184–191. [CrossRef]
38. Ratajczak, P.; Serafin, Z.; Sławińska, A.; Słupski, M.; Leszczyński, W. Improved imaging of colorectal liver metastases using single-source, fast kVp-switching, dual-energy CT: Preliminary results. *Pol. J. Radiol.* **2018**, *83*, e643–e649. [CrossRef]
39. Yamada, Y.; Jinzaki, M.; Tanami, Y.; Abe, T.; Kuribayashi, S. Virtual monochromatic spectral imaging for the evaluation of hypovascular hepatic metastases: The optimal monochromatic level with fast kilovoltage switching dual-energy computed tomography. *Investig. Radiol.* **2012**, *47*, 292–298. [CrossRef]
40. Husarik, D.B.; Gordic, S.; Desbiolles, L.; Krauss, B.; Leschka, S.; Wildermuth, S.; Alkadhi, H. Advanced virtual monoenergetic computed tomography of hyperattenuating and hypoattenuating liver lesions: Ex-vivo and patient experience in various body sizes. *Investig. Radiol.* **2015**, *50*, 695–702. [CrossRef]
41. Agrawal, M.D.; Pinho, D.F.; Kulkarni, N.M.; Hahn, P.F.; Guimaraes, A.R.; Sahani, D.V. Oncologic applications of dual-energy CT in the abdomen. *Radiographics* **2014**, *34*, 589–612. [CrossRef] [PubMed]
42. Patel, B.N.; Rosenberg, M.; Vernuccio, F.; Ramirez-Giraldo, J.C.; Nelson, R.; Farjat, A.; Marin, D. Characterization of Small Incidental Indeterminate Hypoattenuating Hepatic Lesions: Added Value of Single-Phase Contrast-Enhanced Dual-Energy CT Material Attenuation Analysis. *Am. J. Roentgenol.* **2018**, *211*, 571–579. [CrossRef] [PubMed]
43. Sanghavi, P.S.; Jankharia, B.G. Applications of dual energy CT in clinical practice: A pictorial essay. *Indian J. Radiol. Imaging* **2019**, *29*, 289–298. [CrossRef] [PubMed]
44. Wang, N.; Ju, Y.; Wu, J.; Liu, A.; Chen, A.; Liu, J.; Liu, Y.; Li, J. Differentiation of liver abscess from liver metastasis using dual-energy spectral CT quantitative parameters. *Eur. J. Radiol.* **2019**, *113*, 204–208. [CrossRef]
45. Yu, Y.; Guo, L.; Hu, C.; Chen, K. Spectral CT imaging in the differential diagnosis of necrotic hepatocellular carcinoma and hepatic abscess. *Clin. Radiol.* **2014**, *69*, e517–e524. [CrossRef]
46. Kim, J.E.; Kim, H.O.; Bae, K.; Cho, J.M.; Choi, H.C.; Choi, D.S. Differentiation of small intrahepatic mass-forming cholangiocarcinoma from small liver abscess by dual source dual-energy CT quantitative parameters. *Eur. J. Radiol.* **2017**, *92*, 145–152. [CrossRef]
47. Lv, P.; Liu, J.; Yan, X.; Chai, Y.; Chen, Y.; Gao, J.; Pan, Y.; Li, S.; Guo, H.; Zhou, Y. CT spectral imaging for monitoring the therapeutic efficacy of VEGF receptor kinase inhibitor AG-013736 in rabbit VX2 liver tumours. *Eur. Radiol.* **2017**, *27*, 918–926. [CrossRef]

48. Dai, X.; Schlemmer, H.-P.; Schmidt, B.; Höh, K.; Xu, K.; Ganten, T.M.; Ganten, M.-K. Quantitative therapy response assessment by volumetric iodine-uptake measurement: Initial experience in patients with advanced hepatocellular carcinoma treated with sorafenib. *Eur. J. Radiol.* **2013**, *82*, 327–334. [CrossRef]
49. Dai, X.; Schlemmer, H.-P.; Schmidt, B.; Höh, K.; Xu, K.; Ganten, T.M.; Ganten, M.-K. Application of Gemstone CT Spectroscopy in the Evaluation of Abnormal Enhancement of Lesion Margin After Radiofrequency Ablation of Hepatocellular Carcinoma. *Iran. J. Radiol.* **2020**, *17*, e99611. [CrossRef]
50. Li, J.-P.; Zhao, S.; Jiang, H.-J.; Jiang, H.; Zhang, L.-H.; Shi, Z.-X.; Fan, T.-T.; Wang, S. Quantitative dual-energy computed tomography texture analysis predicts the response of primary small hepatocellular carcinoma to radiofrequency ablation. *Hepatobiliary Pancreat. Dis. Int.* **2022**, *21*, 569–576. [CrossRef]
51. Reimer, R.P.; Hokamp, N.G.; Niehoff, J.; Zopfs, D.; Lennartz, S.; Heidar, M.; Wahba, R.; Stippel, D.; Maintz, D.; dos Santos, D.P.; et al. Value of spectral detector computed tomography for the early assessment of technique efficacy after microwave ablation of hepatocellular carcinoma. *PLoS ONE* **2021**, *16*, e0252678. [CrossRef]
52. Bäumler, W.; Beyer, L.P.; Lürken, L.; Wiggermann, P.; Stroszczynski, C.; Dollinger, M.; Schicho, A. Detection of Incomplete Irreversible Electroporation (IRE) and Microwave Ablation (MWA) of Hepatocellular Carcinoma (HCC) Using Iodine Quantification in Dual Energy Computed Tomography (DECT). *Diagnostics* **2022**, *12*, 986. [CrossRef]
53. Xu, Y.; Xiao, A.; Yang, J.; Zhang, Z.; Zhang, G. Assessment of Lipiodol Deposition and Residual Cancer for Hepatocellular Carcinoma After Transcatheter Arterial Chemoembolization via Iodine-Based Material Decomposition Images with Spectral Computed Tomography Imaging: A Preliminary Study. *Iran. J. Radiol.* **2015**, *12*, e26009. [CrossRef]
54. Liu, Y.S.; Chuang, M.T.; Tsai, Y.S.; Tsai, H.M.; Lin, X.Z. Nitroglycerine use in transcatheter arterial (chemo)embolization in patients with hepatocellular carcinoma and dual-energy CT assessment of Lipiodol retention. *Eur. Radiol.* **2012**, *22*, 2193–2200. [CrossRef]
55. Liu, Q.Y.; He, C.D.; Zhou, Y.; Huang, D.; Lin, H.; Wang, Z.; Wang, D.; Wang, J.Q.; Liao, L.P. Application of gemstone spectral imaging for efficacy evaluation in hepatocellular carcinoma after transarterial chemoembolization. *World J. Gastroenterol.* **2016**, *22*, 3242–3251. [CrossRef]
56. Wang, J.; Shen, J.L. Spectral CT in evaluating the therapeutic effect of transarterial chemoembolization for hepatocellular carcinoma: A retrospective study. *Medicine* **2017**, *96*, e9236. [CrossRef]
57. Yue, X.; Jiang, Q.; Hu, X.; Cen, C.; Song, S.; Qian, K.; Lu, Y.; Yang, M.; Li, Q.; Han, P. Quantitative dual-energy CT for evaluating hepatocellular carcinoma after transarterial chemoembolization. *Sci. Rep.* **2021**, *11*, 11127. [CrossRef]
58. Lee, J.A.; Jeong, W.K.; Kim, Y.; Song, S.Y.; Kim, J.; Heo, J.N.; Park, C.K. Dual-energy CT to detect recurrent HCC after TACE: Initial experience of color-coded iodine CT imaging. *Eur. J. Radiol.* **2013**, *82*, 569–576. [CrossRef]
59. Negussie, A.H.; de Ruiter, Q.M.B.; Britton, H.; Donahue, D.R.; Boffi, Q.; Kim, Y.-S.; Pritchard, W.F.; Moonen, C.; Storm, G.; Lewis, A.L.; et al. Synthesis, characterization, and imaging of radiopaque bismuth beads for image-guided transarterial embolization. *Sci. Rep.* **2021**, *11*, 533. [CrossRef]
60. Altenbernd, J.; Wetter, A.; Forsting, M.; Umutlu, L. Treatment response after radioembolisation in patients with hepatocellular carcinoma-An evaluation with dual energy computed-tomography. *Eur. J. Radiol. Open* **2016**, *3*, 230–235. [CrossRef]
61. Bargellini, I.; Crocetti, L.; Turini, F.M.; Lorenzoni, G.; Boni, G.; Traino, A.C.; Caramella, D.; Cioni, R. Response Assessment by Volumetric Iodine Uptake Measurement: Preliminary Experience in Patients with Intermediate-Advanced Hepatocellular Carcinoma Treated with Yttrium-90 Radioembolization. *Cardiovasc. Intervent. Radiol.* **2018**, *41*, 1373–1383. [CrossRef] [PubMed]
62. Apfaltrer, P.; Meyer, M.; Meier, C.; Henzler, T.; Barraza, J.M., Jr.; Dinter, D.J.; Hohenberger, P.; Schoepf, U.J.; Schoenberg, S.O.; Fink, C. Contrast-enhanced dual-energy CT of gastrointestinal stromal tumors: Is iodine-related attenuation a potential indicator of tumor response? *Investig. Radiol.* **2012**, *47*, 65–70. [CrossRef] [PubMed]
63. Meyer, M.; Hohenberger, P.; Overhoff, D.; Bartsch, A.; Henzler, T.; Haubenreisser, H.; Ronald, J.; Schmidt, B.; Flohr, T.; Sedlmair, M.; et al. Dual-Energy CT Vital Iodine Tumor Burden for Response Assessment in Patients with Metastatic GIST Undergoing TKI Therapy: Comparison with Standard CT and FDG PET/CT Criteria. *Am. J. Roentgenol.* **2022**, *218*, 659–669. [CrossRef] [PubMed]
64. Wada, N.; Fujita, N.; Ishimatsu, K.; Takao, S.; Yoshizumi, T.; Miyazaki, Y.; Oda, Y.; Nishie, A.; Ishigami, K.; Ushijima, Y. A novel fast kilovoltage switching dual-energy computed tomography technique with deep learning: Utility for non-invasive assessments of liver fibrosis. *Eur. J. Radiol.* **2022**, *155*, 110461. [CrossRef] [PubMed]
65. Xu, J.J.; Boesen, M.R.; Hansen, S.L.; Ulriksen, P.S.; Holm, S.; Lönn, L.; Hansen, K.L. Assessment of Liver Fat: Dual-Energy CT versus Conventional CT with and without Contrast. *Diagnostics* **2022**, *12*, 708. [CrossRef]
66. Kramer, H.; Pickhardt, P.J.; Kliewer, M.A.; Hernando, D.; Chen, G.H.; Zagzebski, J.A.; Reeder, S.B. Accuracy of Liver Fat Quantification with Advanced CT, MRI, and Ultrasound Techniques: Prospective Comparison with MR Spectroscopy. *Am. J. Roentgenol.* **2017**, *208*, 92–100. [CrossRef]
67. Zheng, X.; Ren, Y.; Phillips, W.T.; Li, M.; Song, M.; Hua, Y.; Zhang, G. Assessment of hepatic fatty infiltration using spectral computed tomography imaging: A pilot study. *J. Comput. Assist. Tomogr.* **2013**, *37*, 134–141. [CrossRef]
68. Corrias, G.; Erta, M.; Sini, M.; Sardu, C.; Saba, L.; Mahmood, U.; Castellanos, S.H.; Bates, D.; Mondanelli, N.; Thomsen, B.; et al. Comparison of Multimaterial Decomposition Fat Fraction with DECT and Proton Density Fat Fraction with IDEAL IQ MRI for Quantification of Liver Steatosis in a Population Exposed to Chemotherapy. *Dose Response* **2021**, *19*, 1559325820984938. [CrossRef]
69. Mendonça, P.R.; Lamb, P.; Kriston, A.; Sasaki, K.; Kudo, M.; Sahani, D.V. Contrast-independent liver-fat quantification from spectral CT exams. *Med. Image Comput. Comput. Assist. Interv.* **2013**, *16 Pt 1*, 324–331. [CrossRef]

70. Molwitz, I.; Campbell, G.M.; Yamamura, J.; Knopp, T.; Toedter, K.D.-C.; Fischer, R.; Wang, Z.J.; Busch, A.; Ozga, A.-K.; Zhang, S.; et al. Fat Quantification in Dual-Layer Detector Spectral Computed Tomography: Experimental Development and First In-Patient Validation. *Investig. Radiol.* **2022**, *57*, 463–469. [CrossRef]
71. Zhang, Q.; Zhao, Y.; Wu, J.; Xie, L.; Chen, A.; Liu, Y.; Song, Q.; Li, J.; Wu, T.; Xie, L.; et al. Quantification of Hepatic Fat Fraction in Patients with Nonalcoholic Fatty Liver Disease: Comparison of Multimaterial Decomposition Algorithm and Fat (Water)-Based Material Decomposition Algorithm Using Single-Source Dual-Energy Computed Tomography. *J. Comput. Assist. Tomogr.* **2021**, *45*, 12–17. [CrossRef] [PubMed]
72. Haji-Momenian, S.; Parkinson, W.; Khati, N.; Brindle, K.; Earls, J.; Zeman, R.K. Single-energy non-contrast hepatic steatosis criteria applied to virtual non-contrast images: Is it still highly specific and positively predictive? *Clin. Radiol.* **2018**, *73*, 594.e7–594.e15. [CrossRef] [PubMed]
73. Zhang, P.P.; Choi, H.H.; Ohliger, M.A. Detection of fatty liver using virtual non-contrast dual-energy CT. *Abdom. Radiol.* **2022**, *47*, 2046–2056. [CrossRef] [PubMed]
74. Choi, M.H.; Lee, Y.J.; Choi, Y.J.; Pak, S. Dual-energy CT of the liver: True noncontrast vs. virtual noncontrast images derived from multiple phases for the diagnosis of fatty liver. *Eur. J. Radiol.* **2021**, *140*, 109741. [CrossRef] [PubMed]
75. Niehoff, J.H.; Woeltjen, M.M.; Saeed, S.; Michael, A.E.; Boriesosdick, J.; Borggrefe, J.; Kroeger, J.R. Assessment of hepatic steatosis based on virtual non-contrast computed tomography: Initial experiences with a photon counting scanner approved for clinical use. *Eur. J. Radiol.* **2022**, *149*, 110185. [CrossRef]
76. Kang, H.J.; Lee, D.H.; Park, S.J.; Han, J.K. Virtual noncontrast images derived from dual-energy CT for assessment of hepatic steatosis in living liver donors. *Eur. J. Radiol.* **2021**, *139*, 109687. [CrossRef]
77. Hong, S.B.; Lee, N.K.; Kim, S.; Um, K.; Kim, K.; Kim, I.J. Hepatic Fat Quantification with the Multi-Material Decomposition Algorithm by Using Low-Dose Non-Contrast Material-Enhanced Dual-Energy Computed Tomography in a Prospectively Enrolled Cohort. *Medicina* **2022**, *58*, 1459. [CrossRef]
78. Beck, S.; Jahn, L.; Deniffel, D.; Riederer, I.; Sauter, A.; Makowski, M.R.; Pfeiffer, D. Iodine Images in Dual-energy CT: Detection of Hepatic Steatosis by Quantitative Iodine Concentration Values. *J. Digit. Imaging* **2022**, *35*, 1738–1747. [CrossRef]
79. Zhang, Y.; Xiao, C.; Li, J.; Song, L.X.; Zhao, Y.S.; Han, S.; Li, Z.W.; Guo, C.; Zhao, J.G.; Chang, C.K. Comparative Study on Iron Content Detection by Energy Spectral CT and MRI in MDS Patients. *Front. Oncol.* **2021**, *11*, 646946. [CrossRef]
80. Ma, Q.; Hu, J.; Yang, W.; Hou, Y. Dual-layer detector spectral CT versus magnetic resonance imaging for the assessment of iron overload in myelodysplastic syndromes and aplastic anemia. *Jpn. J. Radiol.* **2020**, *38*, 374–381. [CrossRef]
81. Luo, X.F.; Xie, X.Q.; Cheng, S.; Yang, Y.; Yan, J.; Zhang, H.; Chai, W.M.; Schmidt, B.; Yan, F.H. Dual-Energy CT for Patients Suspected of Having Liver Iron Overload: Can Virtual Iron Content Imaging Accurately Quantify Liver Iron Content? *Radiology* **2015**, *277*, 95–103. [CrossRef]
82. Elbanna, K.Y.; Mansoori, B.; Mileto, A.; Rogalla, P.; Guimarães, L. Dual-energy CT in diffuse liver disease: Is there a role? *Abdom. Radiol.* **2020**, *45*, 3413–3424. [CrossRef]
83. Jiang, X.; Hintenlang, D.E.; White, R.D. Lower limit of iron quantification using dual-energy CT-a phantom study. *J. Appl. Clin. Med. Phys.* **2021**, *22*, 299–307. [CrossRef]
84. Joe, E.; Kim, S.H.; Lee, K.B.; Jang, J.J.; Lee, J.Y.; Lee, J.M.; Han, J.K.; Choi, B.I. Feasibility and accuracy of dual-source dual-energy CT for noninvasive determination of hepatic iron accumulation. *Radiology* **2012**, *262*, 126–135. [CrossRef]
85. Ma, J.; Song, Z.Q.; Yan, F.H. Separation of hepatic iron and fat by dual-source dual-energy computed tomography based on material decomposition: An animal study. *PLoS ONE* **2014**, *9*, e110964. [CrossRef]
86. Sofue, K.; Tsurusaki, M.; Mileto, A.; Hyodo, T.; Sasaki, K.; Nishii, T.; Chikugo, T.; Yada, N.; Kudo, M.; Sugimura, K.; et al. Dual-energy computed tomography for non-invasive staging of liver fibrosis: Accuracy of iodine density measurements from contrast-enhanced data. *Hepatol. Res.* **2018**, *48*, 1008–1019. [CrossRef]
87. Bottari, A.; Silipigni, S.; Carerj, M.L.; Cattafi, A.; Maimone, S.; Marino, M.A.; Mazziotti, S.; Pitrone, A.; Squadrito, G.; Ascenti, G. Dual-source dual-energy CT in the evaluation of hepatic fractional extracellular space in cirrhosis. *Radiol. Med.* **2020**, *125*, 7–14. [CrossRef]
88. Cicero, G.; Mazziotti, S.; Silipigni, S.; Blandino, A.; Cantisani, V.; Pergolizzi, S.; D'angelo, T.; Stagno, A.; Maimone, S.; Squadrito, G.; et al. Dual-energy CT quantification of fractional extracellular space in cirrhotic patients: Comparison between early and delayed equilibrium phases and correlation with oesophageal varices. *Radiol. Med.* **2021**, *126*, 761–767. [CrossRef]
89. Yoon, J.H.; Lee, J.M.; Kim, J.H.; Lee, K.-B.; Kim, H.; Hong, S.K.; Yi, N.-J.; Lee, K.-W.; Suh, K.-S. Hepatic fibrosis grading with extracellular volume fraction from iodine mapping in spectral liver, C.T. *Eur. J. Radiol.* **2021**, *137*, 109604. [CrossRef]
90. Lv, P.; Lin, X.; Gao, J.; Chen, K. Spectral CT: Preliminary studies in the liver cirrhosis. *Korean J. Radiol.* **2012**, *13*, 434–442. [CrossRef]
91. Marri, U.K.; Das, P.; Shalimar Kalaivani, M.; Srivastava, D.N.; Madhusudhan, K.S. Noninvasive Staging of Liver Fibrosis Using 5-Minute Delayed Dual-Energy CT: Comparison with US Elastography and Correlation with Histologic Findings. *Radiology* **2021**, *298*, 600–608. [CrossRef] [PubMed]
92. Morita, K.; Nishie, A.; Ushijima, Y.; Takayama, Y.; Fujita, N.; Kubo, Y.; Ishimatsu, K.; Yoshizumi, T.; Maehara, J.; Ishigami, K. Noninvasive assessment of liver fibrosis by dual-layer spectral detector CT. *Eur. J. Radiol.* **2021**, *136*, 109575. [CrossRef] [PubMed]
93. Zhao, L.Q.; He, W.; Yan, B.; Wang, H.Y.; Wang, J. The evaluation of haemodynamics in cirrhotic patients with spectral CT. *Br. J. Radiol.* **2013**, *86*, 20130228. [CrossRef] [PubMed]

94. Mastrodicasa, D.; Willemink, M.J.; Duran, C.; Pizzi, A.D.; Hinostroza, V.; Molvin, L.; Khalaf, M.; Jeffrey, R.B.; Patel, B.N. Noninvasive assessment of cirrhosis using multiphasic dual-energy CT iodine maps: Correlation with model for end-stage liver disease score. *Abdom. Radiol.* **2021**, *46*, 1931–1940. [CrossRef]
95. Nagayama, Y.; Kato, Y.; Inoue, T.; Nakaura, T.; Oda, S.; Kidoh, M.; Ikeda, O.; Hirai, T. Liver fibrosis assessment with multiphasic dual-energy CT: Diagnostic performance of iodine uptake parameters. *Eur Radiol.* **2021**, *31*, 5779–5790; Erratum in *Eur Radiol.* **2021**, *31*, 8823–8824. [CrossRef]
96. Hamid, S.; Nicolaou, S.; Khosa, F.; Andrews, G.; Murray, N.; Abdellatif, W.; Qamar, S.R. Dual-Energy CT: A Paradigm Shift in Acute Traumatic Abdomen. *Can. Assoc. Radiol. J.* **2020**, *71*, 371–387. [CrossRef]
97. Sun, E.X.; Wortman, J.R.; Uyeda, J.W.; Lacson, R.; Sodickson, A.D. Virtual monoenergetic dual-energy CT for evaluation of hepatic and splenic lacerations. *Emerg. Radiol.* **2019**, *26*, 419–425. [CrossRef]
98. Marin, D.; Caywood, D.T.; Mileto, A.; Reiner, C.S.; Seaman, D.M.; Patel, B.N.; Boll, D.T.; Nelson, R.C. Dual-Energy Multidetector-Row Computed Tomography of the Hepatic Arterial System: Optimization of Energy and Material-Specific Reconstruction Techniques. *J. Comput. Assist. Tomogr.* **2015**, *39*, 721–729. [CrossRef]
99. Yin, X.-P.; Gao, B.-L.; Li, C.-Y.; Zhou, H.; Zhao, L.; Zheng, Y.-T.; Zhao, Y.-X. Optimal Monochromatic Imaging of Spectral Computed Tomography Potentially Improves the Quality of Hepatic Vascular Imaging. *Korean J. Radiol.* **2018**, *19*, 578–584. [CrossRef]
100. Majeed, N.F.; Ali, S.M.; Therrien, J.; Wald, C.; Wortman, J.R. Virtual Monoenergetic Spectral Detector CT for Preoperative CT Angiography in Liver Donors. *Curr. Probl. Diagn. Radiol.* **2022**, *51*, 517–523. [CrossRef]
101. Zhao, Y.; Wu, Y.; Zuo, Z.; Suo, H.; Zhao, S.; Han, J.; Chang, X.; Cheng, S. Application of low concentration contrast medium in spectral CT imaging for CT portal venography. *J. X-ray Sci. Technol.* **2017**, *25*, 135–143. [CrossRef]
102. Schabel, C.; Bongers, M.; Sedlmair, M.; Korn, A.; Grosse, U.; Mangold, S.; Claussen, C.D.; Thomas, C. Assessment of the hepatic veins in poor contrast conditions using dual energy CT: Evaluation of a novel monoenergetic extrapolation software algorithm. *Rofo* **2014**, *186*, 591–597. [CrossRef]
103. Wang, J.; Gao, F.; Shen, J.L. Noninvasive Assessment of Portal Hypertension Using Spectral Computed Tomography. *J. Clin. Gastroenterol.* **2019**, *53*, e387–e391. [CrossRef]
104. Wang, L.; Wang, R.; Zhang, C.; Yue, Z.; Zhao, H.; Fan, Z.; Wu, Y.; Zhang, Y.; Liu, F.; Dong, J. Hepatic parenchyma and vascular blood flow changes after TIPS with spectral CT iodine density in HBV-related liver cirrhosis. *Sci. Rep.* **2021**, *11*, 10535. [CrossRef]
105. Ascenti, G.; Sofia, C.; Mazziotti, S.; Silipigni, S.; D'Angelo, T.; Pergolizzi, S.; Scribano, E. Dual-energy CT with iodine quantification in distinguishing between bland and neoplastic portal vein thrombosis in patients with hepatocellular carcinoma. *Clin. Radiol.* **2016**, *71*, 938.e1–938.e9. [CrossRef]
106. Martin, S.S.; Kolaneci, J.; Czwikla, R.; Booz, C.; Gruenewald, L.D.; Albrecht, M.H.; Thompson, Z.M.; Lenga, L.; Yel, I.; Vogl, T.J.; et al. Dual-Energy CT for the Detection of Portal Vein Thrombosis: Improved Diagnostic Performance Using Virtual Monoenergetic Reconstructions. *Diagnostics* **2022**, *12*, 1682. [CrossRef]
107. George, E.; Wortman, J.R.; Fulwadhva, U.P.; Uyeda, J.W.; Sodickson, A.D. Dual energy CT applications in pancreatic pathologies. *Br. J. Radiol.* **2017**, *90*, 20170411. [CrossRef]
108. Patel, B.N.; Alexander, L.; Allen, B.; Berland, L.; Borhani, A.; Mileto, A.; Moreno, C.; Morgan, D.; Sahani, D.; Shuman, W.; et al. Dual-energy CT workflow: Multi-institutional consensus on standardization of abdominopelvic MDCT protocols. *Abdom. Radiol.* **2017**, *42*, 676–687. [CrossRef]
109. Homayounieh, F.; Singh, R.; Nitiwarangkul, C.; Lades, F.; Schmidt, B.; Sedlmair, M.; Saini, S.; Kalra, M.K. Semiautomatic Segmentation and Radiomics for Dual-Energy CT: A Pilot Study to Differentiate Benign and Malignant Hepatic Lesions. *Am. J. Roentgenol.* **2020**, *215*, 398–405. [CrossRef]
110. Ebrahimian, S.; Singh, R.; Netaji, A.; Madhusudhan, K.S.; Homayounieh, F.; Primak, A.; Lades, F.; Saini, S.; Kalra, M.K.; Sharma, S. Characterization of Benign and Malignant Pancreatic Lesions with DECT Quantitative Metrics and Radiomics. *Acad. Radiol.* **2022**, *29*, 705–713. [CrossRef]
111. Doda Khera, R.; Homayounieh, F.; Lades, F.; Schmidt, B.; Sedlmair, M.; Primak, A.; Saini, S.; Kalra, M.K. Can Dual-Energy Computed Tomography Quantitative Analysis and Radiomics Differentiate Normal Liver from Hepatic Steatosis and Cirrhosis? *J. Comput. Assist. Tomogr.* **2020**, *44*, 223–229. [CrossRef] [PubMed]
112. Meyer, M.; Ronald, J.; Vernuccio, F.; Nelson, R.C.; Ramirez-Giraldo, J.C.; Solomon, J.; Patel, B.N.; Samei, E.; Marin, D. Reproducibility of CT Radiomic Features within the Same Patient: Influence of Radiation Dose and CT Reconstruction Settings. *Radiology* **2019**, *293*, 583–591. [CrossRef] [PubMed]
113. Lee, T.; Lee, J.M.; Yoon, J.H.; Joo, I.; Bae, J.S.; Yoo, J.; Kim, J.H.; Ahn, C.; Kim, J.H. Deep learning-based image reconstruction of 40-keV virtual monoenergetic images of dual-energy CT for the assessment of hypoenhancing hepatic metastasis. *Eur. Radiol.* **2022**, *32*, 6407–6417. [CrossRef] [PubMed]
114. Sato, M.; Ichikawa, Y.; Domae, K.; Yoshikawa, K.; Kanii, Y.; Yamazaki, A.; Nagasawa, N.; Nagata, M.; Ishida, M.; Sakuma, H. Deep learning image reconstruction for improving image quality of contrast-enhanced dual-energy CT in abdomen. *Eur. Radiol.* **2022**, *32*, 5499–5507. [CrossRef] [PubMed]
115. Seo, J.Y.; Joo, I.; Yoon, J.H.; Kang, H.J.; Kim, S.; Kim, J.H.; Ahn, C.; Lee, J.M. Deep learning-based reconstruction of virtual monoenergetic images of kVp-switching dual energy CT for evaluation of hypervascular liver lesions: Comparison with standard reconstruction technique. *Eur. J. Radiol.* **2022**, *154*, 110390. [CrossRef]

116. Shapira, N.; Fokuhl, J.; Schultheiß, M.; Beck, S.; Kopp, F.K.; Pfeiffer, D.; Dangelmaier, J.; Pahn, G.; Sauter, A.P.; Renger, B.; et al. Liver lesion localisation and classification with convolutional neural networks: A comparison between conventional and spectral computed tomography. *Biomed. Phys. Eng. Express.* **2020**, *6*, 015038. [CrossRef]
117. Mileto, A.; Ananthakrishnan, L.; Morgan, D.E.; Yeh, B.M.; Marin, D.; Kambadakone, A.R. Clinical Implementation of Dual-Energy CT for Gastrointestinal Imaging. *Am. J. Roentgenol.* **2021**, *217*, 651–663. [CrossRef]
118. Ng, Y.S.; Xi, Y.; Qian, Y.; Ananthakrishnan, L.; Soesbe, T.C.; Lewis, M.; Lenkinski, R.; Fielding, J.R. Use of Spectral Detector Computed Tomography to Improve Liver Segmentation and Volumetry. *J. Comput. Assist. Tomogr.* **2020**, *44*, 197–203. [CrossRef]
119. Mongan, J.; Rathnayake, S.; Fu, Y.; Wang, R.; Jones, E.F.; Gao, D.W.; Yeh, B.M. In vivo differentiation of complementary contrast media at dual-energy CT. *Radiology* **2012**, *265*, 267–272. [CrossRef]
120. Esquivel, A.; Ferrero, A.; Mileto, A.; Baffour, F.; Horst, K.; Rajiah, P.S.; Inoue, A.; Leng, S.; McCollough, C.; Fletcher, J.G. Photon-Counting Detector CT: Key Points Radiologists Should Know. *Korean J. Radiol.* **2022**, *23*, 854–865. [CrossRef]
121. Muenzel, D.; Daerr, H.; Proksa, R.; Fingerle, A.A.; Kopp, F.K.; Douek, P.; Herzen, J.; Pfeiffer, F.; Rummeny, E.J.; Noël, P.B. Simultaneous dual-contrast multi-phase liver imaging using spectral photon-counting computed tomography: A proof-of-concept study. *Eur. Radiol. Exp.* **2017**, *1*, 25. [CrossRef]
122. Si-Mohamed, S.; Tatard-Leitman, V.; Laugerette, A.; Sigovan, M.; Pfeiffer, D.; Rummeny, E.J.; Coulon, P.; Yagil, Y.; Douek, P.; Boussel, L.; et al. Spectral Photon-Counting Computed Tomography (SPCCT): In-vivo single-acquisition multi-phase liver imaging with a dual contrast agent protocol. *Sci. Rep.* **2019**, *9*, 8458. [CrossRef]
123. Amato, C.; Klein, L.; Wehrse, E.; Rotkopf, L.T.; Sawall, S.; Maier, J.; Ziener, C.H.; Schlemmer, H.; Kachelrieß, M. Potential of contrast agents based on high-Z elements for contrast-enhanced photon-counting computed tomography. *Med. Phys.* **2020**, *47*, 6179–6190. [CrossRef]

Disclaimer/Publisher's Note: The statements, opinions and data contained in all publications are solely those of the individual author(s) and contributor(s) and not of MDPI and/or the editor(s). MDPI and/or the editor(s) disclaim responsibility for any injury to people or property resulting from any ideas, methods, instructions or products referred to in the content.

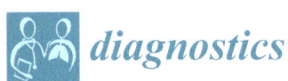

Review

Imaging Diagnosis of Hepatocellular Carcinoma: A State-of-the-Art Review

Gianvito Candita, Sara Rossi, Karolina Cwiklinska, Salvatore Claudio Fanni *, Dania Cioni, Riccardo Lencioni and Emanuele Neri

Department of Translational Research, Academic Radiology, University of Pisa, 56124 Pisa, Italy
* Correspondence: fannisalvatoreclaudio@gmail.com

Abstract: Hepatocellular carcinoma (HCC) remains not only a cause of a considerable part of oncologic mortality, but also a diagnostic and therapeutic challenge for healthcare systems worldwide. Early detection of the disease and consequential adequate therapy are imperative to increase patients' quality of life and survival. Imaging plays, therefore, a crucial role in the surveillance of patients at risk, the detection and diagnosis of HCC nodules, as well as in the follow-up post-treatment. The unique imaging characteristics of HCC lesions, deriving mainly from the assessment of their vascularity on contrast-enhanced computed tomography (CT), magnetic resonance (MR) or contrast-enhanced ultrasound (CEUS), allow for a more accurate, noninvasive diagnosis and staging. The role of imaging in the management of HCC has further expanded beyond the plain confirmation of a suspected diagnosis due to the introduction of ultrasound and hepatobiliary MRI contrast agents, which allow for the detection of hepatocarcinogenesis even at an early stage. Moreover, the recent technological advancements in artificial intelligence (AI) in radiology contribute an important tool for the diagnostic prediction, prognosis and evaluation of treatment response in the clinical course of the disease. This review presents current imaging modalities and their central role in the management of patients at risk and with HCC.

Keywords: hepatocellular carcinoma; computed tomography; ultrasound; magnetic resonance imaging; artificial intelligence

1. Introduction

Liver malignancies undoubtedly represent a global health challenge, with an estimated annual incidence of more than one million cases in 2025 [1]. Primary liver cancer is the sixth most commonly occurring cancer in the world and the third largest contributor to oncologic mortality [1].

Hepatocellular carcinoma (HCC) accounts for a great majority of liver cancer diagnoses and deaths [2].

Although hepatitis B virus (HBV) and hepatitis C virus (HCV) remain the most important global risk factors worldwide, their impact on the rise of HCC will decline in Western countries due to the availability of increasingly efficient antiviral therapies and preventive policies [3]. As overweight will become endemic worldwide, non-alcoholic fatty liver disease (NAFLD) is likely to become the major contributor to the epidemiology of HCC in the coming years, with a higher risk of incidentally detecting large liver nodules also in younger asymptomatic patients [4]. Other established risk factors of HCC are alcohol consumption [5] and idiopathic liver diseases (e.g., hemochromatosis or primary sclerosing cholangitis) [6].

As a result of several studies on HCC pathology published in the past years, hepatocarcinogenesis is well established nowadays. In cirrhotic livers, metabolic and oxidative insults cause an increased turnover of hepatocytes with a progressive accumulation of genetic mutations [7]. Notably, during the progression from cirrhotic nodules through

Citation: Candita, G.; Rossi, S.; Cwiklinska, K.; Fanni, S.C.; Cioni, D.; Lencioni, R.; Neri, E. Imaging Diagnosis of Hepatocellular Carcinoma: A State-of-the-Art Review. *Diagnostics* **2023**, *13*, 625. https://doi.org/10.3390/diagnostics13040625

Academic Editor: Gian Paolo Caviglia

Received: 24 January 2023
Revised: 4 February 2023
Accepted: 6 February 2023
Published: 8 February 2023

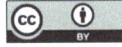

Copyright: © 2023 by the authors. Licensee MDPI, Basel, Switzerland. This article is an open access article distributed under the terms and conditions of the Creative Commons Attribution (CC BY) license (https://creativecommons.org/licenses/by/4.0/).

dysplastic nodules and early HCC to advanced HCC, portal tracts progressively diminish, whereas newly formed unpaired arteries develop due to the tumoral release of vascular endothelial growth factor (VEGF) [7]. Therefore, HCC nodules present a more notable arterial supply as compared to the healthy surrounding parenchyma with the typical greater supply from the portal vein.

Among all the tested serum biomarkers, alpha-fetoprotein (AFP) has proven to improve diagnostic efficiency and to be useful in the evaluation of treatment response in patients with HCC [8].

Unfortunately, the prognosis of patients with HCC remains poor thus far, with an overall ratio of mortality to incidence of 0.91 [9]. However, the accelerated introduction of novel therapeutic modalities is expected to lead to a more favorable scenario. Indeed, due to the recent advances in the oncologic armamentarium, the Barcelona Clinic Liver Cancer (BCLC) treatment strategy was updated in 2022, including the latest evidence of promising medical and interventional therapies [10].

As a matter of fact, in patients at risk, surveillance plays a pivotal role in the detection of small HCC nodules, whose treatment may consist of less invasive and more effective therapies (e.g., percutaneous thermal ablation, surgical excision) [11].

As stated by the latest clinical practice guidelines, published by the European Association for the Study of the Liver (EASL) [12] in 2018, HCC is unique among other cancers in showing typical characteristics on contrast-enhanced computed tomography (CT), magnetic resonance imaging (MRI) or contrast-enhanced ultrasound (CEUS), thus allowing for a highly accurate diagnosis of HCC in patients with cirrhosis. As a result, mini-invasive percutaneous imaging-guided biopsy is strongly recommended for liver nodules with an atypical contrast enhancement [13] or in non-cirrhotic patients [14].

The ability of cross-sectional imaging studies to reliably detect and diagnose HCC in the cirrhotic liver relies primarily on characterizing the enhancement of a suspected lesion as compared to the background liver parenchyma in the hepatic arterial, portal-venous and subsequent phases. The abovementioned differences in the blood flow and extracellular volume between HCC tissue and non-neoplastic cirrhotic liver tissue result in the hallmark imaging characteristics of HCC during the multiphasic flow of contrast, including arterial phase hyperenhancement, subsequent wash-out appearance and capsule appearance [15].

CEUS is a dynamic imaging technique, able to assess the contrast-enhancement pattern of liver nodules in real time, with a considerably higher temporal resolution than that possible to obtain with CT and MRI [16]. CEUS, however, presents some important drawbacks. First of all, CEUS is not a cross-sectional imaging modality, thus not allowing for the detection of distant nodules not seen or included by the operator in the scan after contrast injection. Moreover, ultrasound (US) examination is an operator-dependent modality and may be limited in the detection of nodules in overweight patients or nodules with a difficult location [17].

MRI offers a number of detailed imaging sequences, including T2-weighted and diffusion-weighted images, which may help in the detection of suspicious nodules, although baseline images rarely provide sufficient specificity to enable noninvasive diagnosis. Furthermore, in recent years, two liver-specific contrast agents (gadobenate dimeglumine and gadoxetic acid) have shown to improve the detection of even relatively small and subtle lesions with a hypointense appearance in the hepatobiliary phase [18].

Nevertheless, MRI has some important diagnostic disadvantages, including less availability, greater technical complexity, higher susceptibility to artifacts, higher costs and less consistent image quality. In particular, MRI quality may be compromised in patients with difficulty in breath-holding, trouble keeping still, or large-volume ascites. MRI permits a locoregional evaluation of parenchyma and nodes in the upper abdomen without any information on possible distant metastases. For these reasons, the comparative diagnostic performance of a multiphasic CT and an MRI in real-life practice remains uncertain [19].

In the recent years a rising interest in artificial intelligence (AI) has been observed, and, undeniably, oncologic imaging is one of the most empowered application fields [20–22].

Machine learning (ML) is a branch of AI that focuses on the development of computer algorithms able to learn from structured data to make predictions on decisions without being explicitly programmed to do so. In the oncologic imaging setting, ML is usually combined with radiomics, defined as the process of extracting high-dimensional quantitative features from medical images [23–25]. However, radiomic pipeline consists of numerous steps characterized by several factors, leading to a significant variability between studies affecting their repeatability [26,27].

To overcome the need of prior feature extraction, deep learning (DL) algorithms were developed. DL is a subfield of ML using an artificial neural network (ANN) and has achieved very optimistic performance in image analyses.

Radiomics-based ML and DL have already demonstrated great potential in the diagnosis, staging, survival prediction and tumor response control of HCC [28].

2. Ultrasound

Liver cirrhosis is, thus far, the primary risk factor for HCC, with affected patients requiring periodical imaging surveillance. US is a perfect choice for this purpose due to its safety, wide availability, cost-effectiveness and accuracy in detecting focal liver lesions (FLLs). Once a FLL is detected, US can assist in its characterization using different ultrasonographic techniques, including B-mode, color- and power-Doppler techniques and CEUS [29].

The appearances of HCC nodules on US vary depending on the size and degree of differentiation. The lesion margins are usually relatively well circumscribed in the nodular type but poorly defined in the massive type [30]. HCC nodules smaller than 10 mm are almost hypoechoic or isoechoic, with low-level internal echoes that increase with tissue cellularity. When tumor growth occurs, fatty change is most frequently observed at a tumor diameter of 10–15 mm, and the internal echoes of such nodules are hyperechoic [31]. In HCC nodules greater than 20 mm, typical US patterns such as the "mosaic pattern", "nodule-in-nodule appearance", "peripheral sonolucency" (halo sign) and "lateral shadow" can be more commonly recognized [32].

The evaluation of intranodular vascularity may play a key role in the characterization of FLLs. For this purpose, color Doppler is typically the first-line modality of assessment, even though it encounters different technical limitations such as Doppler angle dependence, operator dependence, low sensitivity to slow flow and overwriting artifacts [30]. Usually, once the tumor increases in size, the "basket" pattern, referring to the presence of a fine network of arterial branches surrounding the lesion, can be appreciated [33]. Using spectral analysis, both pulsatile and continuous waveforms can be recorded, which correspond to the arterial and venous origin of blood supply, respectively. In massive-type HCC, an overall irregular pattern of vascularity, can be appreciated. As a general rule, a continuous portal-like waveform indicates a dysplastic nodule or a well-differentiated HCC; contrarily, a pulsatile arterial waveform is suggestive of advanced HCC [30].

Due to the fact that worldwide ultrasound represents the imaging modality of choice in surveilling patients at risk, the introduction of the US LI-RADS® (Liver Imaging Reporting and Data System), a US-based classification system, was issued by the American College of Radiology in 2017 [34]. Evaluating the size and echogenicity, this system assesses the quality of examination and the potential of a FLL to represent HCC and suggests further management [35].

US, in general, has a reported sensitivity of 98% and specificity of 85% for overall HCC detection. Tumor size is nonetheless a significant factor as the technique's sensitivity reaches approximately 65% for lesions <2 cm [36].

The introduction of CEUS in the evaluation of FLLs certainly represented a turning point in the ultrasonographic diagnosis of HCC. US contrast agents (USCAs) consist of different generations of intravascular gas microbubbles with specific nonlinear acoustic properties [37]. After bolus intravenous injection, USCA allows capillary blood flow to be imaged and contrast enhancement to be assessed, with a much higher temporal resolution compared to CT and MRI [16]. CEUS has proven to be a safe procedure, with low clinical reactions to USCAs reported in the literature and few absolute contraindications (e.g., severe coronary artery disease, pulmonary hypertension). Several studies have stated that CEUS has a significant role as a problem-solving imaging technique for detection of perfusion abnormalities in patients with renal failure and/or at high risk of adverse reaction to CT or MRI contrast agents [17].

In Europe, CEUS is usually performed with SonoVue® (Bracco, Milan, Italy), which is not uptaken by Kupffer cells and hence produces an arterial, portal-venous and late phase [38]. The hallmark of HCC on CEUS using SonoVue® is a homogeneous and intense arterial phase hyper-enhancement (APHE) with mild wash-out starting >60 s after injection [39] (Figure 1).

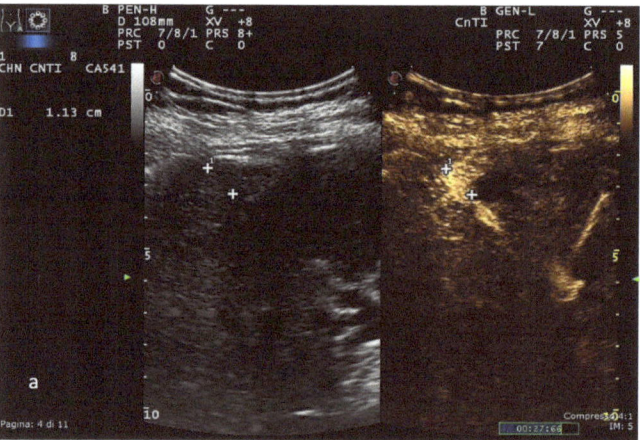

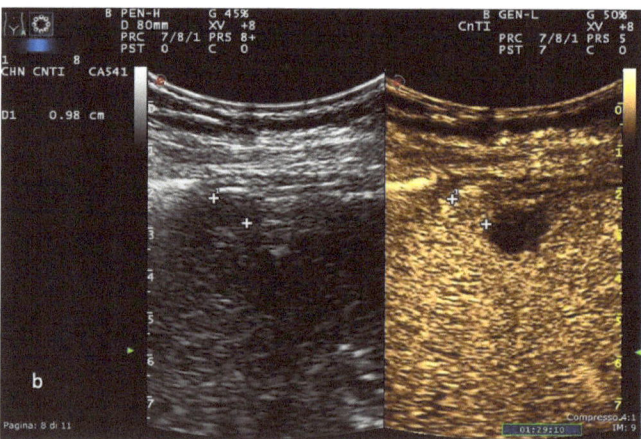

Figure 1. US and CEUS surveillance examination in a patient with HBV-related cirrhosis. Baseline images detect the presence of a centimetric subcapsular hypoechoic nodule. After administration of USCA, the lesion shows arterial hyperenhancement (**a**) with a mild portal-venous wash-out (**b**).

The timing and degree of wash-out are important for the characterization of HCC, which typically shows milder hypo-enhancement compared to metastasis and cholangiocarcinoma. Nodules measuring >5 cm may show heterogeneous enhancement due to necrosis. Both the size and the degree of differentiation affect the enhancement pattern of HCC [40].

Wash-out is less often seen in HCC nodules <2 cm but is more frequent in HCC with poorer grades of differentiation [41].

On the other hand, Sonazoid® (GE Healthcare, Amersham, UK) is a second-generation USCA whose clinical usage was approved in Japan, South Korea and China. As opposed to Sonovue®, Sonazoid® is uptaken by Kupffer cells and produces a late homonym phase in which HCC nodules appear as hypoechoic lesions as compared to the surrounding parenchyma [42].

Moreover, a CEUS LI-RADS® [43] algorithm has been introduced by the American College of Radiology to aid in the accurate characterization of nodules in liver cirrhosis patients. The major criteria are APHE, nodule size and portal-late mild wash-out. A rim APHE and an early (<60 s) or marked wash-out represent LI-RADS M criteria (LR-M), favoring the diagnosis of a non-hepatocellular malignancy [43].

3. Computed Tomography

Nowadays, Multidetector Computed Tomography (MDCT) plays a key role in the diagnostic management of cirrhotic patients who are at an increased risk of developing HCC. According to the majority of guidelines, recognition of a nodule ≥ 10 mm by ultrasonography (US) during HCC surveillance should be followed by a contrast-enhanced CT or MRI examination [44].

MDCT is actually a widely available and rapid imaging modality. Most modern CT scanners have the capability to capture images with wide-detector arrays, typically more than eight-row detectors, allowing for high spatial resolution. Premium CT scanners offer even wider detector arrays with up to 320 detector rows that cover up to 16 cm in the z-axis and fast gantry rotation times down to 0.25 s [45].

As compared to MRI, MDCT is a faster and better-tolerated examination, less prone to motion artifacts, particularly useful in non-cooperative patients or in those who are unable to hold their breath. The main disadvantages of MDCT include radiation exposure and relatively low contrast resolution of tissue, even though iterative reconstruction models have further enabled radiation dose reduction by reducing CT image noise [30].

The baseline pre-contrast phase examination serves as a baseline for determining the extent of liver lesion and is useful to assess background liver disease such as steatosis or cirrhosis [46] For HCC evaluation, the non-contrast phase helps identify subtle areas of arterial phase hyperenhancement and is essential to distinguish hyperdense lipiodol staining and blood products in patients who previously underwent intra-arterial or percutaneous treatments [47].

However, multiphase contrast-enhanced CT and/or MRI examinations consisting of the late arterial, portal-venous and delayed phase are essential for a confident imaging diagnosis of HCC [48].

Whereas the portal-venous phase is sufficient for the detection of hypovascular liver metastases, the late arterial and delayed phases are most important for the evaluation of hypervascular tumors including HCC (Figure 2).

The typical hallmark diagnostic feature of HCC is the combination of non-rim APHE on the late arterial phase and non-peripheral wash-out appearance on the portal-venous and/or delayed phases, thereby reflecting the peculiar vascular derangements induced by hepatocarcinogenesis [49].

As stated by different current guidelines [12], the late hepatic arterial phase (35 s) is considered the most consistent vascular phase for the assessment of HCC, as APHE is an essential finding in making a definitive imaging diagnosis of HCC [50]. The late arterial phase should be characterized by full hepatic arterial enhancement with good portal vein enhancement, but no antegrade enhancement of the hepatic veins. As some HCCs are not conspicuous until the late hepatic arterial phase, earlier arterial phase imaging can result in reduced sensitivity [51]. Moreover, as a favorable late arterial phase occurs during a restricted time interval, individualized CT scan protocols (e.g., test-bolus, bolus-tracking) are recommended.

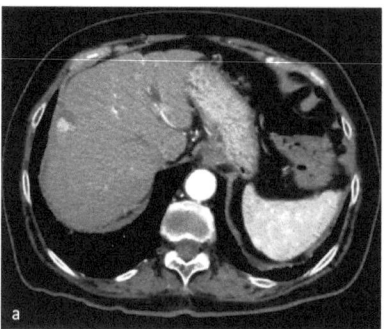
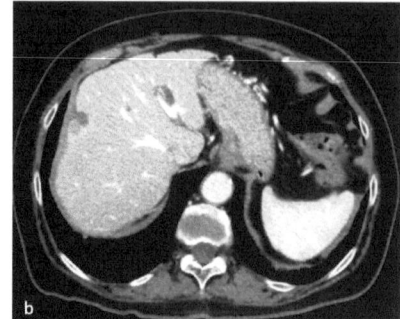
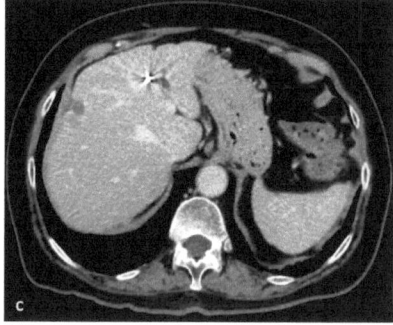

Figure 2. Contrast-enhanced CT of the upper abdomen in the patient discussed in Figure 1. After administration of iodinated contrast agent, the subcapsular lesion showed arterial hyperenhancement (**a**), with progressive wash-out in the portal-venous (**b**) and delayed (**c**) phase.

The portal-venous phase (70–80 s) occurs when enhancement of the portal and hepatic veins is higher and there is peak parenchymal enhancement of the liver. Portal-venous phase FLL imaging best demonstrates the "wash-out appearance" due to the peak enhancement of the surrounding liver [52]. The detection of peripheral washout on the portal phase is not specific for HCC nodules, as intrahepatic cholangiocarcinoma may also show this kind of appearance [53].

The delayed phase (3–5 min) is acquired when overall vessel brightness decreases as compared to the portal-venous phase. A combination of the portal-venous phase and delayed phase can more reliably demonstrate the "wash-out appearance" and "capsule appearance" of the HCC nodule [53]. Conversely, cholangiocarcinoma typically shows peripheral enhancement in the arterial phase, with centripetal progressive reinforcement in the delayed phase [54].

The detection of an "enhancing capsule" [55], with the appearance of a uniformly thick enhancement at the peripheral rim of the nodule on the portal and delayed phase, is another major criterion included in the LI-RADS. The tumor capsule is detected in about 70% of HCCs and is a pathologic feature of progressed disease [30].

Apart from the major imaging features, the LI-RADS CT/MRI contains many ancillary features, including nodule-in-nodule architecture, mosaic appearance and non-enhancing capsule, that may favor the diagnosis of HCC [34].

The nodule-in-nodule architecture consists in the detection of a progressed HCC within a dysplastic nodule or an early HCC. The inner nodule shows APHE, while the parent nodule appears hypo- or iso-attenuated. The nodule-in-nodule appearance presents a poor prognostic value, as the inner hyper-enhancing nodule has a short volume-doubling time [56].

Similarly, the mosaic appearance is the result of a presence of areas within larger nodules in various steps of dedifferentiation. On imaging, similar nodules are composed of compartments with variable enhancements, separated by irregular enhancing septa and necrotic areas [57]. The mosaic pattern is observed in 28–63% nodules of HCCs [30].

The non-enhancing capsule refers to a capsule appearance that is constantly hypodense on dynamic CT/MRI examinations [58].

In recent years, dual-energy CT (DECT) has become increasingly available. DECT can acquire two sets of images of the same tissue using different photon spectra (high and low kVp). By adjusting the photon spectrum, the optimal single energy with an optimized contrast-to-noise ratio (CNR) can be obtained, which, in turn, improves the detection rate of smaller tissue density differences as well as small lesions [59]. As compared to low kVp CT scans, at an equal radiation dose [60], DECT showed higher CNR of HCC and higher image quality, thus allowing the radiologist to evaluate small lesions that were not detectable on conventional CT scan [61].

Furthermore, recently, CT liver perfusion (CTLP) has emerged as a useful imaging modality for quantitative evaluation of tumor angiogenesis. CTLP is based on the analysis of a dataset that includes sequential CT images of the liver acquired over time following intravenous contrast injection, thus measuring the change of attenuation of regions of interest within the liver parenchyma [62]. Conventional CT might mischaracterize small HCC nodules without a clear APHE; CTLP can separate the hepatic arterial from the portal-venous component of blood flow in order to identify the nodules with a still incomplete neo-angiogenesis [63].

In the setting of HCC, CTLP demonstrated fair diagnostic accuracy in the first diagnosis [64] and in assessing treatment response through the evaluation in the arterial perfusion changes [65].

4. Magnetic Resonance Imaging

The introduction of MRI in clinical practice has radically changed the diagnostic algorithm of HCC, since it may achieve a higher contrast resolution and is able to characterize more tissue properties other than tissue density and vascularization [66]. According to recent meta-analyses, the pooled overall sensitivity and specificity of contrast-enhanced MRI are 70% and 94%, respectively, in the detection of HCC nodules [67]. Nevertheless, sensitivity is greater for lesions >2 cm (almost 100%) but drops to 60% for lesions smaller than 2 cm, and it is even lower for lesions smaller than 1 cm [68]. Therefore, MRI has proven to outperform CT for the diagnosis of HCCs smaller than 2 cm, with comparable accuracy for lesions $\geq$2 cm [30]. For this reason, MRI is also a useful imaging modality in the surveillance of cirrhotic patients at risk. Nowadays, a prompt diagnosis of small nodules is mandatory to assure a radical treatment, thus augmenting overall survival [69].

As stated before, large HCC nodules generally show the typical imaging hallmarks ("wash-in/wash-out" appearance) that enable a radiologist to make a definitive diagnosis also in gadolinium-enhanced MRI examinations. However, APHE may not be present in a large percentage of early and poorly differentiated HCCs, which should not be definitively assessed according to the current guidelines [15]. In such cases, MRI plays an indisputable role in finding out the presence of ancillary features in differently weighted images, keeping in mind that lesions <1 cm cannot be definitively characterized as HCC and follow-up is advised [30].

According to LI-RADS, the detection of a capsule is a major finding typically found in progressed HCCs. HCC capsules usually show low T1 and T2 intensity, with a mild enhancement in the portal-venous and delayed phases and are thicker than cirrhotic fibrotic septa [58]. The detection of a disrupted capsule is a negative prognostic factor, as a higher recurrence rate after surgical or interventional treatment is reported [55].

Most large HCCs show moderate hyperintensity on T2-weighted (T2-w) sequences, probably due to a higher cellularity, an increased arterial blood flow and a decreased portal vascularity [70].

Conversely, dysplastic nodules and early HCCs appear iso- or hypo-intense as compared to the background liver [71]. However, mildly increased T2 signal intensity is not a specific imaging feature as it is also imaged in other malignant lesions of the liver [72].

On the other hand, hyperintensity on T1-weighted (T1-w) sequences may be detected if a high amount of fat or glycogen is present within the HCC nodule.

Almost 40% of early HCCs present with intranodular fatty changes, which tend to regress during the tumoral progression to higher histological grades [73]. On chemical shift sequences, fatty areas within the nodule show the characteristic signal drop on the opposed-phase compared to in-phase [74]. Glycogen may be present as a result of the hypercellularity within the nodule [75] and does not show signal drop on chemical shift sequences.

Furthermore, MRI is the preferred imaging modality in surveilling patients with hemochromatosis (liver iron overload), which is itself a risk factor for HCC development [76]. Iron-rich nodules usually appear hypointense on T1-w images and moderately to markedly hypointense on T2-w and T2*-w images [75]. In such parenchymal background, iron-free nodules appear as hyperintense on T1-weighted images and are highly suspicious for a dysplastic or HCC lesion [77].

Since hyperintensity on T1-weighted baseline sequences may produce misinterpretation, subtraction techniques are always recommended in order to correctly detect APHE [78].

In recent years, diffusion-weighted imaging (DWI) has emerged as a baseline MRI sequence that evaluates the reduced diffusivity of water molecules among the closely packed cells within HCC nodules [79]. In general, higher histological grades are associated with higher DWI signal and corresponding lower apparent diffusion coefficient (ADC) values. Early HCCs may be misdiagnosed on DWI due to their relatively low cellular density [80]. However, a restricted diffusion is an ancillary feature that favors the diagnosis of liver malignancy, but it is not specific for HCC [81]; evaluating the appearance on different MRI sequences, including contrast-enhanced images, may support the diagnosis of HCC. DWI is useful in corroborating the suspicion in typical and atypical HCC nodules or in patients that cannot undergo intravenous contrast injection (e.g., for a previous allergic reaction), thus increasing the overall sensitivity of HCC detection [82].

In the last decade, several meta-analyses have established that MRI paired with gadoxetic acid-based hepatobiliary contrast agents presents a higher sensitivity than MRI paired with extracellular agents, in particular in the setting of small HCCs that may not show the typical APHE [83]. Hepatobiliary contrast agents (gadobenate dimeglumine, gadoxetate disodium) are selectively taken up by normal hepatocytes through specific organic anion transporting polypeptide (OATP) transporters, allowing the acquisition of hepatobiliary phase (HBP) images at 20–40 min [84]. Nodules with a lack of hepatocytes (angiomas) or degenerated hepatocytes lacking OATP (malignancies) are hypointense on HBP [85], while lesions with a higher number of functioning hepatocytes (focal nodular hyperplasia, low-grade dysplastic nodules) may appear hyperintense on HBP [86].

Since up to 90% of HCCs demonstrate hypointensity in the HBP, this ancillary feature may contribute to the differentiation of HCC from benign nodules developed in chronic liver diseases (Figure 3) [87].

However, until now, there has been no established consensus regarding the value of HBP hypointensity during liver MRI. In East Asia, some guidelines attribute importance to the use of HBP hypointense appearance, thus permitting the diagnosis of smaller HCCs [88]. Meanwhile, in the Western countries, where liver transplantation is one of the major treatment options [89], the practice guidelines suggest that wash-out should be determined in the portal phase, thus obtaining the highest specificity [12]. In fact, recent studies have suggested that HBP hypointense appearance is highly sensitive and specific for HCC when combining with non-rim APHE [84].

In addition, in MRI, perfusion imaging is a quantitative technique that provides information about tissue microcirculation. In the liver, the most used approach is dynamic contrast-enhanced (DCE) MRI, which requires gadolinium contrast administration as a tracer, followed by consequential acquisition of signal-time curves that quantify changes in contrast concentrations over time [90]. DCE consists of free-breathing 3D perfusion sequences covering the entire liver with a short acquisition time (1–2 s) repeated for up to 5 min after contrast administration [91].

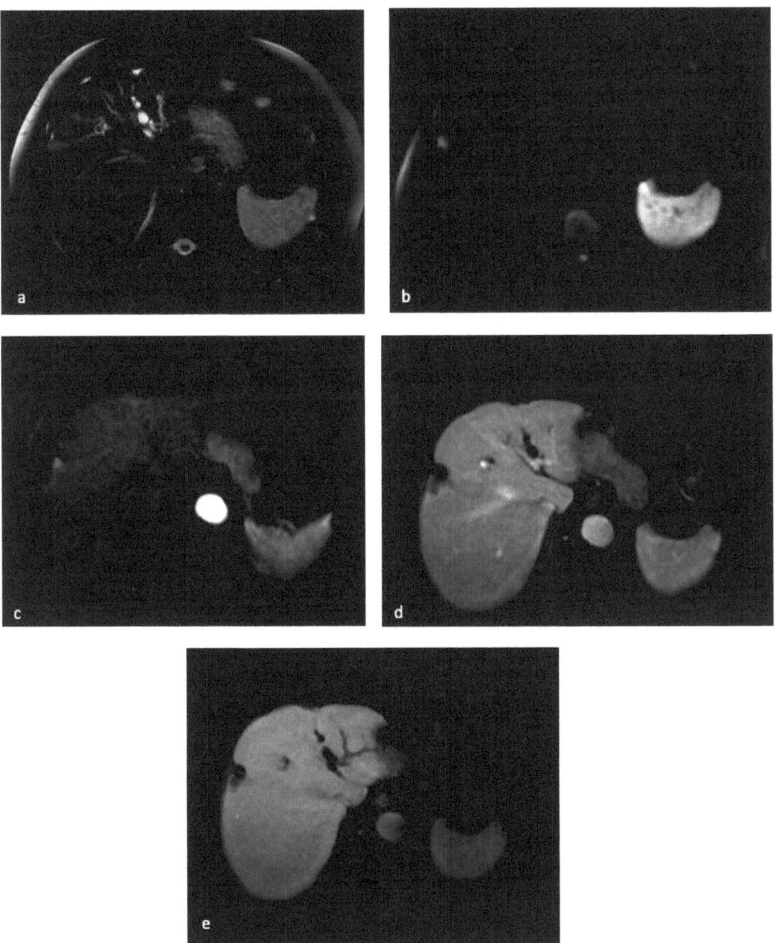

Figure 3. MR examination of the patient discussed in Figures 1 and 2. On T2-weighted images, the centimetric subcapsular appeared as hyperintense (**a**). On DWI with a b-value of 1000, the lesion showed signal restriction (**b**). After administration of a hepatobiliary contrast agent, the lesion showed arterial hyperenhancement (**c**) with hypointensity in the portal-venous phase (**d**) and in the hepatobiliary phase. (**e**) The lesion appeared hypointense.

DCE-MRI provides information based on the intralesional temporal distribution of contrast agents in lesions that often present with a heterogeneous vascular network. Time-to-peak enhancement (time between arrival of the tracer and maximum enhancement), area under the curve (amount of enhancement during a specific time interval), maximum enhancement (peak height) and maximum slope are semi-quantitative analyses affected by acquisition parameters, injection protocols and the patient's physical conditions [92]. On the other hand, true quantitative models evaluate the change in concentrations of the contrast agent using pharmacokinetic modeling techniques [93].

5. PET/CT

Though HCC diagnosis is primarily based on the typical characteristics of contrast hyperenhancement and wash-out on CT and MRI, some of the biologic features of HCC can be appreciated fully only with the 18F-fluorodeoxyglucose positron-emission tomography (FDG-PET)/CT. This imaging modality provides some additional information on primary HCC lesions and extrahepatic metastases which aids clinicians with treatment selection [94]. FDG-PET/CT is an extremely useful tool in the evaluation of many oncologic patients, yet it is not routinely used for HCC as it is limited by low sensitivity due to the high physiologic uptake of liver tissue and the variable expression of glucose transporters and glycolytic activity in HCC nodules [95]. In fact, FDG usually accumulates in poorly differentiated HCCs but not in well-differentiated ones. Furthermore, since a poorly differentiated HCC is more likely to metastasize, FDG-PET/CT may be useful to detect distant metastasis and complete the staging in uncertain cases [96].

However, tracers based on choline recently showed improved detection rates of well-differentiated HCCs [97]. Dual-tracer PET/CT combining choline and FDG as tracers has shown high overlap between well- and less-differentiated HCCs, thus making it possible to classify lesions in proliferative (poorly differentiated nodules) and non-proliferative (well-differentiated nodules) [98].

FDG-PET/CT can be used to monitor treatment response and provide prognostic information on the risk of HCC recurrence after surgery or interventional treatment, as the scans reflect high tissue metabolism that may be indicative of recurrent disease even in areas of increased tissue rearrangement due to the treatment [94].

6. Artificial Intelligence

Artificial intelligence (AI) represents the ability of machines to emulate the intelligence of human beings [99]. Radiomics-based ML and DL could potentially assist radiologists in HCC imaging by overcoming some of the main limitations presented by imaging modalities that were described above. Indeed, the human eye, especially with low expertise, could lead to wrong or indefinite diagnoses, leading to several other investigations with various modalities. This is particularly true in US imaging, which hugely relies on the radiologist's expertise and which represents the primary technique used to follow-up patients suffering from liver cirrhosis—remaining one of the principal risk factors for HCC development. Indeed, AI could empower the role of US imaging, being a safe, non-invasive and rapid modality; decreasing the use of second-level imaging techniques generally based on contrast media; and attenuating the limitations of US. The advantages of AI use for patients with HCC could be represented by the time reduction needed to identify the malignant lesion and, thus, faster treatment; its differential diagnosis between benign and malignant conditions to avoid unnecessary CT/MRI studies; and, finally, the ability of AI to differentiate HCC from other primary or secondary malignancies [100].

AI has already been demonstrated to reduce the time-to-diagnosis of HCC by US using ML and DL algorithms, with the latter characterized by superior accuracy, sensitivity and area under the curve (AUC) [101].

Regarding the differential diagnosis between benign entities (cysts or hemangiomas) and malignancies, Schmauch developed an artificial neural network (ANN) that achieved an AUC of 0.924 [102]. Accordingly, Guo et al. implemented a computer aided diagnosis (CAD) system for three-phase CEUS to differentiate between benign and malignant liver lesions and found an overall accuracy of $93.56 \pm 5.90\%$ [103].

HCC, as previously mentioned, can sometimes have characteristics of other malignant lesions, and differentiating between HCC and other primitive lesions or secondary ones may become challenging. AI may help in this setting, as demonstrated by Mao et al., who reported an accuracy of 0.843 ± 0.078 in differentiating between primary and metastatic liver cancer (AUC, 0.816 ± 0.088; sensitivity, 0.768 ± 0.232; specificity, 0.880 ± 0.117) [104].

Another challenge for radiologists is to differentiate HCC from cholangiocarcinoma, or a combination of the two (hepato-cholangiocarcinoma), as the two pathologies have the same risk factors and, especially in US imaging, lack particular characteristics to distinguish between them. Currently, AFP and carbohydrate antigen 19-9 are considered the ideal serum tumor markers for HCC and intrahepatic cholangiocarcinoma, yet they are generally deemed unsatisfactory in diagnostic sensitivity or specificity [104]. The two tumor markers are especially unreliable if the diagnosis is made based on them alone [1]. Ichikawa et al. determined the imaging hallmarks for distinguishing intrahepatic mass-forming biliary carcinomas from HCC, and the diagnostic value was further verified by Bayesian statistics (AUC = 0.960) [105].

US imaging is also suitable for radiomics-based approaches, and its utility has already been proven in distinguishing between low- and high-grade HCC. This differentiation is important to establish patients' prognosis and to estimate the probability of recurrence or metastasis after treatment [106], especially because patients with high-grade HCC have poor prognosis. According to Ren et al., grayscale ultrasomics features can be used to distinguish high- and low-grade HCC with a p value of <0.05, providing information on tumor heterogeneity which cannot be identified by human eye in normal US images [107]. Radiomics-based model benefit from the combination with clinical data, as demonstrated by Wang et al., who combined radiomics features extracted from CEUS with clinical variables to improve the tumor grading performance.

The use of AI on CT images could enhance its diagnostic potential for HCC and aid differentiating its different aspects (i.e., nodular, diffuse or massive), as well as distinguish HCC from other benign and malignant liver lesions and estimate a grading scale.

Convolutional neural networks (CNN) are able to automatically perform liver and tumor segmentation and classify lesions as nodular, diffuse or massive type. Studies have demonstrated the superiority of this fully automated method over the semi-automated one [108].

As mentioned before, to distinguish HCC from other liver lesions, the use of contrast media aids the study of vascular patterns of different kinds of lesions. CNN is a potential method to diagnose and differentiate HCC using the Liver Imaging-Reporting and Data System (LI-RADS). The use of CNN can reduce radiation dose to patients because it is able to diagnose HCC based on a three-phase CT without the pre-contrast phase. In fact, this protocol shows similar diagnostic accuracy compared to the four-phase protocol, limiting the radiation dose to patients, especially as these patients need multiple CTs in the course of follow-up [109]. Radiomic-based ML could also assist radiologists in diagnosing HCC when it shows indeterminate or doubtful aspects without the specific wash-in and wash-out imaging features [110]. It is based on different tumor aspect during arterial and portal phase, such as, for example, wash-out without a clear wash-in. This technique is used for images taken with different protocols, so it can be used for images taken at different institutes. Nevertheless, the features extracted often overlap between HCC and other malignant lesions. This is a limit of radiomics that is able to well differentiate benignity from malignancy, yet may not always identify the malignant lesion as HCC.

AI could also help to estimate patients' prognosis, evaluating, for example, the recurrence risk or microvascular invasion (MVI) tumor pattern. Studies have shown that MVI is an independent histopathological prognostic factor associated with survival in all-stage HCC patients [111]. MVI has been reported to be a better predictor of tumor recurrence and overall survival than the Milan criteria [112]. Patients with a poor prognosis need a more aggressive treatment approach. Different features are evaluated to distinguish MVI, such as the smooth and irregular margin of lesions, presence of internal tumor arteries, hypodense halo, peritumoral enhancement and lobes involved. In the study published by Jiang et al., the median recurrence-free survival (RFS) of the entire cohort was 22 months while the RFS of patients with MVI was 6 months, and a CNN was able to accurately differentiate MVI pre-operatively [113].

MVI invasion is also important to evaluate recurrence risk after trans-arterial chemoembolization [114].

Studies on AI and MRI are still limited compared to US and CT. AI in MRI can differentiate LI-RADS 3 grade from LI-RADS 4-5, which is extremely important for clinical decision and patient management. In fact, LI-RADS 3 needs no or less invasive management. Many LR-3 lesions are benign hyper-enhancing pseudolesions which can be followed for stability with imaging, whereas 80% of biopsied LR-4 lesions are HCC, and 68% of untreated LR-4 lesions become LR-5 lesions within two years [50]. LR-4 lesions may be biopsied, while an LR-5 score indicates HCC diagnostic certainty and biopsy is usually not needed before treatment [115].

The results demonstrated that tumor size and shape, associated with its contrast aspect, are important factors for HCC diagnosis. In addition, it is demonstrated that the late contrast phase does not contribute to the LI-RADS classification performance of CNN model and it can be avoided [116]. This condition makes it possible to reduce time for MRI imaging, limiting patients' artifacts. CNN improves the recognition of this classification and reduces misdiagnosis by radiologists.

7. Conclusions

Imaging plays a pivotal role in the multidisciplinary management of patients at risk or suffering from HCC and in the radiological evaluation of response to treatment.

US is the most recognized imaging modality for HCC surveillance, even though MRI has been recently proved to be a useful tool in surveilling cirrhotic patients.

However, non-invasive diagnosis of HCC mainly relies on CT and MR examination. Different radiological hallmarks have been described, with APHE being an essential finding in making a definitive diagnosis of HCC. The recent introduction of hepatobiliary contrast agent in liver MRI has shown to increase sensitivity and specificity in assessing HCC nodules, as well as in the absence of typical APHE, and may change the diagnostic imaging algorithm in the coming years.

Furthermore, recent applications of AI, including radiomics and machine learning, have shown interesting results in the setting of liver imaging in patients with HCC. AI has proven to empower the role of imaging diagnosis, helping the radiologist to distinguish HCC from other liver malignancies in atypical or doubtful cases or to evaluate microvascular invasion that heavily modify patients' prognosis. Through AI applications, it will be reasonably possible in the upcoming years to reduce the time and number of examinations needed to characterize malignant lesions, thus allowing for faster diagnosis, better prognosis and reduced medical costs.

Author Contributions: Conceptualization, G.C., D.C., R.L. and E.N.; methodology, G.C. and S.C.F.; writing—original draft preparation, G.C., S.R., K.C., S.C.F. and D.C.; writing—review and editing, S.C.F., D.C., R.L. and E.N.; supervision, D.C., R.L. and E.N. All authors have read and agreed to the published version of the manuscript.

Funding: This research received no external funding.

Institutional Review Board Statement: Not applicable.

Informed Consent Statement: Not applicable.

Data Availability Statement: Not applicable.

Conflicts of Interest: The authors declare no conflict of interest.

References

1. Sung, H.; Ferlay, J.; Siegel, R.L.; Laversanne, M.; Soerjomataram, I.; Jemal, A.; Bray, F. Global Cancer Statistics 2020: GLOBOCAN Estimates of Incidence and Mortality Worldwide for 36 Cancers in 185 Countries. *CA Cancer J. Clin.* **2021**, *71*, 209–249. [CrossRef]
2. Singal, A.G.; Lampertico, P.; Nahon, P. Epidemiology and surveillance for hepatocellular carcinoma: New trends. *J. Hepatol.* **2020**, *72*, 250–261. [CrossRef]
3. Alberts, C.J.; Clifford, G.M.; Georges, D.; Negro, F.; Lesi, O.A.; Hutin, Y.J.-F.; de Martel, C. Worldwide prevalence of hepatitis B virus and hepatitis C virus among patients with cirrhosis at country, region, and global levels: A systematic review. *Lancet Gastroenterol. Hepatol.* **2022**, *7*, 724–735. [CrossRef] [PubMed]

4. Onzi, G.; Moretti, F.; Balbinot, S.S.; Balbinot, R.A.; Soldera, J. Hepatocellular carcinoma in non-alcoholic fatty liver disease with and without cirrhosis. *Hepatoma Res.* **2019**, *2019*. [CrossRef]
5. Testino, G.; Leone, S.; Borro, P. Alcohol and hepatocellular carcinoma: A review and a point of view. *World J. Gastroenterol.* **2014**, *20*, 15943–15954. [CrossRef]
6. Kowdley, K.V. Iron, hemochromatosis, and hepatocellular carcinoma. *Gastroenterology* **2004**, *127*, S79–S86. [CrossRef]
7. Takeda, H.; Takai, A.; Eso, Y.; Takahashi, K.; Marusawa, H.; Seno, H. Genetic Landscape of Multistep Hepatocarcinogenesis. *Cancers* **2022**, *14*, 568. [CrossRef] [PubMed]
8. Muscari, F.; Maulat, C. Preoperative alpha-fetoprotein (AFP) in hepatocellular carcinoma (HCC): Is this 50-year biomarker still up-to-date? *Transl. Gastroenterol. Hepatol.* **2020**, *5*, 46. [CrossRef]
9. Markakis, G. The changing epidemiology of hepatocellular carcinoma in Greece. *Ann. Gastroenterol.* **2022**, *35*, 88–94. [CrossRef] [PubMed]
10. Reig, M.; Forner, A.; Rimola, J.; Ferrer-Fàbrega, J.; Burrel, M.; Garcia-Criado, Á.; Kelley, R.K.; Galle, P.R.; Mazzaferro, V.; Salem, R.; et al. BCLC strategy for prognosis prediction and treatment recommendation Barcelona Clinic Liver Cancer (BCLC) staging system: The 2022 update. *J. Hepatol.* **2021**, *76*, 681–693. [CrossRef] [PubMed]
11. Harris, P.S.; Hansen, R.M.; Gray, M.E.; Massoud, O.I.; McGuire, B.M.; Shoreibah, M.G. Hepatocellular carcinoma surveillance: An evidence-based approach. *World J. Gastroenterol.* **2019**, *25*, 1550–1559. [CrossRef] [PubMed]
12. European Association for the Study of the Liver. EASL Clinical Practice Guidelines: Management of Hepatocellular Carcinoma. *J. Hepatol.* **2018**, *69*, 182–236. [CrossRef]
13. Russo, F.P.; Imondi, A.; Lynch, E.N.; Farinati, F. When and how should we perform a biopsy for HCC in patients with liver cirrhosis in 2018? A review. *Dig. Liver Dis.* **2018**, *50*, 640–646. [CrossRef] [PubMed]
14. Desai, A.; Sandhu, S.; Lai, J.-P.; Sandhu, D.S. Hepatocellular carcinoma in non-cirrhotic liver: A comprehensive review. *World J. Hepatol.* **2019**, *11*, 1–18. [CrossRef]
15. Kim, J.H.; Joo, I.; Lee, J.M. Atypical Appearance of Hepatocellular Carcinoma and Its Mimickers: How to Solve Challenging Cases Using Gadoxetic Acid-Enhanced Liver Magnetic Resonance Imaging. *Korean J. Radiol.* **2019**, *20*, 1019–1041. [CrossRef]
16. Eisenbrey, J.R.; Gabriel, H.; Savsani, E.; Lyshchik, A. Contrast-enhanced ultrasound (CEUS) in HCC diagnosis and assessment of tumor response to locoregional therapies. *Abdom. Imaging* **2021**, *46*, 3579–3595. [CrossRef]
17. Bartolotta, T.V.; Taibbi, A.; Midiri, M.; Lagalla, R. Contrast-enhanced ultrasound of hepatocellular carcinoma: Where do we stand? *Ultrasonography* **2019**, *38*, 200–214. [CrossRef] [PubMed]
18. Francisco, F.A.F.; De Araújo, A.L.E.; Neto, J.A.O.; Parente, D.B. Contraste hepatobiliar: Diagnóstico diferencial das lesões hepáticas focais, armadilhas e outras indicações. *Radiol. Bras.* **2014**, *47*, 301–309. [CrossRef] [PubMed]
19. Roberts, L.R.; Sirlin, C.B.; Zaiem, F.; Almasri, J.; Prokop, L.J.; Heimbach, J.K.; Murad, M.H.; Mohammed, K. Imaging for the diagnosis of hepatocellular carcinoma: A systematic review and meta-analysis. *Hepatology* **2018**, *67*, 401–421. [CrossRef]
20. Romei, C.; Fanni, S.C.; Volpi, F.; Milazzo, A.; D'Amore, C.A.; Colligiani, L.; Neri, E.; De Liperi, A.; Stella, G.M.; Bortolotto, C. New Updates of the Imaging Role in Diagnosis, Staging, and Response Treatment of Malignant Pleural Mesothelioma. *Cancers* **2021**, *13*, 4377. [CrossRef] [PubMed]
21. Chiu, H.-Y.; Chao, H.-S.; Chen, Y.-M. Application of Artificial Intelligence in Lung Cancer. *Cancers* **2022**, *14*, 1370. [CrossRef] [PubMed]
22. Gabelloni, M.; Faggioni, L.; Borgheresi, R.; Restante, G.; Shortrede, J.; Tumminello, L.; Scapicchio, C.; Coppola, F.; Cioni, D.; Gómez-Rico, I.; et al. Bridging gaps between images and data: A systematic update on imaging biobanks. *Eur. Radiol.* **2022**, *32*, 3173–3186. [CrossRef] [PubMed]
23. Lambin, P.; Leijenaar, R.T.H.; Deist, T.M.; Peerlings, J.; de Jong, E.E.C.; van Timmeren, J.; Sanduleanu, S.; Larue, R.T.H.M.; Even, A.J.G.; Jochems, A.; et al. Radiomics: The bridge between medical imaging and personalized medicine. *Nat. Rev. Clin. Oncol.* **2017**, *14*, 749–762. [CrossRef]
24. Spadarella, G.; Stanzione, A.; D'Antonoli, T.A.; Andreychenko, A.; Fanni, S.C.; Ugga, L.; Kotter, E.; Cuocolo, R. Systematic review of the radiomics quality score applications: An EuSoMII Radiomics Auditing Group Initiative. *Eur. Radiol.* **2022**, 1–11. [CrossRef] [PubMed]
25. Scapicchio, C.; Gabelloni, M.; Barucci, A.; Cioni, D.; Saba, L.; Neri, E. A deep look into radiomics. *La Radiol. Medica* **2021**, *126*, 1296–1311. [CrossRef]
26. Aringhieri, G.; Fanni, S.C.; Febi, M.; Colligiani, L.; Cioni, D.; Neri, E. The Role of Radiomics in Salivary Gland Imaging: A Systematic Review and Radiomics Quality Assessment. *Diagnostics* **2022**, *12*, 3002. [CrossRef] [PubMed]
27. Koçak, B.; Cuocolo, R.; dos Santos, D.P.; Stanzione, A.; Ugga, L. Must-have Qualities of Clinical Research on Artificial Intelligence and Machine Learning. *Balk. Med. J.* **2023**, *40*, 3–12. [CrossRef]
28. Yao, S.; Ye, Z.; Wei, Y.; Jiang, H.-Y.; Song, B. Radiomics in hepatocellular carcinoma: A state-of-the-art review. *World J. Gastrointest. Oncol.* **2021**, *13*, 1599–1615. [CrossRef]
29. Sparchez, Z.; Craciun, R.; Caraiani, C.; Horhat, A.; Nenu, I.; Procopet, B.; Sparchez, M.; Stefanescu, H.; Mocan, T. Ultrasound or Sectional Imaging Techniques as Screening Tools for Hepatocellular Carcinoma: Fall Forward or Move Forward? *J. Clin. Med.* **2021**, *10*, 903. [CrossRef] [PubMed]
30. Chartampilas, E.; Rafailidis, V.; Georgopoulou, V.; Kalarakis, G.; Hatzidakis, A.; Prassopoulos, P. Current Imaging Diagnosis of Hepatocellular Carcinoma. *Cancers* **2022**, *14*, 3997. [CrossRef] [PubMed]

31. Tanaka, H. Current role of ultrasound in the diagnosis of hepatocellular carcinoma. *J. Med. Ultrason.* **2020**, *47*, 239–255. [CrossRef] [PubMed]
32. Minami, Y.; Kudo, M. Hepatic malignancies: Correlation between sonographic findings and pathological features. *World J. Radiol.* **2010**, *2*, 249–256. [CrossRef]
33. Yang, F.; Zhao, J.; Liu, C.; Mao, Y.; Mu, J.; Wei, X.; Jia, J.; Zhang, S.; Xin, X.; Tan, J. Superb microvascular imaging technique in depicting vascularity in focal liver lesions: More hypervascular supply patterns were depicted in hepatocellular carcinoma. *Cancer Imaging* **2019**, *19*, 92. [CrossRef] [PubMed]
34. Ren, A.-H.; Du, J.-B.; Yang, D.-W.; Zhao, P.-F.; Wang, Z.-C.; Yang, Z.-H. The role of ancillary features for diagnosing hepatocellular carcinoma on CT: Based on the Liver Imaging Reporting and Data System version 2017 algorithm. *Clin. Radiol.* **2020**, *75*, 478.e25–478.e35. [CrossRef]
35. Chernyak, V.; Fowler, K.J.; Kamaya, A.; Kielar, A.Z.; Elsayes, K.M.; Bashir, M.R.; Kono, Y.; Do, R.K.; Mitchell, D.G.; Singal, A.G.; et al. Liver Imaging Reporting and Data System (LI-RADS) Version 2018: Imaging of Hepatocellular Carcinoma in At-Risk Patients. *Radiology* **2018**, *289*, 816–830. [CrossRef]
36. Sangiovanni, A.; Del Ninno, E.; Fasani, P.; De Fazio, C.; Ronchi, G.; Romeo, R.; Morabito, A.; De Franchis, R.; Colombo, M. Increased survival of cirrhotic patients with a hepatocellular carcinoma detected during surveillance. *Gastroenterology* **2004**, *126*, 1005–1014. [CrossRef]
37. Beckmann, S.; Simanowski, J.H. Update in Contrast-Enhanced Ultrasound. *Visc. Med.* **2020**, *36*, 476–486. [CrossRef]
38. Dietrich, C.F.; Nolsøe, C.P.; Barr, R.G.; Berzigotti, A.; Burns, P.N.; Cantisani, V.; Chammas, M.C.; Chaubal, N.; Choi, B.I.; Clevert, D.-A.; et al. Guidelines and Good Clinical Practice Recommendations for Contrast-Enhanced Ultrasound (CEUS) in the Liver–Update 2020 WFUMB in Cooperation with EFSUMB, AFSUMB, AIUM, and FLAUS. *Ultrasound Med. Biol.* **2020**, *46*, 2579–2604. [CrossRef]
39. Fraquelli, M.; Nadarevic, T.; Colli, A.; Manzotti, C.; Giljaca, V.; Miletic, D.; Štimac, D.; Casazza, G. Contrast-enhanced ultrasound for the diagnosis of hepatocellular carcinoma in adults with chronic liver disease. *Cochrane Database Syst. Rev.* **2022**, *2022*, CD013483. [CrossRef]
40. Dietrich, C.F.; Bamber, J.; Berzigotti, A.; Bota, S.; Cantisani, V.; Castera, L.; Cosgrove, D.; Ferraioli, G.; Friedrich-Rust, M.; Gilja, O.H.; et al. EFSUMB Guidelines and Recommendations on the Clinical Use of Liver Ultrasound Elastography, Update 2017 (Long Version). *Ultraschall Med.-Eur. J. Ultrasound* **2017**, *38*, e16–e47. [CrossRef]
41. Yang, H.K.; Burns, P.N.; Jang, H.-J.; Kono, Y.; Khalili, K.; Wilson, S.R.; Kim, T.K. Contrast-enhanced ultrasound approach to the diagnosis of focal liver lesions: The importance of washout. *Ultrasonography* **2019**, *38*, 289–301. [CrossRef] [PubMed]
42. Minami, Y.; Kudo, M. Contrast-enhanced ultrasonography with Sonazoid in hepatocellular carcinoma diagnosis. *Hepatoma Res.* **2020**, *2020*. [CrossRef]
43. Bartolotta, T.V.; Terranova, M.C.; Gagliardo, C.; Taibbi, A. CEUS LI-RADS: A pictorial review. *Insights Imaging* **2020**, *11*, 9. [CrossRef]
44. Tang, A.; Cruite, I.; Mitchell, D.G.; Sirlin, C.B. Hepatocellular carcinoma imaging systems: Why they exist, how they have evolved, and how they differ. *Abdom. Imaging* **2017**, *43*, 3–12. [CrossRef]
45. Kulkarni, N.M.; Fung, A.; Kambadakone, A.R.; Yeh, B.M. Computed Tomography Techniques, Protocols, Advancements, and Future Directions in Liver Diseases. *Magn. Reson. Imaging Clin. N. Am.* **2021**, *29*, 305–320. [CrossRef] [PubMed]
46. Hennedige, T.; Yang, Z.J.; Ong, C.K.; Venkatesh, S.K. Utility of non-contrast-enhanced CT for improved detection of arterial phase hyperenhancement in hepatocellular carcinoma. *Abdom. Imaging* **2014**, *39*, 1247–1254. [CrossRef] [PubMed]
47. Burgio, M.D.; Sartoris, R.; Libotean, C.; Zappa, M.; Sibert, A.; Vilgrain, V.; Ronot, M. Lipiodol retention pattern after TACE for HCC is a predictor for local progression in lesions with complete response. *Cancer Imaging* **2019**, *19*, 75. [CrossRef] [PubMed]
48. Santillan, C. CT and MRI of the liver for hepatocellular carcinoma. *Hepatoma Res.* **2020**, *2020*. [CrossRef]
49. Lee, Y.; Wang, J.J.; Zhu, Y.; Agopian, V.G.; Tseng, H.; Yang, J.D. Diagnostic Criteria and LI-RADS for Hepatocellular Carcinoma. *Clin. Liver Dis.* **2021**, *17*, 409–413. [CrossRef] [PubMed]
50. Marrero, J.A.; Kulik, L.; Sirlin, C.B.; Zhu, A.X.; Finn, R.S.; Abecassis, M.M.; Roberts, L.R.; Heimbach, J.K. Diagnosis, Staging, and Management of Hepatocellular Carcinoma: 2018 Practice Guidance by the American Association for the Study of Liver Diseases. *Hepatology* **2018**, *68*, 723–750. [CrossRef] [PubMed]
51. Chan, R.; Kumar, G.; Abdullah, B.; Ng, K.; Vijayananthan, A.; Nor, H.M.; Liew, Y.W. Optimising the scan delay for arterial phase imaging of the liver using the bolus tracking technique. *Biomed. Imaging Interv. J.* **2011**, *7*. [CrossRef]
52. Kitzing, Y.X.; Ng, B.H.K.; Kitzing, B.; Waugh, R.; Kench, J.; Strasser, S.I.; McCormack, S. Washout of hepatocellular carcinoma on portal venous phase of multidetector computed tomography in a pre-transplant population. *J. Med. Imaging Radiat. Oncol.* **2015**, *59*, 673–680. [CrossRef] [PubMed]
53. Han, J.; Liu, Y.; Han, F.; Li, Q.; Yan, C.; Zheng, W.; Wang, J.; Guo, Z.; Wang, J.; Li, A.; et al. The Degree of Contrast Washout on Contrast-Enhanced Ultrasound in Distinguishing Intrahepatic Cholangiocarcinoma from Hepatocellular Carcinoma. *Ultrasound Med. Biol.* **2015**, *41*, 3088–3095. [CrossRef] [PubMed]
54. Joo, I.; Lee, J.M.; Yoon, J.H. Imaging Diagnosis of Intrahepatic and Perihilar Cholangiocarcinoma: Recent Advances and Challenges. *Radiology* **2018**, *288*, 7–13. [CrossRef]

55. Cannella, R.; Ronot, M.; Sartoris, R.; Cauchy, F.; Hobeika, C.; Beaufrere, A.; Trapani, L.; Paradis, V.; Bouattour, M.; Bonvalet, F.; et al. Enhancing capsule in hepatocellular carcinoma: Intra-individual comparison between CT and MRI with extracellular contrast agent. *Diagn. Interv. Imaging* **2021**, *102*, 735–742. [CrossRef]
56. Giambelluca, D.; Cannella, R.; Caruana, G.; Brancatelli, G. "Nodule-in-nodule" architecture of hepatocellular carcinoma. *Abdom. Imaging* **2019**, *44*, 2671–2673. [CrossRef]
57. Cannella, R.; Furlan, A. Mosaic architecture of hepatocellular carcinoma. *Abdom. Radiol.* **2017**, *43*, 1847–1848.
58. Kim, B.; Lee, J.H.; Kim, J.K.; Kim, H.J.; Kim, Y.B.; Lee, D. The capsule appearance of hepatocellular carcinoma in gadoxetic acid-enhanced MR imaging. *Medicine* **2018**, *97*, e11142. [CrossRef]
59. Li, J.; Zhao, S.; Ling, Z.; Li, D.; Jia, G.; Zhao, C.; Lin, X.; Dai, Y.; Jiang, H.; Wang, S. Dual-Energy Computed Tomography Imaging in Early-Stage Hepatocellular Carcinoma: A Preliminary Study. *Contrast Media Mol. Imaging* **2022**, *2022*, 2146343. [CrossRef]
60. Marin, D.; Boll, D.T.; Mileto, A.; Nelson, R.C. State of the Art: Dual-Energy CT of the Abdomen. *Radiology* **2014**, *271*, 327–342. [CrossRef]
61. Yoo, J.; Lee, J.M.; Yoon, J.H.; Joo, I.; Lee, E.S.; Jeon, S.K.; Jang, S. Comparison of low kVp CT and dual-energy CT for the evaluation of hypervascular hepatocellular carcinoma. *Abdom. Imaging* **2021**, *46*, 3217–3226. [CrossRef]
62. Hatzidakis, A.; Perisinakis, K.; Kalarakis, G.; Papadakis, A.; Savva, E.; Ippolito, D.; Karantanas, A. Perfusion-CT analysis for assessment of hepatocellular carcinoma lesions: Diagnostic value of different perfusion maps. *Acta Radiol.* **2018**, *60*, 561–568. [CrossRef]
63. Shalaby, M.H.; Shehata, K.A.A. CT perfusion in hepatocellular carcinoma: Is it reliable? *Egypt. J. Radiol. Nucl. Med.* **2017**, *48*, 791–798. [CrossRef]
64. Kalarakis, G.; Perisinakis, K.; Akoumianakis, E.; Karageorgiou, I.; Hatzidakis, A. CT liver perfusion in patients with hepatocellular carcinoma: Can we modify acquisition protocol to reduce patient exposure? *Eur. Radiol.* **2020**, *31*, 1410–1419. [CrossRef]
65. Osman, M.F.; Shawali, I.H.; Metwally, L.I.A.; Kamel, A.H.; Ibrahim, M.E.S. CT perfusion for response evaluation after interventional ablation of hepatocellular carcinoma: A prospective study. *Egypt. J. Radiol. Nucl. Med.* **2021**, *52*, 281. [CrossRef]
66. Chan, M.V.; Huo, Y.R.; Trieu, N.; Mitchelle, A.; George, J.; He, E.; Lee, A.U.; Chang, J.; Yang, J. Noncontrast MRI for Hepatocellular Carcinoma Detection: A Systematic Review and Meta-analysis—A Potential Surveillance Tool? *Clin. Gastroenterol. Hepatol.* **2021**, *20*, 44–56.e2. [CrossRef]
67. Zhao, C.; Dai, H.; Shao, J.; He, Q.; Su, W.; Wang, P.; Tang, Q.; Zeng, J.; Xu, S.; Zhao, J.; et al. Accuracy of Various Forms of Contrast-Enhanced MRI for Diagnosing Hepatocellular Carcinoma: A Systematic Review and Meta-Analysis. *Front. Oncol.* **2021**, *11*, 680691. [CrossRef]
68. Semaan, S.; Violi, N.V.; Lewis, S.; Chatterji, M.; Song, C.; Besa, C.; Babb, J.S.; Fiel, M.I.; Schwartz, M.; Thung, S.; et al. Hepatocellular carcinoma detection in liver cirrhosis: Diagnostic performance of contrast-enhanced CT vs. MRI with extracellular contrast vs. gadoxetic acid. *Eur. Radiol.* **2019**, *30*, 1020–1030. [CrossRef]
69. Kim, D.H.; Choi, S.H.; Shim, J.H.; Kim, S.Y.; Lee, S.S.; Byun, J.H.; Kim, K.W.; Choi, J.-I. Magnetic Resonance Imaging for Surveillance of Hepatocellular Carcinoma: A Systematic Review and Meta-Analysis. *Diagnostics* **2021**, *11*, 1665. [CrossRef]
70. Shinmura, R.; Matsui, O.; Kobayashi, S.; Terayama, N.; Sanada, J.; Ueda, K.; Gabata, T.; Kadoya, M.; Miyayama, S. Cirrhotic Nodules: Association between MR Imaging Signal Intensity and Intranodular Blood Supply. *Radiology* **2005**, *237*, 512–519. [CrossRef]
71. Cho, E.-S.; Choi, J.-Y. MRI Features of Hepatocellular Carcinoma Related to Biologic Behavior. *Korean J. Radiol.* **2015**, *16*, 449–464. [CrossRef] [PubMed]
72. Granata, V.; Fusco, R.; Avallone, A.; Catalano, O.; Filice, F.; Leongito, M.; Palaia, R.; Izzo, F.; Petrillo, A. Major and ancillary magnetic resonance features of LI-RADS to assess HCC: An overview and update. *Infect. Agents Cancer* **2017**, *12*, 23. [CrossRef] [PubMed]
73. Matondang, S.B.R.E.; Karismaputri, K.S.; Suharlim, E.; Yonathan, I.W.M. Hepatocellular Carcinoma with Macroscopic Fat Metamorphosis: A Case Series. *J. Clin. Imaging Sci.* **2021**, *11*, 36. [CrossRef] [PubMed]
74. Shetty, A.S.; Sipe, A.L.; Zulfiqar, M.; Tsai, R.; Raptis, D.A.; Raptis, C.A.; Bhalla, S. In-Phase and Opposed-Phase Imaging: Applications of Chemical Shift and Magnetic Susceptibility in the Chest and Abdomen. *Radiographics* **2019**, *39*, 115–135. [CrossRef] [PubMed]
75. Park, H.J.; Choi, B.I.; Lee, E.S.; Bin Park, S.; Lee, J.B. How to Differentiate Borderline Hepatic Nodules in Hepatocarcinogenesis: Emphasis on Imaging Diagnosis. *Liver Cancer* **2017**, *6*, 189–203. [CrossRef] [PubMed]
76. Jayachandran, A.; Shrestha, R.; Bridle, K.R.; Crawford, D.H.G. Association between hereditary hemochromatosis and hepatocellular carcinoma: A comprehensive review. *Hepatoma Res.* **2020**, *2020*. [CrossRef]
77. Pecorelli, A.; Franceschi, P.; Braccischi, L.; Izzo, F.; Renzulli, M.; Golfieri, R. MRI Appearance of Focal Lesions in Liver Iron Overload. *Diagnostics* **2022**, *12*, 891. [CrossRef]
78. Kim, S.-S.; Lee, S.; Bae, H.; Chung, Y.E.; Choi, J.-Y.; Park, M.-S.; Kim, M.-J. Extended application of subtraction arterial phase imaging in LI-RADS version 2018: A strategy to improve the diagnostic performance for hepatocellular carcinoma on gadoxetate disodium–enhanced MRI. *Eur. Radiol.* **2020**, *31*, 1620–1629. [CrossRef]
79. Shankar, S.; Kalra, N.; Bhatia, A.; Srinivasan, R.; Singh, P.; Dhiman, R.K.; Khandelwal, N.; Chawla, Y. Role of Diffusion Weighted Imaging (DWI) for Hepatocellular Carcinoma (HCC) Detection and its Grading on 3T MRI: A Prospective Study. *J. Clin. Exp. Hepatol.* **2016**, *6*, 303–310. [CrossRef]

80. De Gaetano, A.M.; Catalano, M.; Pompili, M.; Marini, M.G.; Rodríguez, C.P.; Gullì, C.; Infante, A.; Iezzi, R.; Ponziani, F.R.; Cerrito, L.; et al. Critical analysis of major and ancillary features of LI-RADS v2018 in the differentiation of small (≤2 cm) hepatocellular carcinoma from dysplastic nodules with gadobenate dimeglumine-enhanced magnetic resonance imaging. *Eur. Rev. Med. Pharmacol. Sci.* **2019**, *23*, 7786–7801.
81. Ablefoni, M.; Surup, H.; Ehrengut, C.; Schindler, A.; Seehofer, D.; Denecke, T.; Meyer, H.-J. Diagnostic Benefit of High b-Value Computed Diffusion-Weighted Imaging in Patients with Hepatic Metastasis. *J. Clin. Med.* **2021**, *10*, 5289. [CrossRef] [PubMed]
82. Park, M.J.; Kim, Y.K.; Lee, M.W.; Lee, W.J.; Kim, Y.-S.; Kim, S.H.; Choi, N.; Rhim, H. Small Hepatocellular Carcinomas: Improved Sensitivity by Combining Gadoxetic Acid–enhanced and Diffusion-weighted MR Imaging Patterns. *Radiology* **2012**, *264*, 761–770. [CrossRef] [PubMed]
83. Kim, D.K.; An, C.; Chung, Y.E.; Choi, J.-Y.; Lim, J.S.; Park, M.-S.; Kim, M.-J. Hepatobiliary versus Extracellular MRI Contrast Agents in Hepatocellular Carcinoma Detection: Hepatobiliary Phase Features in Relation to Disease-free Survival. *Radiology* **2019**, *293*, 594–604. [CrossRef] [PubMed]
84. Li, Y.; Chen, J.; Weng, S.; Yan, C.; Ye, R.; Zhu, Y.; Wen, L.; Cao, D.; Hong, J. Hepatobiliary phase hypointensity on gadobenate dimeglumine- enhanced magnetic resonance imaging may improve the diagnosis of hepatocellular carcinoma. *Ann. Transl. Med.* **2021**, *9*, 55. [CrossRef]
85. Xiao, Y.-D.; Ma, C.; Liu, J.; Li, H.-B.; Zhang, Z.S.; Zhou, S.-K. Evaluation of hypointense liver lesions during hepatobiliary phase MR imaging in normal and cirrhotic livers: Is increasing flip angle reliable? *Sci. Rep.* **2016**, *6*, 18942. [CrossRef]
86. Fujita, N.; Nishie, A.; Asayama, Y.; Ishigami, K.; Ushijima, Y.; Kakihara, D.; Nakayama, T.; Morita, K.; Ishimatsu, K.; Honda, H. Hyperintense Liver Masses at Hepatobiliary Phase Gadoxetic Acid–enhanced MRI: Imaging Appearances and Clinical Importance. *Radiographics* **2020**, *40*, 72–94. [CrossRef]
87. Kovac, J.D.; Ivanovic, A.; Milovanovic, T.; Micev, M.; Alessandrino, F.; Gore, R.M. An overview of hepatocellular carcinoma with atypical enhancement pattern: Spectrum of magnetic resonance imaging findings with pathologic correlation. *Radiol. Oncol.* **2021**, *55*, 130–143. [CrossRef]
88. Omata, M.; Cheng, A.-L.; Kokudo, N.; Kudo, M.; Lee, J.M.; Jia, J.; Tateishi, R.; Han, K.-H.; Chawla, Y.K.; Shiina, S.; et al. Asia–Pacific clinical practice guidelines on the management of hepatocellular carcinoma: A 2017 update. *Hepatol. Int.* **2017**, *11*, 317–370. [CrossRef]
89. Otto, F.G.; Pitton, M.B.; Hoppe-Lotichius, M.; Weinmann, A. Liver transplantation and BCLC classification: Limitations impede optimum treatment. *Hepatobiliary Pancreat. Dis. Int.* **2020**, *20*, 6–12. [CrossRef]
90. Cannella, R.; Sartoris, R.; Grégory, J.; Garzelli, L.; Vilgrain, V.; Ronot, M.; Burgio, M.D. Quantitative magnetic resonance imaging for focal liver lesions: Bridging the gap between research and clinical practice. *Br. J. Radiol.* **2021**, *94*, 20210220. [CrossRef]
91. Hectors, S.J.; Wagner, M.; Besa, C.; Bane, O.; Dyvorne, H.A.; Fiel, M.I.; Zhu, H.; Donovan, M.; Taouli, B. Intravoxel incoherent motion diffusion-weighted imaging of hepatocellular carcinoma: Is there a correlation with flow and perfusion metrics obtained with dynamic contrast-enhanced MRI? *J. Magn. Reson. Imaging* **2016**, *44*, 856–864. [CrossRef] [PubMed]
92. Donato, H.; França, M.; Candelária, I.; Caseiro-Alves, F. Liver MRI: From basic protocol to advanced techniques. *Eur. J. Radiol.* **2017**, *93*, 30–39. [CrossRef] [PubMed]
93. Pahwa, S.; Liu, H.; Chen, Y.; Dastmalchian, S.; O'Connor, G.; Lu, Z.; Badve, C.; Yu, A.; Wright, K.; Chalian, H.; et al. Quantitative perfusion imaging of neoplastic liver lesions: A multi-institution study. *Sci. Rep.* **2018**, *8*, 4990. [CrossRef]
94. Lu, R.-C.; She, B.; Gao, W.-T.; Ji, Y.-H.; Xu, D.-D.; Wang, Q.-S.; Wang, S.-B. Positron-emission tomography for hepatocellular carcinoma: Current status and future prospects. *World J. Gastroenterol.* **2019**, *25*, 4682–4695. [CrossRef]
95. Izuishi, K.; Yamamoto, Y.; Mori, H.; Kameyama, R.; Fujihara, S.; Masaki, T.; Suzuki, Y. Molecular mechanisms of [18F]fluorodeoxyglucose accumulation in liver cancer. *Oncol. Rep.* **2013**, *31*, 701–706. [CrossRef] [PubMed]
96. Cho, K.J.; Choi, N.K.; Shin, M.H.; Chong, A.R. Clinical usefulness of FDG-PET in patients with hepatocellular carcinoma undergoing surgical resection. *Ann. Hepato-Biliary-Pancreatic Surg.* **2017**, *21*, 194–198. [CrossRef]
97. Signore, G.; Nicod-Lalonde, M.; Prior, J.O.; Bertagna, F.; Muoio, B.; Giovanella, L.; Furlan, C.; Treglia, G. Detection rate of radiolabelled choline PET or PET/CT in hepatocellular carcinoma: An updated systematic review and meta-analysis. *Clin. Transl. Imaging* **2019**, *7*, 237–253. [CrossRef]
98. Ghidaglia, J.; Golse, N.; Pascale, A.; Sebagh, M.; Besson, F.L. 18F-FDG /18F-Choline Dual-Tracer PET Behavior and Tumor Differentiation in HepatoCellular Carcinoma. A Systematic Review. *Front. Med.* **2022**, *9*, 924824. [CrossRef]
99. Dos Santos, D.P.; Baessler, B. Big data, artificial intelligence, and structured reporting. *Eur. Radiol. Exp.* **2018**, *2*, 1–5. [CrossRef]
100. Yang, Q.; Wei, J.; Hao, X.; Kong, D.; Yu, X.; Jiang, T.; Xi, J.; Cai, W.; Luo, Y.; Jing, X.; et al. Improving B-mode ultrasound diagnostic performance for focal liver lesions using deep learning: A multicentre study. *eBiomedicine* **2020**, *56*, 102777. [CrossRef]
101. Brehar, R.; Mitrea, D.-A.; Vancea, F.; Marita, T.; Nedevschi, S.; Lupsor-Platon, M.; Rotaru, M.; Badea, R.I. Comparison of Deep-Learning and Conventional Machine-Learning Methods for the Automatic Recognition of the Hepatocellular Carcinoma Areas from Ultrasound Images. *Sensors* **2020**, *20*, 3085. [CrossRef]
102. Schmauch, B.; Herent, P.; Jehanno, P.; Dehaene, O.; Saillard, C.; Aubé, C.; Luciani, A.; Lassau, N.; Jégou, S. Diagnosis of focal liver lesions from ultrasound using deep learning. *Diagn. Interv. Imaging* **2019**, *100*, 227–233. [CrossRef]
103. Guo, L.-H.; Wang, D.; Qian, Y.-Y.; Zheng, X.; Zhao, C.-K.; Li, X.-L.; Bo, X.-W.; Yue, W.-W.; Zhang, Q.; Shi, J.; et al. A two-stage multi-view learning framework based computer-aided diagnosis of liver tumors with contrast enhanced ultrasound images. *Clin. Hemorheol. Microcirc.* **2018**, *69*, 343–354. [CrossRef]

104. Mao, B.; Ma, J.; Duan, S.; Xia, Y.; Tao, Y.; Zhang, L. Preoperative classification of primary and metastatic liver cancer via machine learning-based ultrasound radiomics. *Eur. Radiol.* **2021**, *31*, 4576–4586. [CrossRef] [PubMed]
105. Ichikawa, S.; Isoda, H.; Shimizu, T.; Tamada, D.; Taura, K.; Togashi, K.; Onishi, H.; Motosugi, U. Distinguishing intrahepatic mass-forming biliary carcinomas from hepatocellular carcinoma by computed tomography and magnetic resonance imaging using the Bayesian method: A bi-center study. *Eur. Radiol.* **2020**, *30*, 5992–6002. [CrossRef]
106. Wang, W.; Wu, S.-S.; Zhang, J.-C.; Xian, M.-F.; Huang, H.; Li, W.; Zhou, Z.-M.; Zhang, C.-Q.; Wu, T.-F.; Li, X.; et al. Preoperative Pathological Grading of Hepatocellular Carcinoma Using Ultrasomics of Contrast-Enhanced Ultrasound. *Acad. Radiol.* **2020**, *28*, 1094–1101. [CrossRef]
107. Ren, S.; Qi, Q.; Liu, S.; Duan, S.; Mao, B.; Chang, Z.; Zhang, Y.; Wang, S.; Zhang, L. Preoperative prediction of pathological grading of hepatocellular carcinoma using machine learning-based ultrasomics: A multicenter study. *Eur. J. Radiol.* **2021**, *143*. [CrossRef]
108. Nayak, A.; Kayal, E.B.; Arya, M.; Culli, J.; Krishan, S.; Agarwal, S.; Mehndiratta, A. Computer-aided diagnosis of cirrhosis and hepatocellular carcinoma using multi-phase abdomen CT. *Int. J. Comput. Assist. Radiol. Surg.* **2019**, *14*, 1341–1352. [CrossRef]
109. Shi, W.; Kuang, S.; Cao, S.; Hu, B.; Xie, S.; Chen, S.; Chen, Y.; Gao, D.; Chen, Y.; Zhu, Y.; et al. Deep learning assisted differentiation of hepatocellular carcinoma from focal liver lesions: Choice of four-phase and three-phase CT imaging protocol. *Abdom. Imaging* **2020**, *45*, 2688–2697. [CrossRef]
110. Mokrane, F.-Z.; Lu, L.; Vavasseur, A.; Otal, P.; Peron, J.-M.; Luk, L.; Yang, H.; Ammari, S.; Saenger, Y.; Rousseau, H.; et al. Radiomics machine-learning signature for diagnosis of hepatocellular carcinoma in cirrhotic patients with indeterminate liver nodules. *Eur. Radiol.* **2019**, *30*, 558–570. [CrossRef] [PubMed]
111. Ünal, E.; Idilman, I.S.; Akata, D.; Özmen, M.N.; Karçaaltıncaba, M. Microvascular invasion in hepatocellular carcinoma. *Diagn. Interv. Radiol.* **2016**, *22*, 125–132. [CrossRef]
112. Mazzaferro, V.M.; Llovet, J.M.; Miceli, R.; Bhoori, S.; Schiavo, M.; Mariani, L.; Camerini, T.; Roayaie, S.; Schwartz, M.E.; Grazi, G.L.; et al. Predicting survival after liver transplantation in patients with hepatocellular carcinoma beyond the Milan criteria: A retrospective, exploratory analysis. *Lancet Oncol.* **2009**, *10*, 35–43. [CrossRef] [PubMed]
113. Jiang, Y.-Q.; Cao, S.-E.; Cao, S.; Chen, J.-N.; Wang, G.-Y.; Shi, W.-Q.; Deng, Y.-N.; Cheng, N.; Ma, K.; Zeng, K.-N.; et al. Preoperative identification of microvascular invasion in hepatocellular carcinoma by XGBoost and deep learning. *J. Cancer Res. Clin. Oncol.* **2020**, *147*, 821–833. [CrossRef]
114. Qi, Y.-P.; Zhong, J.-H.; Liang, Z.-Y.; Zhang, J.; Chen, B.; Chen, C.-Z.; Li, L.-Q.; Xiang, B.-D. Adjuvant transarterial chemoembolization for patients with hepatocellular carcinoma involving microvascular invasion. *Am. J. Surg.* **2019**, *217*, 739–744. [CrossRef]
115. Choi, J.-Y.; Cho, H.C.; Sun, M.; Kim, H.C.; Sirlin, C.B. Indeterminate Observations (Liver Imaging Reporting and Data System Category 3) on MRI in the Cirrhotic Liver: Fate and Clinical Implications. *Am. J. Roentgenol.* **2013**, *201*, 993–1001. [CrossRef]
116. Wu, Y.; White, G.M.; Cornelius, T.; Gowdar, I.; Ansari, M.H.; Supanich, M.P.; Deng, J. Deep learning LI-RADS grading system based on contrast enhanced multiphase MRI for differentiation between LR-3 and LR-4/LR-5 liver tumors. *Ann. Transl. Med.* **2020**, *8*, 701. [CrossRef]

Disclaimer/Publisher's Note: The statements, opinions and data contained in all publications are solely those of the individual author(s) and contributor(s) and not of MDPI and/or the editor(s). MDPI and/or the editor(s) disclaim responsibility for any injury to people or property resulting from any ideas, methods, instructions or products referred to in the content.

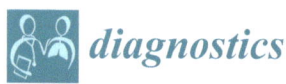

Review

Principles and Applications of Dual-Layer Spectral CT in Gastrointestinal Imaging

Paolo Niccolò Franco [1,†], Chiara Maria Spasiano [2,†], Cesare Maino [1,*], Elena De Ponti [3], Maria Ragusi [1], Teresa Giandola [1], Simone Terrani [4], Marta Peroni [4], Rocco Corso [1] and Davide Ippolito [1,5]

1. Department of Diagnostic Radiology, Fondazione IRCCS San Gerardo dei Tintori, Via Pergolesi 33, 20900 Monza, Italy; francopaoloniccolo@gmail.com (P.N.F.); maria.ragusi@gmail.com (M.R.); teresagiandola1990@gmail.com (T.G.); r.corso@asst-monza.it (R.C.); davide.atena@tiscali.it (D.I.)
2. Department of Diagnostic Radiology, Istituti Clinici Zucchi, Via Zucchi 24, 20900 Monza, Italy; chiaraspasiano@gmail.com
3. Department of Medical Physics, Fondazione IRCCS San Gerardo dei Tintori, Via Pergolesi 33, 20900 Monza, Italy; elena.deponti@unimib.it
4. Philips Healtcare, Viale Sarca 54, 20126 Milano, Italy; simone.terrani@philips.it (S.T.); marta.peroni@philips.it (M.P.)
5. School of Medicine, Università Milano-Bicocca, Piazza dell'Ateneo Nuovo, 1, 20100 Milano, Italy
* Correspondence: mainocesare@gmail.com; Tel.: +39-347-5735853
† These authors contributed equally to this work.

Abstract: The advance in technology allows for the development of different CT scanners in the field of dual-energy computed tomography (DECT). In particular, a recently developed detector-based technology can collect data from different energy levels, thanks to its layers. The use of this system is suited for material decomposition with perfect spatial and temporal registration. Thanks to post-processing techniques, these scanners can generate conventional, material decomposition (including virtual non-contrast (VNC), iodine maps, Z-effective imaging, and uric acid pair images) and virtual monoenergetic images (VMIs). In recent years, different studies have been published regarding the use of DECT in clinical practice. On these bases, considering that different papers have been published using the DECT technology, a review regarding its clinical application can be useful. We focused on the usefulness of DECT technology in gastrointestinal imaging, where DECT plays an important role.

Keywords: image interpretation; computer-assisted; tomography; X-ray-computed; diagnostic techniques; digestive system

1. Introduction

Conventional single-energy computed tomography (SECT) is a diagnostic imaging technique that uses a polyenergetic X-ray beam from a single source that rotates around the patient's body and a panel of detectors that records the radiation attenuated by the different densities of tissues, expressed in terms of Hounsfield Unit (HU).

Due to its fast acquisition and diagnostic accuracy, SECT has become the gold standard for the detection and assessment of different pathological entities. One of the limits of conventional SECT is that the characterization of tissues with a similar density is not always straightforward as, for instance, in the case of calcified plaques and iodinated blood within arterial vessels in angiographic studies. Moreover, SECT protocols frequently consist of repeated scanning before, during and after contrast injection, resulting in high-dose exposures.

Dual-energy CT (DECT) is a more recent technology that helps to overcome these limitations by acquiring data at two different energy levels to derive different tissue attenuations. Data obtained can be combined to generate images for routine clinical interpretation or more accurate material characterization [1].

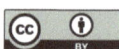

The main contributors to attenuation coefficients during CT scanning are the photoelectric effect and the Compton scattering. Whereas the latter is minimally dependent on photon energy and is mainly related to a material's electron density, the photoelectric effect is strongly X-ray-energy-dependent and increases with a higher element's atomic number (Z). The photoelectric effect can be calculated by comparing attenuation levels derived from two energy levels. Because of its dependency on Z, it is crucial for distinguishing different materials with similar attenuation in any energy level. This characteristic is defined as material decomposition and represents the basis for spectral proprieties in DECT imaging [2]. Elements with high Z, such as iodine (Z = 53) or calcium (Z = 20), are susceptible to the photoelectric effect and have strong spectral properties. These elements present similar CT attenuation values in SECT due to their relative density.

Conversely, when exposed to different energy levels via DECT scanning, they interact in different ways, regardless of their density. This capability of differentiating structures with similar densities but different elemental compositions underlie multiple clinical applications of DECT scanning [3]. On the contrary, soft-tissue anatomic structures, including muscles or parenchyma, have a low photoelectric effect and consequently demonstrate less variability in their attenuation values at different energy levels.

The datasets of the two energy levels can be obtained using multiple acquisition techniques [4]. Depending upon how the two different X-ray energies are generated, DECTs are divided into two major groups: tube-based and detector-based. Two of the three leading DECT platforms currently in the market are tube-based: dual-source DECT (ds-DECT) (Somatom Drive/Somatom Definition Flash, Siemens Medical Solutions, Forchheim, Germany) and rapid kV-switching DECT (rs-DECT) (Revolution CT, GE Healthcare, Milwaukee, WI, USA; Aquilion ONE GENESIS Edition, Canon Medical Systems, Otawara, Japan). In the detector-based category, the dual-layer detector DECT (dl-DECT) (IQon spectral CT, Philips Healthcare, Eindhoven, The Netherlands) is the only currently available platform.

The first DECT scanner approved for clinical use was introduced into the market in 2006 and was based on a dual-source technique. These scanners consist of two detectors and two X-ray sources, a low-kV and a high-kV tube, with 90° orientation differences that scan simultaneously to achieve two energy spectra. Conversely, rs-DECT uses a single X-ray tube that rapidly alternates between low and high kV during its rotation (fast switching) and a single detector that registers information from both energies. The most recent technology is the ds-DECT, which was commercially introduced in 2016. It is based on a single energetic radiation tube associated with a detector panel, constituting two layers (sandwich detector) that simultaneously detect two energy levels.

This review aims to summarize the technical features of CT scanners with dual-layer detector technology, showing the added diagnostic value in daily practice of this approach via a review of the most recent literature on gastrointestinal applications.

1.1. Dual-Layer Detector Dual-Energy CT Technology

As mentioned before, in the dl-DECT scanner system, spectral separation is achieved at the detector level. This system takes advantage of the polychromatic nature of the beam produced with a single-energy source, combined with highly specialized detectors that consist of two layers with maximal sensitivity for different energies. The top (inner) layer preferentially absorbs low-energy photons by design, approximately 50% of the total incident photon flux. In contrast, the bottom (outer) layer absorbs the remaining photons, which are primarily high-energy ones [5,6] (Figure 1).

A significant advantage of this system is, firstly, its excellent temporal registration. This system is well suited for material decomposition in the projection domain, making it quantitatively accurate and robust for possible patient motion. Another advantage is the perfect spatial registration of the acquired data to create a complete spectral dataset. The tube always operates at a high kVp, resulting in a high total X-ray power, which is advantageous for larger patients. Moreover, with this approach, scanning is performed at the full field of view of 50 cm. The last advantage is the dl-DECT retrospective acquisition mode: a dl-DECT scanner always acquires scans in the DECT mode, allowing one to gain spectral information for all scans performed, and hence there is no need to prospectively decide which scans perform in spectral mode, which is mandatory in other currently available dual-energy technologies. Retrospective on-demand spectral data of a region of interest allow radiologists to further investigate incidental findings without additional radiation exposure [5,7].

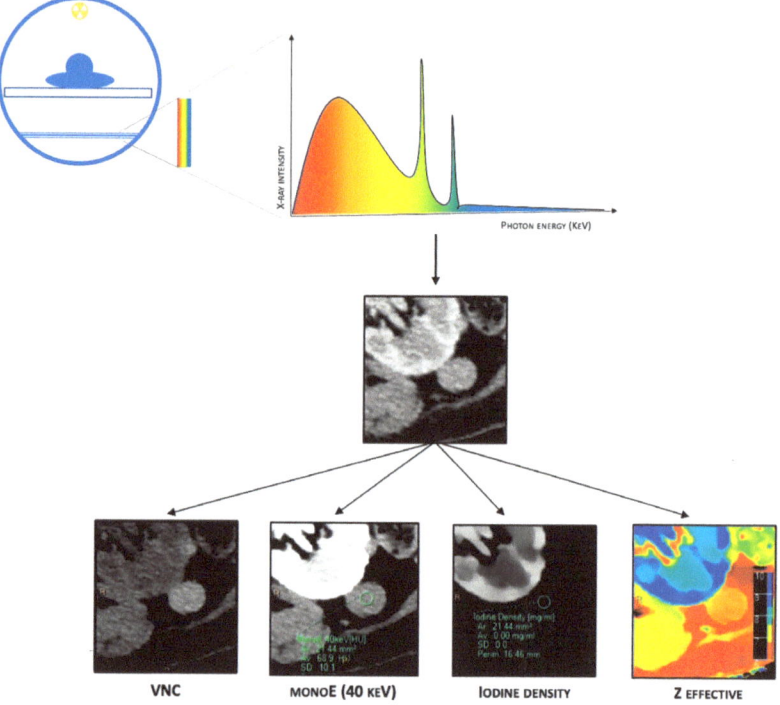

Figure 1. Schematic representation of DECT. It is based on a single energetic radiation tube associated with a detector panel constituted of two layers (sandwich detector) that simultaneously detect two energy levels. Different post-processing techniques are available due to spectral properties, such as material composition images (virtual non-contrast (VNC)), iodine maps, Z-effective imaging, and virtual monoenergetic images (VMIs).

The main disadvantage of this system is its lower energy separation because the scintillator absorption properties do not offer a sharp distinction between lower- and higher-energy photons. As a result, the material differentiation contrast is decreased unless a higher radiation dose is used.

1.2. Dual-Layer CT Post-Processing

Combining data from both layers of detectors, dl-DECT scanners can generate conventional images comparable to those obtained from SECT, providing morphological details and material-specific image sets. Furthermore, plenty of different post-processing techniques are available due to spectral properties, such as material composition images (virtual non-contrast (VNC), iodine maps, Z-effective imaging, and uric acid pair images) and virtual monoenergetic images (VMIs). VNC images, also called "water-based", are similar to conventional unenhanced CT images but are obtained via a dedicated algorithm that subtracts iodine-containing pixels from enhanced phases, allowing to create virtual plane images. Iodine concentration (IC) images (iodine maps) are material decomposition maps obtained via an algorithm that enhances only the pixels containing iodine. Iodine maps allow for identifying the presence or absence of iodine and its uptake in several tissues, which is particularly helpful in evaluating the contrast enhancement. Z-effective imaging consists of colorimetric maps that visually enhance the differences between tissues: the average atomic numbers of elements in each pixel are translated into color-coded images that provide a higher degree of discrimination than HU attenuation in conventional CT. Z-effective mapping is also used to define the peak enhancement (PE), which expresses the maximal concentration of the contrast agent with time in a tissue, according to the acquisition phase. Uric acid pair images show only pixels containing uric acid with original HU values, while all others appear dark, which is extremely useful for assessing urinary calculi composition and gout.

Finally, VMIs are a set of monochromatic images that simulate the appearance of images acquired using a monoenergetic X-ray beam at a selected energy level. VMIs can be obtained at discrete energy levels ranging from 40 to 190 keV with dl-DECT. Due to the approximation of the energy with the K-edge of iodine, low-keV VMIs show increased iodine conspicuity, which results in attenuation values equivalent to conventional images at a 120-kVp, but with a significant reduction in noise. Conversely, higher energy levels in VMIs reveal decreased iodine conspicuity and a drop in beam hardening artifacts, a physical phenomenon of the beam itself that produces an artifact that typically appears in the presence of metallic implants.

1.3. Radiation Dose

The White Paper of the Society of Computed Body Tomography on Dual-Energy CT published in 2016 stated that DECT acquisitions, even if using different X-ray spectra, do not provide additional radiation dose exposure in patients [8].

In the literature, various studies have demonstrated similar or lower radiation dose exposure via DECT acquisitions compared to SECT [9–12]. One investigation revealed that DECT imaging at 80 and 140 kVp resulted in a decrease in the dose-length product and CT dose index values of 10% and 12%, respectively, compared to standard SECT (120 kVp) imaging using the same dual-source scanner, with no significant difference in objective image noise or subjective image quality [9]. Duan et al. compared radiation dose and image quality for abdominal CT imaging performed on dl-DECT and conventional SECT scanners in patients of different sizes. The volume CT dose index (CTDIvol) during dl-DECT was similar to one measured on a conventional SECT for average-size patients, lower for smaller patients, and slightly higher for larger patients [11].

Furthermore, VNC imaging allows one to reconstruct plain images from enhanced phases, reducing the number of scans and, consequently, the radiation dose [13]. This tool is particularly advantageous in oncologic patients, who usually undergo repeated follow-up CT examinations, and pediatric patients.

Finally, a potential radiation dose reduction can be achieved by avoiding additional CT studies for further incidental lesion characterization.

2. Clinical Applications

Table 1 gathers published papers regarding current evidence on the utility of dl-DECT for gastrointestinal imaging.

2.1. Liver

The added value of DECT technology in hepatic imaging mainly consists of helping radiologists visualize and correctly characterize lesions and quantify the degree of diffuse hepatic diseases.

Regarding focal liver lesions, it has been shown that DECT low-energy VMIs facilitate and improve the assessment of hypervascular lesions [14,15]. Preliminary research on dl-DECT platforms has demonstrated similar results. Große Hokamp et al. observed that, throughout the entire keV spectrum, VMIs at 40 keV had the highest detectability of arterially hyper-enhancing lesions in phantoms and in vivo due to an increase in lesion contrast without an increase in image noise [16]. Furthermore, in a more recent investigation, low-energy VMIs also improved the wash-out assessment of arterially hyper-enhancing liver lesions in contrast-enhanced dl-DECT scans. The authors evaluated a population of patients undergoing CT scans for hepatocellular carcinoma (HCC) screening. Both wash-out assessment and image quality parameters resulted in significantly better VMIs at 40 kV compared to higher-energy VMIs and conventional CT imaging [17]. The significant advantage of low-energy VMIs was also proven concerning the assessment of hypovascular liver metastases. Nagayama et al. demonstrated that both the tumor-to-liver contrast and contrast-to-noise ratio (CNR) increased as the energy decreased. At the same time, 40 kV VMIs overcame higher-energy VMIs and PEI in lesion detectability [18].

Table 1. Overview of the reviewed sources regarding dl-DECT applications in gastrointestinal imaging.

Author	Year	Country	Study Nature	Pathology	Number of Subjects
Liver					
GroßeHokamp	2018	Germany	Retrospective	Arterially hyper-enhancing liver lesions	20
Reimer	2021	Germany	Retrospective	Arterially hyper-enhancing liver lesions	31
Nagayama	2019	Japan	Retrospective	Hypovascular liver metastases	81
Morita	2021	Japan	Retrospective	Liver fibrosis	68
Ma	2020	China	Prospective	Liver iron overload	31
Gallbladder and biliary tree					
Saito	2018	Japan	Retrospective	Iso-dense biliary gallstones	3
Soesbe	2019	USA	Prospective	Iso-dense biliary gallstones	105
Huda	2021	USA	Retrospective	Acute cholecystitis	57
Pancreas					
El Kayal	2019	Germany	Retrospective	Pancreatic lesions (PDAC, cyst lesions, IPMN, MCN, NET, lymphomas, metastasis, chronic pancreatitis)	61
Nagayama	2019	Japan	Retrospective	PDAC	48
Wang	2022	China	Retrospective	Neuroendocrine neoplasms	104
Gastrointestinal tract					
Chen	2022	China	Retrospective	Colorectal cancer	131
Wang	2021	China	Retrospective	Colonic wall thickening	80
Lee	2018	Korea	Retrospective	Crohn's disease	76
Kim	2018	Korea	Retrospective	Crohn's disease	39
Taguchi	2018	Japan	Retrospective	Electronic cleansing	35

Dl-DECT: dual-layer detector dual-energy computed tomography; PDAC: pancreatic ductal adenocarcinoma; IPMN: intraductal papillary mucinous neoplasm; MCN: mucinous cystic neoplasm; NET: neuroendocrine tumor.

DECT can also be considered as a helpful approach for diffuse liver diseases. An accurate evaluation of liver fibrosis is clinically significant due to its correlation with carcinogenesis and prognosis. The degree of fibrosis is conventionally assessed via blood tests, ultrasonography-based transient elastography, and magnetic resonance elastography [19]. Many studies have investigated the applications of tube-based DECTs in the assessment of liver fibrosis, mainly via the measurement of parenchymal IC on equilibrium imaging and the quantification of liver extracellular volume (ECV) [20–22]. In 2021, Morita et al. evaluated these measurements for the first time using a dl-DECT platform. The authors demonstrated that the iodine density ratio (calculated by dividing the iodine density of the liver parenchyma by the iodine density of the aorta) and the CT-ECV increased significantly as the fibrosis stage advanced ($p < 0.01$ for both). The CT-ECV showed better diagnostic accuracy for the degree of fibrosis. In the case of advanced-stage fibrosis, the sensitivity ranged from 90% to 95%, and the specificity ranged from 72.9% to 85.4% among two readers [23].

Dl-DECT may also improve the assessment of iron overload. Ma et al. compared the evaluation of liver and cardiac iron overload with T2*-weighted unenhanced MRI to unenhanced dl-DECT scans in patients with myelodysplastic syndromes and aplastic anemia. The two techniques were comparable in the case of iron overload in the liver [24].

The capability of DECT to derive VNC images from contrast-enhanced examinations by identifying and subtracting iodine potentially underlies many applications in liver imaging, particularly concerning liver steatosis. Different studies have compared the performance in diagnosing fatty liver between true non-contrast (TNC) images and VNC images generated from DECT scanners [25,26]. In their study, Choi et al. proved that, even if liver densities in VNC images were significantly different from those in TNC images, various parameters (liver and spleen densities, liver-minus-spleen density, and liver-to-spleen ratio) would be significantly higher in healthy liver patients than in fatty liver patients in TNC images as well as in VNC images from multiple phases. Additionally, the diagnostic performances of all parameters for fatty liver diagnosis in VNC images were not significantly different to those in TNC images [25].

To our knowledge, there is a lack of publications regarding the application of dl-DECT to assess liver steatosis. However, the value of VNC imaging obtained using a dl-DECT platform for the assessment of liver attenuation has been compared to conventional TNC images. Laukamp and colleagues demonstrated that VNC images from various enhanced phases were not significantly different from the TNC ones in terms of liver attenuation and image noise. However, the accuracy decreased in the early arterial phases of the liver when only a small quantity of contrast media was present in the parenchyma [27,28].

Finally, in recently published research, the authors described another technical advantage of dl-DECT platforms. They found that peristalsis-related artifacts were significantly less frequent and less relevant when the liver was evaluated with iodine image reconstructions than with conventional 120 kVp images in both qualitative and quantitative analysis [29].

2.2. Gallbladder and Biliary Tree

In CT diagnosis, gallbladder stones are indicated directly via high-density or low-density stones and indirectly via the dilation of the intrahepatic biliary duct, left and right hepatic ducts, biliary duct, and gallbladder [30]. Based on density, gallbladder stones are classified into high-, iso-, low-, and mixed-density stones, relative to the density of the surrounding bile. Conventional SECT has high accuracy in diagnosing high-density or low-density gallbladder stones [31]. However, it is challenging to diagnose iso-density stones, such as those made of cholesterol, due to their similar attenuation value with the bile (Figure 2).

DECT provides a new approach for the differential diagnosis of gallbladder stones and reliable information for their clinical treatment. In 2018, Saito et al. applied the property of dl-DECT to provide on-demand retrospective spectral analysis to detect iso-dense biliary stones that were not detected using conventional CT scans. Using magnetic resonance cholangiopancreatography (MRCP) or endoscopic retrograde cholangiopancreatography (ERCP) as the reference standard, the authors found that in two out of three cases, the stones were readily detected in VMIs at 40 keV. In contrast, only a small stone (<5 mm) remained undetected during spectral dataset evaluation [32].

In their prospective ex vivo study, Soesbe and colleagues devised a method for detecting iso-dense stones using a dl-DECT scanner. They compared it with previously reported methods built using tube-based DECT images. After placing iso-dense gallstones inside vials containing ox bile, six readers evaluated the presence of isodose gallstones via conventional PEI at 120 kVp, VNC images, VMIs at 40 and 200 keV 120 kVp, and segmented images obtained using a two-dimensional histogram of Compton and photoelectric X-ray attenuation derived from dl-DECT. The authors found that for gallstones measuring less than 9 mm, the segmented images had the highest overall AUC ($p < 0.01$) compared to VMIs [33].

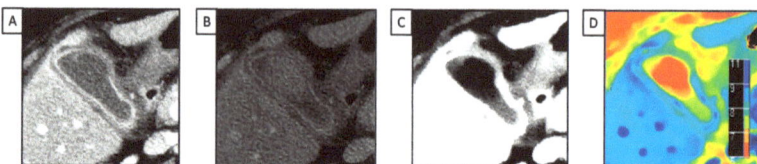

Figure 2. A 42 y-o patient with right upper pain underwent abdominal CT with a final diagnosis of cholecystitis. (**A**) Conventional CT image acquired after intravenous contrast media injection shows diffuse thickening of the gallbladder wall, without evidence of any calcific stone; (**B**) low mono-energetic map shows a hypoattenuating round stone, due to cholesteric composition; (**C**) opposite that, the high mono-energetic map demonstrates the hyperattenuating mass consistent with the cholesteric gallstone; (**D**) the Z-effective map allows us to better define the different structures of the images via the different atomic values of the gallbladder: blue (contrast agent), red (lipid content), and green (fluid).

Only one study published in the literature evaluated the potential role of dl-DECT technology in evaluating acute cholecystitis. In this research, spectral imaging obtained using a dl-DECT and an rs-DECT were compared with SECT imaging for the detection of multiple individual findings associated with acute cholecystitis, such as gallbladder fossa hyperemia, gangrene, and heterogeneous wall enhancement. During the evaluation of two readers, DECT showed increased sensitivity (R1, 86%; R2, 89.5%) compared with conventional CT (R1, 77.2%; R2, 70.2%) for the diagnosis of acute cholecystitis and the assessment of the aforementioned related findings [34].

2.3. Pancreas

The CT appearance of most focal pancreatic lesions usually ranges from mildly hypo- to iso-attenuating in comparison with the normal pancreatic parenchyma, making the differential diagnosis a radiological dilemma [35]. Several investigations demonstrated that spectral imaging could improve the diagnosis of pancreatic tumors in terms of lesion conspicuity, extension, and vascular invasion [36,37].

Even despite its more recent commercialization, some studies have already focused on the application of dl-DECT technology for diagnosing pancreatic lesions. In a cohort of 61 patients with different types of pancreatic lesions, El Kayal et al. found that, compared to conventional poly-energetic imaging (PEI), low-energy VMIs and iodine maps facilitated subjective lesion delineation, because of the increased attenuation of iodine at energy levels close to its maximum absorption (33 keV). Moreover, dl-DECT imaging increased reader diagnostic confidence, assessed using a five-point Likert scale by two radiologists [38]. In patients with pancreatic ductal adenocarcinoma (PDAC), detector-based MVI at 40 KeV yielded better quality lesion assessment in each enhancement phase than PEI due to its high pancreas tumor contrast and vascular opacification without a relevant increase in image noise [39]. In a more recent publication, Han and colleagues compared portal-venous-phase VMIs obtained using a dl-DECT scanner with the traditional polychromatic pancreatic phase scan for the diagnosis of PDAC. The authors found that low-energy VMIs at 40 and 55 KeV had a higher tumor-to-pancreas contrast-to-noise ratio (CNR), attenuation difference, and higher peripancreatic vascular CNR and signal-to-noise ratio (SNR) than the pancreatic phase image ($p < 0.001$). Furthermore, in a subjective analysis, VMIs at 55 KeV showed the best tumor conspicuity [40].

Not so many studies have been performed to evaluate neuroendocrine neoplasms (NENs) of the pancreas. In their research, Wang et al. analyzed both DECT (NIC, tumor attenuation, and effective Z) and SECT features in a cohort of 104 patients with pathologically confirmed NEN. The authors found that combining DECT metrics (NIC, tumor attenuation, and effective Z) with qualitative SECT features improved the differential diagnosis between neuroendocrine tumors and neuroendocrine carcinomas [41].

2.4. Gastrointestinal Tract

DECT has proven to have many applications, including in the evaluation of gastrointestinal tract diseases. In emergency settings, CECT is typically the preferred imaging tool when acute bowel ischemia is suspected to assess a decreased or lack of bowel parietal enhancement. However, detecting these findings is not always straightforward, especially in the case of early ischemia [42]. DECT can improve confidence in diagnosing bowel ischemia due to its capability in enabling a quantitative measure of wall enhancement via iodine mapping. In addition, a low-keV VMI can highlight the attenuation differences between perfused and non-perfused walls [43,44] (Figure 3).

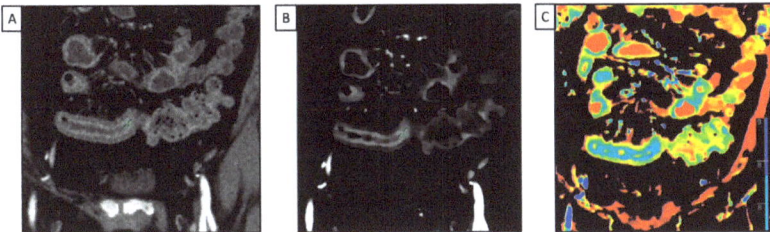

Figure 3. A 49 y-o male with known Crohn's disease, diffuse abdominal pain, and suspected relapse of disease underwent abdominal CT. (**A**) Conventional CT images on the coronal plane acquired after intravenous contrast media injection show a poor layered enhancement appearance of the distal ileum; (**B**) iodine map enhances iodine's uptake by the mucosa layer, and the hypoattenuating appearance of the submucosa one, consistent with edema; (**C**) the Z-effective map allows us to define the pattern of enhancement due to the atomic number of iodine.

Among the different spectral technologies, dl-DECT is particularly useful because it allows for the simultaneous acquisition of low- and high-KeV information at the same spatial position, facilitating the visualization of the un-enhanced bowel, and because the spectral dataset is always retrospectively available for every scan [45].

Possible applications of DECT, iodine mapping, and VMIs for the evaluation of gastrointestinal cancers have been explored in various pieces of research [46]. In Chen and colleagues' investigation, quantitative parameters extracted via dl-DECT imaging (iodine concentration (NIC), slope of the spectral HU curve, and effective Z) showed a significant correlation with both pT stages and two histologic-grade groups of colorectal adenocarcinomas [47]. Wang et al. verified that the IC and NIC generated from dl-DECT imaging could help to detect local colonic wall thickening caused by colon neoplasia among radiologically indeterminate colonic wall thickenings, with no specific requirement for bowel distension or luminal insufflation [48].

Even if MRI is considered the gold standard in evaluating small intestine inflammatory bowel diseases [Maaser2019], DECT has proven to have high diagnostic accuracy in assessing inflammation activity and severity in those with Crohn's disease [49–51] (Figure 4).

In particular, it has been demonstrated that a quantitative assessment of DECT parameters, including NIC and slope of the HU curve (which represents the X-ray attenuation coefficient at different energy levels), had higher accuracy in predicting intestinal activity and severity in ileocolonic Crohn's disease when compared to conventional SECT parameters [49]. Further investigations corroborated these results and proved that the walls of the bowel segments with active inflammation show a higher NIC value than those without inflammation, using histopathologic results from either ileocolonic resection or biopsy of the terminal ileum as the reference standard [51].

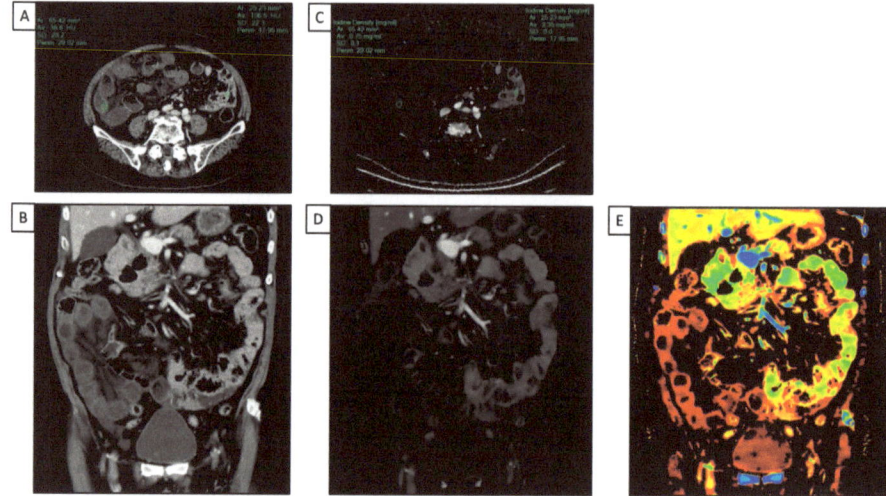

Figure 4. A 66 y-o male with diffuse abdominal pain underwent abdominal CT with a final diagnosis of distal ileum bowel ischemia. (**A,C**) Axial and coronal conventional CT images acquired after intravenous contrast media injection show a slight difference in attenuation value (HU) of the small bowel walls, with reduced enhancement in the distal ileum and regular enhancement in jejunum and proximal ileum; (**B,D**) iodine maps clearly show the difference in iodine uptake between the normal walls of the jejunum and proximal ileum and the poor iodine uptake of the distal tract of the ileum; (**E**) the Z-effective map allows us to better and more simply define the different enhancement in terms of colors between healthy and ischemic bowels due to the atomic number of iodine.

With regard to detector-based platforms, Kim et al. evaluated various qualitative and quantitative dl-DECT features in a population of thirty-nine patients with Crohn's disease at different stages, ranging from remission to severe activity state. Due to its ability to quantify the contrast distribution across intestine walls at a single point in time, the iodine concentration measured on the iodine map was the only independent variable associated with the Crohn's disease activity index [52]. Active disease qualitative assessment may also be improved because of the increased hyper-enhancement seen in low-keV images. Lee et al. demonstrated that low-energy (40 keV) VMIs on a dl-DECT scan provided the best CNR for both healthy and pathologic small bowel walls. Moreover, the diagnostic performance in assessing active Crohn's disease of three radiologists with different levels of experience was significantly improved with the addition of low-energy VMIs, compared to only the conventional PEI at 120 kVp [53].

CT colonography is a low-dose and minimally invasive method for diagnosing clinically relevant lesions within the colon lumen. However, electronic fecal cleansing is often needed to correct inadequate bowel preparation using fecal tagging with iodine or barium. In the literature, a possible advantage of the tube-based DECT approach for electronic cleansing in CT colonography imaging has been proposed [54]. Nevertheless, tube-based technology may lead to an increase in radiation dose and image noise at a lower keV. Conversely, dl-DECT allows for VMIs in the projection domain without the need for temporal and angular interpolation because it measures low- and high-energy projection information in the two layers of the detector at the same spatial and angular location. This may theoretically yield more accurate beam hardening artifact correction. In addition, since spectral data are always available, using dl-DECT fecal tagging density can be calibrated to a precise level after scanning. Taguchi et al. investigated these aspects, demonstrating that both the mean tagging density and the number of colon segments with appropriate tagging density were significantly higher in dl-DECT VMIs than that in conventional 120 kVp images ($p < 0.01$ for both) [55]. A more recent investigation further strengthened these promising results. The authors found that 40-keV monoenergetic images showed higher overall sensitivity in polyp detection compared with conventional 120 kVp PEI (58.8% vs. 42.1%, $p < 0.001$) and improved reader confidence at different fecal tagging levels ($p < 0.001$) in a colon phantom [56].

3. Conclusions

Dual-layer DECT has several applications in gastrointestinal imaging and has already demonstrated utility above that of conventional SECT in various pathologies. Particularly, virtual monoenergetic images can improve vascular contrast and lesion conspicuity at low energy levels. Iodine concentration measurements may help to characterize different lesions by highlighting their contrast enhancement. Virtual non-contrast imaging can provide pre-contrast information and potentially eliminate true non-contrast series in multiphasic studies, saving radiation doses and additional studies. Lastly, a significant advantage of this dual-layer DECT is that the spectral information is provided retrospectively for all patients, without the need for prospectively screening the patient to determine whether the dual-energy mode must be turned on.

Author Contributions: Conceptualization, D.I.; methodology, D.I.; software, M.P. and S.T.; validation, C.M.; formal analysis, P.N.F., C.M.S., C.M. and D.I.; investigation, P.N.F. and C.M.S.; resources, E.D.P., M.P. and S.T.; data curation, M.R. and T.G.; writing—original draft preparation, P.N.F. and C.M.S.; writing—review and editing, P.N.F., C.M.S. and D.I.; supervision, R.C.; project administration, C.M. All authors have read and agreed to the published version of the manuscript.

Funding: This research received no external funding.

Institutional Review Board Statement: Ethical review and approval were waived for this study due to nature of the study.

Informed Consent Statement: Not applicable.

Data Availability Statement: Not applicable.

Conflicts of Interest: The authors declare no conflict of interest.

References

1. Forghani, R.; De Man, B.; Gupta, R. Dual-Energy Computed Tomography: Physical Principles, Approaches to Scanning, Usage, and Implementation: Part 1. *Neuroimaging Clin. N. Am.* **2017**, *27*, 371–384. [CrossRef] [PubMed]
2. Yoshizumi, T. Dual Energy CT in Clinical Practice. *Med. Phys.* **2011**, *38*, 6346. [CrossRef]
3. McCollough, C.H.; Leng, S.; Yu, L.; Fletcher, J.G. Dual- and Multi-Energy CT: Principles, Technical Approaches, and Clinical Applications. *Radiology* **2015**, *276*, 637–653. [CrossRef]
4. Rajiah, P.; Parakh, A.; Kay, F.; Baruah, D.; Kambadakone, A.R.; Leng, S. Update on Multienergy CT: Physics, Principles, and Applications. *Radiographics* **2020**, *40*, 1284–1308. [CrossRef] [PubMed]
5. Rassouli, N.; Etesami, M.; Dhanantwari, A.; Rajiah, P. Detector-Based Spectral CT with a Novel Dual-Layer Technology: Principles and Applications. *Insights Imaging* **2017**, *8*, 589–598. [CrossRef]
6. Große Hokamp, N.; Maintz, D.; Shapira, N.; Chang, D.H.; Noël, P.B. Technical Background of a Novel Detector-Based Approach to Dual-Energy Computed Tomography. *Diagn. Interv. Radiol.* **2020**, *26*, 68–71. [CrossRef] [PubMed]
7. Demirler Simsir, B.; Danse, E.; Coche, E. Benefit of Dual-Layer Spectral CT in Emergency Imaging of Different Organ Systems. *Clin. Radiol.* **2020**, *75*, 886–902. [CrossRef]
8. Siegel, M.J.; Kaza, R.K.; Bolus, D.N.; Boll, D.T.; Rofsky, N.M.; De Cecco, C.N.; Foley, W.D.; Morgan, D.E.; Schoepf, U.J.; Sahani, D.V.; et al. White Paper of the Society of Computed Body Tomography and Magnetic Resonance on Dual-Energy CT, Part 1: Technology and Terminology. *J. Comput. Assist. Tomogr.* **2016**, *40*, 841–845. [CrossRef]
9. Tawfik, A.M.; Kerl, J.M.; Razek, A.A.; Bauer, R.W.; Nour-Eldin, N.E.; Vogl, T.J.; Mack, M.G. Image Quality and Radiation Dose of Dual-Energy CT of the Head and Neck Compared with a Standard 120-KVp Acquisition. *AJNR Am. J. Neuroradiol.* **2011**, *32*, 1994–1999. [CrossRef] [PubMed]
10. Grajo, J.R.; Sahani, D.V. Dual-Energy CT of the Abdomen and Pelvis: Radiation Dose Considerations. *J. Am. Coll. Radiol.* **2018**, *15*, 1128–1132. [CrossRef]

11. Duan, X.; Ananthakrishnan, L.; Guild, J.B.; Xi, Y.; Rajiah, P. Radiation Doses and Image Quality of Abdominal CT Scans at Different Patient Sizes Using Spectral Detector CT Scanner: A Phantom and Clinical Study. *Abdom. Radiol.* 2020, *45*, 3361–3368. [CrossRef] [PubMed]
12. Dubourg, B.; Caudron, J.; Lestrat, J.-P.; Bubenheim, M.; Lefebvre, V.; Godin, M.; Tron, C.; Eltchaninoff, H.; Bauer, F.; Dacher, J.-N. Single-Source Dual-Energy CT Angiography with Reduced Iodine Load in Patients Referred for Aortoiliofemoral Evaluation before Transcatheter Aortic Valve Implantation: Impact on Image Quality and Radiation Dose. *Eur. Radiol.* 2014, *24*, 2659–2668. [CrossRef] [PubMed]
13. Zhang, X.; Zhang, G.; Xu, L.; Bai, X.; Lu, X.; Yu, S.; Sun, H.; Jin, Z. Utilisation of Virtual Non-Contrast Images and Virtual Mono-Energetic Images Acquired from Dual-Layer Spectral CT for Renal Cell Carcinoma: Image Quality and Radiation Dose. *Insights Imaging* 2022, *13*, 12. [CrossRef] [PubMed]
14. Husarik, D.B.; Gordic, S.; Desbiolles, L.; Krauss, B.; Leschka, S.; Wildermuth, S.; Alkadhi, H. Advanced Virtual Monoenergetic Computed Tomography of Hyperattenuating and Hypoattenuating Liver Lesions: Ex-Vivo and Patient Experience in Various Body Sizes. *Investig. Radiol.* 2015, *50*, 695–702. [CrossRef]
15. Lv, P.; Lin, X.Z.; Chen, K.; Gao, J. Spectral CT in Patients with Small HCC: Investigation of Image Quality and Diagnostic Accuracy. *Eur. Radiol.* 2012, *22*, 2117–2124. [CrossRef]
16. Große Hokamp, N.; Höink, A.J.; Doerner, J.; Jordan, D.W.; Pahn, G.; Persigehl, T.; Maintz, D.; Haneder, S. Assessment of Arterially Hyper-Enhancing Liver Lesions Using Virtual Monoenergetic Images from Spectral Detector CT: Phantom and Patient Experience. *Abdom. Radiol.* 2018, *43*, 2066–2074. [CrossRef]
17. Reimer, R.P.; Große Hokamp, N.; Fehrmann Efferoth, A.; Krauskopf, A.; Zopfs, D.; Kröger, J.R.; Persigehl, T.; Maintz, D.; Bunck, A.C. Virtual Monoenergetic Images from Spectral Detector Computed Tomography Facilitate Washout Assessment in Arterially Hyper-Enhancing Liver Lesions. *Eur. Radiol.* 2021, *31*, 3468–3477. [CrossRef]
18. Nagayama, Y.; Iyama, A.; Oda, S.; Taguchi, N.; Nakaura, T.; Utsunomiya, D.; Kikuchi, Y.; Yamashita, Y. Dual-Layer Dual-Energy Computed Tomography for the Assessment of Hypovascular Hepatic Metastases: Impact of Closing k-Edge on Image Quality and Lesion Detectability. *Eur. Radiol.* 2019, *29*, 2837–2847. [CrossRef]
19. Horowitz, J.M.; Venkatesh, S.K.; Ehman, R.L.; Jhaveri, K.; Kamath, P.; Ohliger, M.A.; Samir, A.E.; Silva, A.C.; Taouli, B.; Torbenson, M.S.; et al. Evaluation of Hepatic Fibrosis: A Review from the Society of Abdominal Radiology Disease Focus Panel. *Abdom. Radiol.* 2017, *42*, 2037–2053. [CrossRef]
20. Sofue, K.; Tsurusaki, M.; Mileto, A.; Hyodo, T.; Sasaki, K.; Nishii, T.; Chikugo, T.; Yada, N.; Kudo, M.; Sugimura, K.; et al. Dual-Energy Computed Tomography for Non-Invasive Staging of Liver Fibrosis: Accuracy of Iodine Density Measurements from Contrast-Enhanced Data. *Hepatol. Res.* 2018, *48*, 1008–1019. [CrossRef]
21. Bak, S.; Kim, J.E.; Bae, K.; Cho, J.M.; Choi, H.C.; Park, M.J.; Choi, H.Y.; Shin, H.S.; Lee, S.M.; Kim, H.O. Quantification of Liver Extracellular Volume Using Dual-Energy CT: Utility for Prediction of Liver-Related Events in Cirrhosis. *Eur. Radiol.* 2020, *30*, 5317–5326. [CrossRef] [PubMed]
22. Lamb, P.; Sahani, D.V.; Fuentes-Orrego, J.M.; Patino, M.; Ghosh, A.; Mendonça, P.R.S. Stratification of Patients with Liver Fibrosis Using Dual-Energy CT. *IEEE Trans. Med. Imaging* 2015, *34*, 807–815. [CrossRef] [PubMed]
23. Morita, K.; Nishie, A.; Ushijima, Y.; Takayama, Y.; Fujita, N.; Kubo, Y.; Ishimatsu, K.; Yoshizumi, T.; Maehara, J.; Ishigami, K. Noninvasive Assessment of Liver Fibrosis by Dual-Layer Spectral Detector CT. *Eur. J. Radiol.* 2021, *136*, 109575. [CrossRef] [PubMed]
24. Ma, Q.; Hu, J.; Yang, W.; Hou, Y. Dual-Layer Detector Spectral CT versus Magnetic Resonance Imaging for the Assessment of Iron Overload in Myelodysplastic Syndromes and Aplastic Anemia. *Jpn. J. Radiol.* 2020, *38*, 374–381. [CrossRef] [PubMed]
25. Choi, M.H.; Lee, Y.J.; Choi, Y.J.; Pak, S. Dual-Energy CT of the Liver: True Noncontrast vs. Virtual Noncontrast Images Derived from Multiple Phases for the Diagnosis of Fatty Liver. *Eur. J. Radiol.* 2021, *140*, 109741. [CrossRef] [PubMed]
26. Xu, J.J.; Boesen, M.R.; Hansen, S.L.; Ulriksen, P.S.; Holm, S.; Lönn, L.; Hansen, K.L. Assessment of Liver Fat: Dual-Energy CT versus Conventional CT with and without Contrast. *Diagnostics* 2022, *12*, 708. [CrossRef]
27. Laukamp, K.R.; Ho, V.; Obmann, V.C.; Herrmann, K.; Gupta, A.; Borggrefe, J.; Lennartz, S.; Große Hokamp, N.; Ramaiya, N. Virtual Non-Contrast for Evaluation of Liver Parenchyma and Vessels: Results from 25 Patients Using Multi-Phase Spectral-Detector CT. *Acta Radiol.* 2020, *61*, 1143–1152. [CrossRef]
28. Laukamp, K.R.; Lennartz, S.; Ho, V.; Große Hokamp, N.; Zopfs, D.; Gupta, A.; Graner, F.P.; Borggrefe, J.; Gilkeson, R.; Ramaiya, N. Evaluation of the Liver with Virtual Non-Contrast: Single Institution Study in 149 Patients Undergoing TAVR Planning. *Br. J. Radiol.* 2020, *93*, 20190701. [CrossRef]
29. Grosu, S.; Wang, Z.J.; Obmann, M.M.; Sugi, M.D.; Sun, Y.; Yeh, B.M. Reduction of Peristalsis-Related Streak Artifacts on the Liver with Dual-Layer Spectral CT. *Diagnostics* 2022, *12*, 782. [CrossRef]
30. Gandhi, D.; Ojili, V.; Nepal, P.; Nagar, A.; Hernandez-Delima, F.J.; Bajaj, D.; Choudhary, G.; Gupta, N.; Sharma, P. A Pictorial Review of Gall Stones and Its Associated Complications. *Clin. Imaging* 2020, *60*, 228–236. [CrossRef]
31. Kim, C.W.; Chang, J.H.; Lim, Y.S.; Kim, T.H.; Lee, I.S.; Han, S.W. Common Bile Duct Stones on Multidetector Computed Tomography: Attenuation Patterns and Detectability. *World J. Gastroenterol.* 2013, *19*, 1788–1796. [CrossRef]
32. Saito, H.; Noda, K.; Ogasawara, K.; Atsuji, S.; Takaoka, H.; Kajihara, H.; Nasu, J.; Morishita, S.; Matsushita, I.; Katahira, K. Usefulness and Limitations of Dual-Layer Spectral Detector Computed Tomography for Diagnosing Biliary Stones Not Detected by Conventional Computed Tomography: A Report of Three Cases. *Clin. J. Gastroenterol.* 2018, *11*, 172–177. [CrossRef] [PubMed]

33. Soesbe, T.C.; Lewis, M.A.; Xi, Y.; Browning, T.; Ananthakrishnan, L.; Fielding, J.R.; Lenkinski, R.E.; Leyendecker, J.R. A Technique to Identify Isoattenuating Gallstones with Dual-Layer Spectral CT: An Ex Vivo Phantom Study. *Radiology* **2019**, *292*, 400–406. [CrossRef]
34. Huda, F.; LeBedis, C.A.; Qureshi, M.M.; Anderson, S.W.; Gupta, A. Acute Cholecystitis: Diagnostic Value of Dual-Energy CT-Derived Iodine Map and Low-KeV Virtual Monoenergetic Images. *Abdom. Radiol.* **2021**, *46*, 5125–5133. [CrossRef] [PubMed]
35. Ishigami, K.; Yoshimitsu, K.; Irie, H.; Tajima, T.; Asayama, Y.; Nishie, A.; Hirakawa, M.; Ushijima, Y.; Okamoto, D.; Nagata, S.; et al. Diagnostic Value of the Delayed Phase Image for Iso-Attenuating Pancreatic Carcinomas in the Pancreatic Parenchymal Phase on Multidetector Computed Tomography. *Eur. J. Radiol.* **2009**, *69*, 139–146. [CrossRef]
36. Macari, M.; Spieler, B.; Kim, D.; Graser, A.; Megibow, A.J.; Babb, J.; Chandarana, H. Dual-Source Dual-Energy MDCT of Pancreatic Adenocarcinoma: Initial Observations with Data Generated at 80 KVp and at Simulated Weighted-Average 120 KVp. *AJR Am. J. Roentgenol.* **2010**, *194*, W27–W32. [CrossRef]
37. Bhosale, P.; Le, O.; Balachandran, A.; Fox, P.; Paulson, E.; Tamm, E. Quantitative and Qualitative Comparison of Single-Source Dual-Energy Computed Tomography and 120-KVp Computed Tomography for the Assessment of Pancreatic Ductal Adenocarcinoma. *J. Comput. Assist. Tomogr.* **2015**, *39*, 907–913. [CrossRef]
38. El Kayal, N.; Lennartz, S.; Ekdawi, S.; Holz, J.; Slebocki, K.; Haneder, S.; Wybranski, C.; Mohallel, A.; Eid, M.; Grüll, H.; et al. Value of Spectral Detector Computed Tomography for Assessment of Pancreatic Lesions. *Eur. J. Radiol.* **2019**, *118*, 215–222. [CrossRef] [PubMed]
39. Nagayama, Y.; Tanoue, S.; Inoue, T.; Oda, S.; Nakaura, T.; Utsunomiya, D.; Yamashita, Y. Dual-Layer Spectral CT Improves Image Quality of Multiphasic Pancreas CT in Patients with Pancreatic Ductal Adenocarcinoma. *Eur. Radiol.* **2020**, *30*, 394–403. [CrossRef]
40. Han, Y.E.; Park, B.J.; Sung, D.J.; Kim, M.J.; Han, N.Y.; Sim, K.C.; Cho, Y.; Kim, H. Dual-Layer Spectral CT of Pancreas Ductal Adenocarcinoma: Can Virtual Monoenergetic Images of the Portal Venous Phase Be an Alternative to the Pancreatic-Phase Scan? *J. Belg. Soc. Radiol.* **2022**, *106*, 83. [CrossRef]
41. Wang, Y.; Hu, X.; Shi, S.; Song, C.; Wang, L.; Yuan, J.; Lin, Z.; Cai, H.; Feng, S.-T.; Luo, Y. Utility of Quantitative Metrics From Dual-Layer Spectral-Detector CT for Differentiation of Pancreatic Neuroendocrine Tumor and Neuroendocrine Carcinoma. *AJR Am. J. Roentgenol.* **2022**, *218*, 999–1009. [CrossRef] [PubMed]
42. Firetto, M.C.; Lemos, A.A.; Marini, A.; Avesani, E.C.; Biondetti, P.R. Acute Bowel Ischemia: Analysis of Diagnostic Error by Overlooked Findings at MDCT Angiography. *Emerg. Radiol.* **2013**, *20*, 139–147. [CrossRef]
43. Potretzke, T.A.; Brace, C.L.; Lubner, M.G.; Sampson, L.A.; Willey, B.J.; Lee, F.T. Early Small-Bowel Ischemia: Dual-Energy CT Improves Conspicuity Compared with Conventional CT in a Swine Model. *Radiology* **2015**, *275*, 119–126. [CrossRef] [PubMed]
44. Lourenco, P.D.M.; Rawski, R.; Mohammed, M.F.; Khosa, F.; Nicolaou, S.; McLaughlin, P. Dual-Energy CT Iodine Mapping and 40-KeV Monoenergetic Applications in the Diagnosis of Acute Bowel Ischemia. *Am. J. Roentgenol.* **2018**, *211*, 564–570. [CrossRef] [PubMed]
45. Oda, S.; Nakaura, T.; Utsunomiya, D.; Funama, Y.; Taguchi, N.; Imuta, M.; Nagayama, Y.; Yamashita, Y. Clinical Potential of Retrospective On-Demand Spectral Analysis Using Dual-Layer Spectral Detector-Computed Tomography in Ischemia Complicating Small-Bowel Obstruction. *Emerg. Radiol.* **2017**, *24*, 431–434. [CrossRef] [PubMed]
46. Chen, C.-Y.; Hsu, J.-S.; Jaw, T.-S.; Wu, D.-C.; Shih, M.-C.P.; Lee, C.-H.; Kuo, C.-H.; Chen, Y.-T.; Lai, M.-L.; Liu, G.-C. Utility of the Iodine Overlay Technique and Virtual Nonenhanced Images for the Preoperative T Staging of Colorectal Cancer by Dual-Energy CT with Tin Filter Technology. *PLoS ONE* **2014**, *9*, e113589. [CrossRef]
47. Chen, W.; Ye, Y.; Zhang, D.; Mao, L.; Guo, L.; Zhang, H.; Du, X.; Deng, W.; Liu, B.; Liu, X. Utility of Dual-Layer Spectral-Detector CT Imaging for Predicting Pathological Tumor Stages and Histologic Grades of Colorectal Adenocarcinoma. *Front. Oncol.* **2022**, *12*, 1002592. [CrossRef]
48. Wang, G.; Fang, Y.; Wang, Z.; Jin, Z. Quantitative Assessment of Radiologically Indeterminate Local Colonic Wall Thickening on Iodine Density Images Using Dual-Layer Spectral Detector CT. *Acad. Radiol.* **2021**, *28*, 1368–1374. [CrossRef] [PubMed]
49. Peng, J.C.; Feng, Q.; Zhu, J.; Shen, J.; Qiao, Y.Q.; Xu, J.R.; Ran, Z.H. Usefulness of Spectral Computed Tomography for Evaluation of Intestinal Activity and Severity in Ileocolonic Crohn's Disease. *Therap. Adv. Gastroenterol.* **2016**, *9*, 795–805. [CrossRef]
50. Taguchi, N.; Oda, S.; Kobayashi, T.; Naoe, H.; Sasaki, Y.; Imuta, M.; Nakaura, T.; Yamashita, Y. Advanced Parametric Imaging for Evaluation of Crohn's Disease Using Dual-Energy Computed Tomography Enterography. *Radiol. Case Rep.* **2018**, *13*, 709–712. [CrossRef]
51. Dane, B.; Sarkar, S.; Nazarian, M.; Galitzer, H.; O'Donnell, T.; Remzi, F.; Chang, S.; Megibow, A. Crohn Disease Active Inflammation Assessment with Iodine Density from Dual-Energy CT Enterography: Comparison with Histopathologic Analysis. *Radiology* **2021**, *301*, 144–151. [CrossRef] [PubMed]
52. Kim, Y.S.; Kim, S.H.; Ryu, H.S.; Han, J.K. Iodine Quantification on Spectral Detector-Based Dual-Energy CT Enterography: Correlation with Crohn's Disease Activity Index and External Validation. *Korean J. Radiol.* **2018**, *19*, 1077. [CrossRef] [PubMed]
53. Lee, S.M.; Kim, S.H.; Ahn, S.J.; Kang, H.-J.; Kang, J.H.; Han, J.K. Virtual Monoenergetic Dual-Layer, Dual-Energy CT Enterography: Optimization of KeV Settings and Its Added Value for Crohn's Disease. *Eur. Radiol.* **2018**, *28*, 2525–2534. [CrossRef] [PubMed]
54. Cai, W.; Zhang, D.; Lee, J.-G.; Shirai, Y.; Kim, S.H.; Yoshida, H. Dual-Energy Index Value of Luminal Air in Fecal-Tagging Computed Tomography Colonography: Findings and Impact on Electronic Cleansing. *J. Comput. Assist. Tomogr.* **2013**, *37*, 183–194. [CrossRef]

55. Taguchi, N.; Oda, S.; Imuta, M.; Yamamura, S.; Yokota, Y.; Nakaura, T.; Nagayama, Y.; Kidoh, M.; Utsunomiya, D.; Funama, Y.; et al. Dual-Energy Computed Tomography Colonography Using Dual-Layer Spectral Detector Computed Tomography: Utility of Virtual Monochromatic Imaging for Electronic Cleansing. *Eur. J. Radiol.* **2018**, *108*, 7–12. [CrossRef]
56. Obmann, M.M.; An, C.; Schaefer, A.; Sun, Y.; Wang, Z.J.; Yee, J.; Yeh, B.M. Improved Sensitivity and Reader Confidence in CT Colonography Using Dual-Layer Spectral CT: A Phantom Study. *Radiology* **2020**, *297*, 99–107. [CrossRef] [PubMed]

Disclaimer/Publisher's Note: The statements, opinions and data contained in all publications are solely those of the individual author(s) and contributor(s) and not of MDPI and/or the editor(s). MDPI and/or the editor(s) disclaim responsibility for any injury to people or property resulting from any ideas, methods, instructions or products referred to in the content.

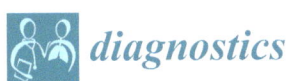

Article

Multi-Slice CT Features Predict Pathological Risk Classification in Gastric Stromal Tumors Larger Than 2 cm: A Retrospective Study

Sikai Wang [1], Ping Dai [1], Guangyan Si [1,*], Mengsu Zeng [2] and Mingliang Wang [2,*]

[1] Department of Radiology, The Affiliated Traditional Chinese Medicine Hospital of Southwest Medical University, No. 182 Chunhui Road, Longmatan District, Luzhou 646000, China; qiuzhi2010@163.com (S.W.); daipbb0830@163.com (P.D.)
[2] Department of Radiology, Zhongshan Hospital, Fudan University, No. 180 Fenglin Road, Xuhui District, Shanghai 200032, China; zeng.mengsu@zs-hospital.sh.cn
* Correspondence: siguangyan@126.com (G.S.); wang.mingliang@zs-hospital.sh.cn (M.W.)

Abstract: Background: The Armed Forces Institute of Pathology (AFIP) had higher accuracy and reliability in prognostic assessment and treatment strategies for patients with gastric stromal tumors (GSTs). The AFIP classification is frequently used in clinical applications. But the risk classification is only available for patients who are previously untreated and received complete resection. We aimed to investigate the feasibility of multi-slice MSCT features of GSTs in predicting AFIP risk classification preoperatively. Methods: The clinical data and MSCT features of 424 patients with solitary GSTs were retrospectively reviewed. According to pathological AFIP risk criteria, 424 GSTs were divided into a low-risk group ($n = 282$), a moderate-risk group ($n = 72$), and a high-risk group ($n = 70$). The clinical data and MSCT features of GSTs were compared among the three groups. Those variables ($p < 0.05$) in the univariate analysis were included in the multivariate analysis. The nomogram was created using the rms package. Results: We found significant differences in the tumor location, morphology, necrosis, ulceration, growth pattern, feeding artery, vascular-like enhancement, fat-positive signs around GSTs, CT value in the venous phase, CT value increment in the venous phase, longest diameter, and maximum short diameter (all $p < 0.05$). Two nomogram models were successfully constructed to predict the risk of GSTs. Low- vs. high-risk group: the independent risk factors of high-risk GSTs included the location, ulceration, and longest diameter. The area under the receiver operating characteristic curve (AUC) of the prediction model was 0.911 (95% CI: 0.872–0.951), and the sensitivity and specificity were 80.0% and 89.0%, respectively. Moderate- vs. high-risk group: the morphology, necrosis, and feeding artery were independent risk factors of a high risk of GSTs, with an AUC value of 0.826 (95% CI: 0.759–0.893), and the sensitivity and specificity were 85.7% and 70.8%, respectively. Conclusions: The MSCT features of GSTs and the nomogram model have great practical value in predicting pathological AFIP risk classification between high-risk and non-high-risk groups before surgery.

Keywords: gastric stromal tumors; X-ray computed; risk classification; Armed Forces Institute of Pathology; nomogram model

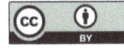

1. Introduction

Gastrointestinal stromal tumors (GISTs) are very rare but are the most common mesenchymal tumors of the digestive tract. GISTs occur most frequently in the stomach (50–60%) and small intestine (20–30%) [1]. Gastric stromal tumors (GSTs) differ in the range of biological behavior from benign to extremely malignant. With the development of targeted drug therapy, accurate risk stratification for GSTs has become increasingly important. Presently, different risk classification standards are used for GSTs. The 2008 modified version of the National Institutes of Health (NIH) classification and the Armed Forces Institute of Pathology (AFIP) classification are frequently used in clinical applications [2,3].

Previous studies [3–6] showed that AFIP criteria had higher accuracy and reliability in prognostic assessment and treatment strategies for patients with GSTs.

AFIP risk stratification was typically based on the tumor location, size, and mitotic count [7]. However, due to tumor stroma changes induced by treatment with tyrosine kinase inhibitor (TKI) before surgery, the mitotic count and tumor size cannot be accurately evaluated using post-operative specimens. Preoperative puncture biopsy may also not provide accurate measurements of mitotic count when samples are few and for more heterogeneous tumors. Moreover, puncture biopsy may cause the tumor to rupture, bleed, or seed, spreading cancer cells along the needle path. Therefore, the risk classification is only available for patients who were previously untreated and received complete resection.

MSCT has emerged as a clinically preferred imaging modality for its ability to provide a differential diagnosis, an evaluation of metastasis and therapy, and a prediction of rupture and follow-up after surgery [1,8,9]. Previous comparative studies [8,10,11] reported different risk classification and prognosis evaluations of GISTs using CT or other inspection methods. However, most of these studies included all GISTs and had fewer samples. Liu et al. [12,13] reported that CT and clinical features differed between GSTs and non-GSTs. In addition, GSTs account for more than half of GISTs. Accurate preoperative risk assessment of GSTs using MSCT has important clinical significance in guiding treatment and predicting prognosis. Therefore, this study aims to investigate the feasibility of MSCT features in predicting pathological AFIP risk classification of GSTs before treatment.

2. Methods

2.1. Study Population

The clinical data and MSCT features of 476 patients with GSTs confirmed by surgical and post-operative pathological examination at Zhongshan Hospital, Fudan University and the Affiliated Traditional Chinese Medicine Hospital of Southwest Medical University were retrospectively reviewed from November 2014 to November 2021.

The inclusion criteria: (1) GSTs were resected completely and were confirmed by the post-operative pathological examination; (2) patients underwent abdominal triple-phase (non-contrast CT, arterial, and venous phases) CT scan before surgery; and (3) longest diameter of tumor specimen > 2 cm.

The exclusion criteria: (1) tumor rupture (preoperative or intraoperative tumor rupture; tumor specimens were several pieces or incomplete); (2) severe CT artifacts; (3) treatment with TKI before surgery; (4) distant metastasis (including lymph node metastasis, visceral metastases, peritoneal metastases) was confirmed by biopsy; and (5) the number of GSTs ≥ 2 in the same patient (Figure 1).

After screening, a total of 424 patients with solitary GSTs were included in this study. According to the AFIP criteria [7] (Table 1), 424 GSTs were categorized as a low-risk group (including very low and low risk), a moderate-risk group, and a high-risk group.

Table 1. AFIP criteria of GSTs.

Tumor Parameters		Characterization of Risk for Metastasis	Proportion of Patients with Progressive Disease (%)
Size	Mitotic Count		
>2 cm $\leq$ 5 cm	$\leq$5 per 50 HPFs	Very low	1.9
>2 cm $\leq$ 5 cm	>5 per 50 HPFs	Moderate	16
>5 cm $\leq$ 10 cm	$\leq$5 per 50 HPFs	Low	3.6
>5 cm $\leq$ 10 cm	>5 per 50 HPFs	High	55
>10 cm	$\leq$5 per 50 HPFs	Moderate	12
>10 cm	>5 per 50 HPFs	High	86

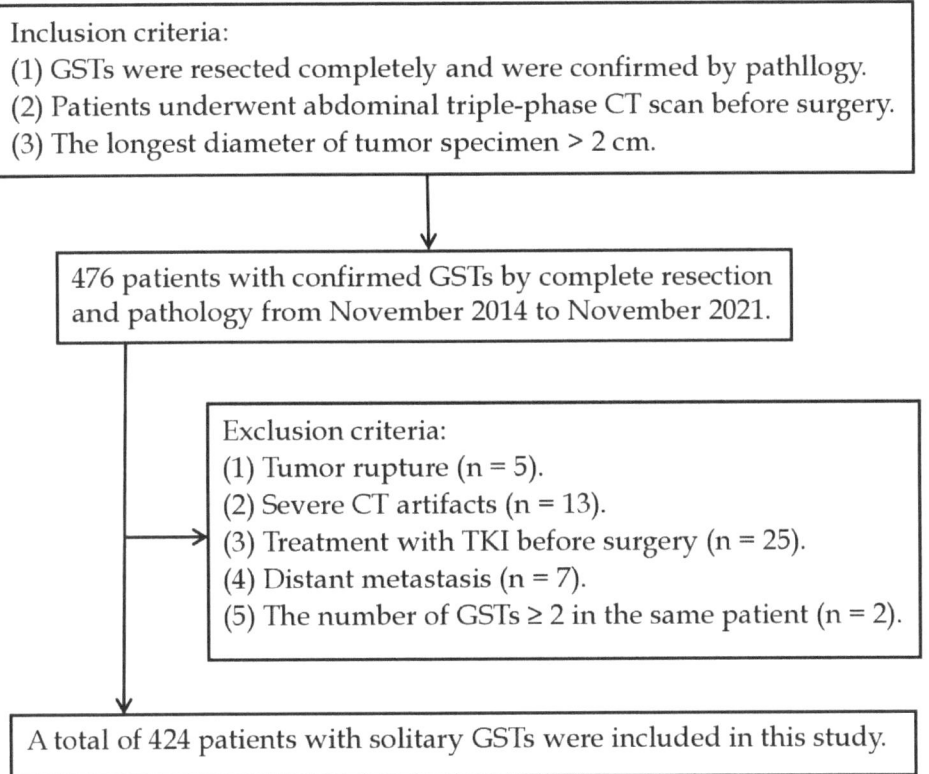

Figure 1. Flow diagram of the study population.

2.2. CT Technique

All the patients drank 500–800 mL of water 15 min before the CT examination to expand the stomach and were trained in breathing. All the patients underwent a triple-phase (non-contrast, arterial, and venous phases) CT scan using one of the following MSCT scanners: 64-slice spiral CT (Siemens Medical Solutions, Forchheim, Germany), second Dual Source CT (Siemens Medical Solutions, Forchheim, Germany), or UIH 40 CT (United Imaging Healthcare, Shanghai, China) scanner. The scanning parameters were as follows: 120-kV tube voltage, adaptive tube current, and axial images of 5 mm slice thickness. An 80–100 mL dose of non-ionic contrast agent (iopromide, 370 mgI/mL iodine, Bayer Schering Company, Guangzhou, China; or iohexol, 300 mgI/mL iodine, GE Healthcare, Shanghai, China) was injected into the cubital vein at a rate of 2.5–3 mL/s using a dual-barrel power injector. The scan of the arterial and venous phases was initiated at about 25 s and 80 s after starting the contrast injection, respectively.

2.3. Imaging Interpretation

Two radiologists with more than 10 years of clinical experience in abdominal CT diagnosis reviewed the CT images using a single-blinded comparison to reach an agreement through consultation, without prior knowledge of the pathological results. A consensus was reached between a third senior abdominal radiologist and the two radiologists when there was any disagreement between the two radiologists.

The following quantitative parameters were used in this study: (1) longest diameter on axial image, maximal short diameter (perpendicular to longest diameter on the same axial image); (2) CT value in non-contrast CT, arterial phase, and venous phase. More than

20 mm², circular regions of interest (ROI) of triple-phase CT value were drawn on the same solid parts of lesions while avoiding necrotic cystic areas, calcification, and vascular areas; (3) CT value increment in arterial phase ($\Delta CT_{arterial}$) was calculated by subtracting the CT value in non-contrast CT from the CT value in the arterial phase; (4) CT value increment in venous phase (ΔCT_{venous}) was calculated by subtracting the CT value in the non-contrast CT scan from the CT value in the venous phase.

The qualitative parameters were as follows: (1) morphology (regular was defined as smooth-walled, round, or oval; irregular otherwise); (2) growth pattern (endophytic vs. exophytic vs. mixed); (3) calcification (defined as extremely high-density imaging in the non-contrast CT); (4) ulceration (defined as superficial defects of tumor); (5) necrosis (defined as unenhanced regions in arterial and venous phase); (6) location (gastric fundus vs. gastric cardia vs. gastric body vs. gastric antrum); (7) feeding artery (larger arteries enter the tumor in the arterial phase); (8) vascular-like enhancement (striated vascular shadow was seen in the arterial phase or venous phase inside the tumor); (9) fat-positive signs around the lesion (increased fat density).

2.4. Statistical Analyses

SPSS statistical software (version: 26.0) and R software (version: 4.0.3) were used to process and analyze all the data. All the continuous variables that did not always follow a normal distribution were presented as the median (first quartile, third quartile). The quantitative data were statistically analyzed using the Kruskal–Wallis H test, and the least significant difference (LSD) test was used for pairwise comparisons. The categorical variables were expressed as frequencies (percentages). The categorical variables were statistically analyzed using the chi-square test and Bonferroni method for pairwise comparisons. Those variables ($p < 0.05$) in the univariate analysis were included in the multivariate analysis. Multivariate analysis was performed with stepwise logistic regression based on the Akaike information criterion. The nomogram was created using the rms package. The calibration curve (the Brier score) and receiver operating characteristic (ROC) curve were used to evaluate the predictive performance of the nomogram model. A smaller value of the Brier score (<0.2) suggests a better model. The bootstrap resampling method (1000 samples) was used for internal validation and the stability of the model. The random seed was set to 123,456. $p < 0.05$ was considered statistically significant.

3. Results

3.1. Clinical Information (Table 2)

A total of 424 patients (223 men and 201 women) with a median age of 61.0 (range, 14–85) years were included in the study. In total, 424 GSTs were divided into a low-risk group ($n = 282$), a moderate-risk group ($n = 72$), and a high-risk group ($n = 70$). We found no significant differences in age, gender, and gastrointestinal bleeding among the three groups ($p > 0.05$).

Table 2. Comparison of clinical information.

Groups	Gender		Age (Years Old)	Gastrointestinal Bleeding	
	Male ($n = 223$)	Female ($n = 201$)		Yes ($n = 96$)	No ($n = 328$)
Low-risk group ($n = 282$)	146(51.8)	138 (48.2)	61.00 (54.00, 69.00)	55 (19.5)	227 (80.5)
Moderate-risk group ($n = 72$)	32 (44.4)	40 (55.6)	60.50 (52.50, 68.00)	19 (26.4)	53 (73.6)
High-risk group ($n = 70$)	45 (64.3)	25 (35.7)	60.00 (52.00, 67.00)	22 (31.4)	48 (68.6)
Statistical Value	5.832 #		1.181 *	5.248 #	
p value	0.054		0.554	0.072	

Note: * represents H value, # represents χ^2 value.

3.2. CT Features (Table 3, Figure 2)

There were significant differences in the longest diameter, maximum short diameter, tumor location, morphology, necrosis, ulceration, growth pattern, feeding artery, vascular-like enhancement, fat-positive signs around the lesion, the venous phase CT value, and the ΔCT_{venous} among the three groups ($p < 0.05$). However, we found no significant differences in the CT value in the non-contrast and arterial phase, $\Delta CT_{arterial}$, and calcification ($p > 0.05$).

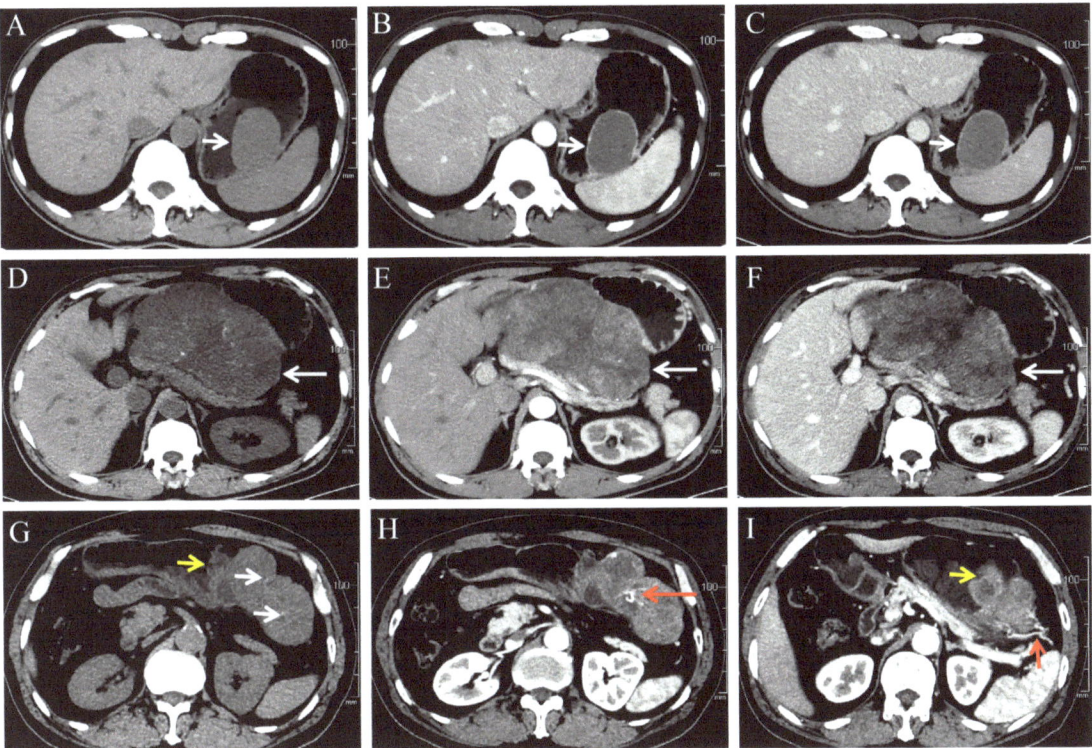

Figure 2. (**A**–**C**) A 46-year-old male patient with very low-risk GSTs in gastric body (white arrow). The non-contrast (**A**), arterial phase (**B**), and venous phase (**C**) CT images showed endophytic growth tumor with regular morphology, homogeneous enhancement and no necrosis. (**D**–**F**) A 59-year-old male patient with moderate-risk GSTs in gastric body (white arrow). The non-contrast (**D**), arterial phase (**E**), and venous phase (**F**) CT images showed exophytic growth lesion with irregular morphology, thin dotted calcification (**D**), heterogeneous enhancement, and necrosis. (**G**–**I**) A 57-year-old male patient with high-risk GSTs in gastric fundus. The non-contrast (**G**), arterial phase (**H**,**I**) CT images showed a mixed growth tumor with irregular morphology, thin dotted calcification ((**G**), white arrow), heterogeneous enhancement and necrosis area, feeding artery ((**I**), short red arrow), vascular-like enhancement ((**H**), long red arrow), and ulceration ((**G**,**I**), short yellow arrow).

Table 3. Comparison of MSCT features of GSTs.

Parameters	Low-Risk Group (n = 282)	Moderate-Risk Group (n = 72)	High-Risk Group (n = 70)	Statistical Value	p Value
Morphology				41.629 #	<0.001
Regular (n = 239)	178 (63.1) [a]	46 (63.9) [a]	15 (21.4) [b]		
Irregular (n = 185)	104 (36.9)	26 (36.1)	55 (78.6)		
Calcification				44.338 #	0.338
No (n = 346)	232 (82.3)	61 (84.7)	53 (75.7)		
Yes (n = 78)	50 (17.7)	11 (15.3)	17 (24.3)		
Ulceration				48.116 #	<0.001
No (n = 299)	228 (80.9) [a]	42 (58.3) [b]	29 (41.4) [c]		
Yes (n = 125)	54 (19.1)	30 (41.7)	41 (58.6)		
Feeding artery				52.490 #	<0.001
No (n = 294)	216 (76.6) [a]	55 (76.4) [a]	23 (32.9) [b]		
Yes (n = 130)	66 (23.4)	17 (23.6)	47 (67.1)		
Vascular-like enhancement				45.383 #	<0.001
No (n = 321)	233 (82.6) [a]	57 (79.2) [a]	31 (44.3) [b]		
Yes (n = 103)	49 (17.4)	15 (20.8)	39 (55.7)		
Fat-positive sign around lesion				59.171 #	<0.001
No (n = 394)	275 (97.5) [a]	69 (95.8) [a]	50 (71.4) [b]		
Yes (n = 30)	7 (2.5)	3 (4.2)	20 (28.6)		
Necrosis				44.338 #	<0.001
No (n = 183)	142 (50.4) [a]	36 (50.0) [a]	5 (7.1) [b]		
Yes (n = 241)	140 (49.6)	36 (50.0)	65 (92.9)		
Location				29.563 #	<0.001
Gastric fundus (n = 157)	90 (31.9) [a]	38 (52.8) [b]	29 (41.4) [ab]		
Gastric cardi (n = 10)	4 (1.4) [a]	1 (1.4) [ab]	5 (7.1) [b]		
Gastric body (n = 215)	149 (52.8) [a]	31 (43.1) [a]	35 (50.0) [a]		
Gastric antrum (n = 42)	39 (13.8) [a]	2 (2.8) [b]	1 (1.4) [b]		
Growth pattern				19.755 #	0.001
Endophytic (n = 133)	81 (28.7) [a]	25 (34.7) [a]	7 (10.0) [b]		
Exophytic (n = 179)	124 (44.0) [a]	27 (37.5) [a]	28 (40.0) [a]		
Mixed (n = 132)	77 (27.3) [a]	20 (27.8) [a]	35 (50.0) [b]		
Maximal short diameter (cm)	2.87 (2.30, 3.84) [a]	3.07 (2.36, 3.99) [a]	6.06 (4.34, 8.29) [b]	98.088 *	<0.001
CT value in non-contrast (HU)	32.45 (29.00, 36.00)	32.85 (29.45, 34.60)	33.55 (30.30, 36.00)	1.740 *	0.419
CT value in arterial phase (HU)	52.75 (46.00, 60.70)	48.95 (46.13, 57.15)	49.95 (44.40, 58.00)	3.504 *	0.173
CT value in venous phase (HU)	64.10 (57.40, 74.20) [a]	61.05 (54.80, 67.75) [b]	59.50 (54.05, 69.40) [b]	9.208 *	0.010
ΔCT$_{arterial}$	19.50 (13.39, 26.70)	17.83 (12.65, 24.38)	16.50 (11.75, 23.93)	4.193 *	0.123
ΔCT$_{venous}$	31.00 (24.60, 41.49) [a]	27.55 (21.50, 37.60) [b]	26.25 (21.12, 36.15) [b]	8.557 *	0.014

Note: * represents H value, # represents χ^2 value, Different letters ([a, b, c]) indicate statistical differences.

3.3. Construction of Binary Logistic Regression and Nomogram Model

Low- vs. high-risk group: with the low-risk group as a reference, the independent risk factors of high-risk GSTs included location, ulceration, and the longest diameter based on multivariate logistic regression analysis (Table 4). A nomogram model was constructed to predict the high-risk GSTs using R software (Figure 3A). The AUC value of the predictive model was 0.911 (95% CI: 0.872–0.951), and the sensitivity and specificity were 80.0% and 89.0%, respectively. The AUC obtained from the internal validation using the bootstrap method was 0.913 (95% CI: 0.870–0.947), and the sensitivity and specificity were 84.3% and 84.0%, respectively. The optimal cut-off value of the total score was 54 (Figure 3B). The

ROC curve and the calibration curve (Brier value = 0.083, Figure 3C) both suggested that the nomogram model had good predictive performance.

Table 4. Results of binary logistic regression analysis of low- vs. high-risk group.

Risk Factor		β Value	Standard Error	Wald Value	p Value	OR Value (95% CI)
Location	Gastric antrum *					
Gastric fundus		2.476	1.146	4.671	0.031	11.895 (1.259, 112.345)
Gastric cardia		4.135	1.572	6.914	0.009	62.467 (2.865, 1361.919)
Gastric body		2.191	1.135	3.728	0.054	8.946 (0.967, 82.716)
Ulceration	No *					
	Yes	1.190	0.384	9.586	0.002	3.286 (1.547, 6.980)
Longest diameter	No *					
	Yes	0.569	0.090	40.251	<0.001	1.767 (1.482, 2.106)
Vascular-like enhancement	No *					
	Yes	0.658	0.419	2.468	0.116	1.931 (0.850, 4.390)

Note: * represents refer.

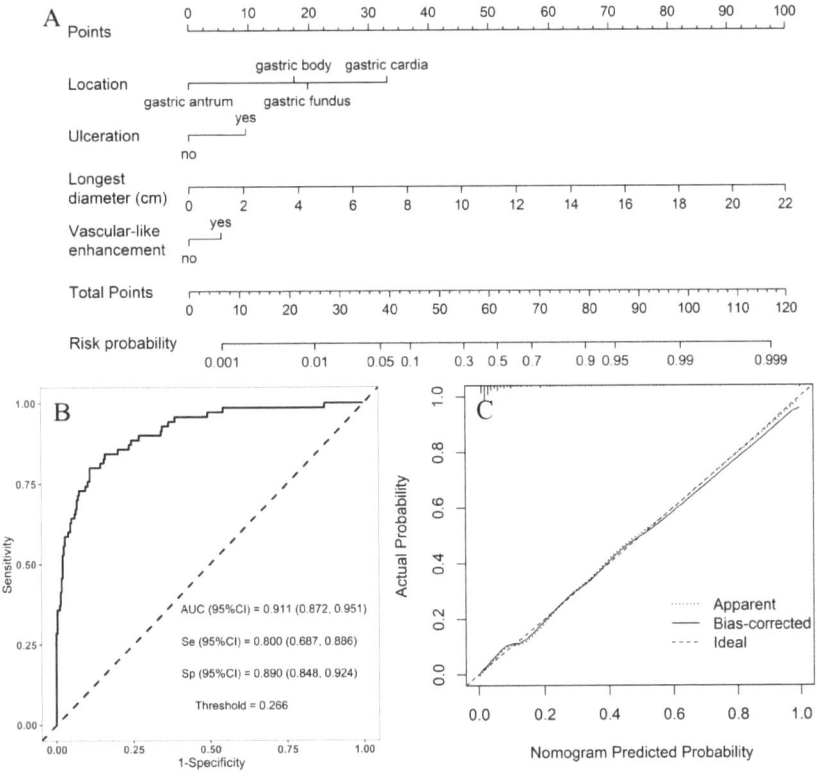

Figure 3. Using low-risk group as a reference, construction of predicting high-risk GSTs nomogram model. (A) Construction of nomogram based on the binary logistic regression analysis. The risk score was calculated using a nomogram. The optimal cut-off value of the total score was 54. (B) ROC curve of the prediction model; the sensitivity and specificity suggested that the nomogram model had good predictive performance. (C) Calibration curve of nomogram; the closer the bias-corrected line was to the ideal line, the more predictive accuracy of the nomogram model was (Brier value = 0.083).

Moderate- vs. high-risk group: using the moderate-risk group as a reference, multivariate logistic regression analysis showed that morphology, necrosis, and feeding artery were independent risk factors of high-risk GSTs (Table 5). A nomogram model was constructed to predict the high-risk GSTs using R software (Figure 4A). The AUC value of the predictive model was 0.826 (95% CI: 0.759–0.893), and the sensitivity and specificity were 85.7% and 70.8%, respectively (Figure 4B). The AUC obtained from the internal validation using the bootstrap method was 0.828 (95% CI: 0.761–0.892), and the sensitivity and specificity were 85.7% and 70.8%, respectively. The optimal cut-off value of the total score was 111. The ROC curve and the calibration curve (Brier value = 0.163, Figure 4C) both suggested that the nomogram model had good predictive performance.

Table 5. Results of binary logistic regression analysis of moderate- vs. high-risk group.

Risk Factor		β Value	Standard Error	Wald Value	p Value	OR Value (95% CI)
Morphology	Regular *					
	Irregular	1.256	0.436	8.288	0.004	3.511 (1.493, 8.255)
Necrosis	No *					
	Yes	1.994	0.554	12.938	<0.001	7.342 (2.478, 1.757)
Feeding artery	No *					
	Yes	1.173	0.433	7.357	0.007	3.233 (1.385, 7.549)

Note: * represents refer.

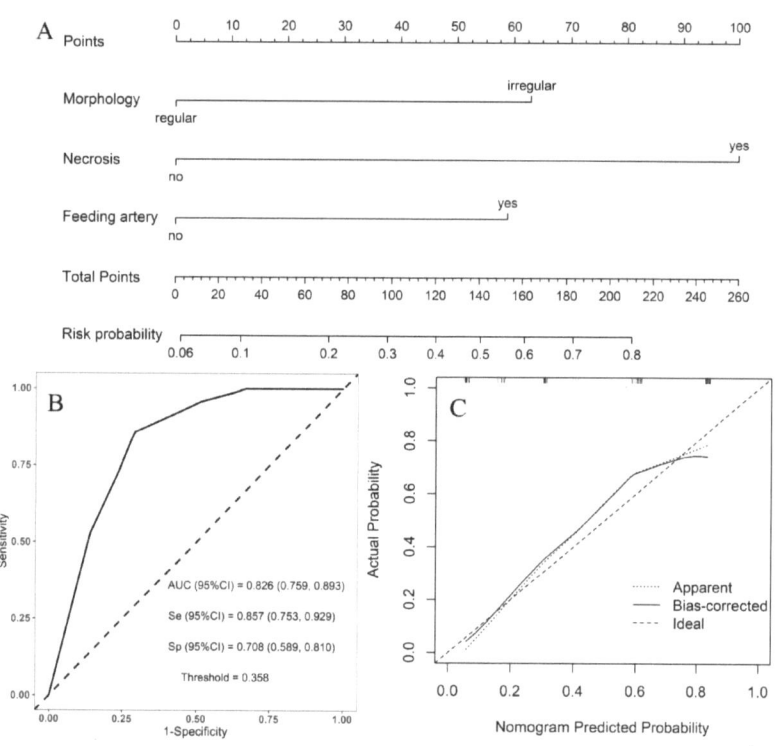

Figure 4. Using moderate-risk group as a reference, construction of predicting high-risk GSTs nomogram model. (**A**) Construction of nomogram based on the binary logistic regression analysis. The risk score was calculated by nomogram. The optimal cut-off value of the total score was 111. (**B**) ROC curve of the prediction model; the sensitivity and specificity suggested that the nomogram model had good predictive performance. (**C**) Calibration curve of nomogram; the closer the bias-corrected line was to the ideal line, the more predictive accuracy of the nomogram model was (Brier value = 0.163).

4. Discussion

GSTs develop from the Cajal mesenchymal cells or their common stem cells and are potentially malignant. They could occur at any age but mainly in middle-aged and seniors, exhibiting similar incidence in men and women [14], which agrees with our study.

In this study, the tumor size in the high-risk group was larger than the other two groups. Using the low-risk group as a reference, the multivariable analysis indicated that the longest diameter was the independent risk factor for high-risk GSTs. Previous studies [8,15] indicate a correlation between larger tumor size and a worse patient prognosis, which is consistent with our results. The characteristics of tumor rapid growth are indicative of malignant tumors. The tumor size in the low-risk group was similar to that of the moderate-risk group. Therefore, tumor size could not be used to differentiate low- from moderate-risk GSTs.

In the present study, we found that the incidence of ulceration increased with increasing risk classification, with significant differences between different groups. Meanwhile, ulceration was the independent risk factor for high-risk GSTs. We speculated that GSTs with a higher risk classification were probably more invasive and easily destroyed gastric mucosa. The incidence of feeding artery and vascular-like enhancement in the high-risk group was about three times higher than in the other two groups. Research by Xu et al. [16] also showed that feeding artery and vascular-like enhancement were more likely to occur in high-risk GSTs. Neovascularization is an essential step in tumor metastasis and the invasion of malignant tumors. A relatively larger tumor in the high-risk group likely accounted for this result because larger tumors would need more neovascularization to provide nutrition for tumor growth.

The necrosis rate (92.9%) of tumors in the high-risk group was significantly higher than that in the low- and moderate-risk groups. Grazzini et al. [11] also found that the necrosis rate of the tumor was 99% in the high-risk group. High-risk tumors grew faster and disproportionately to the relatively slow growth rate of neovascularization, leading to ischemic necrosis. Previous studies [16,17] reported that the degree of enhancement in the venous phase reduced as the risk stratification increased, which is in agreement with the results of the present study. A possible explanation for this outcome is that the growth rate of neovascularization in the moderate- and high-risk groups was lower than that of the tumor, resulting in relatively few contrast agents entering the tumor. In addition, the high-risk tumor is accessible to myxoid change and ischemic necrosis, which resulted in a reduced CT value in the venous phase. A previous study by Jumniensuk et al. [18] showed that GISTs with myxoid change likely exhibit recurrence and metastasis.

The growth patterns of the high-risk lesions were mainly mixed and exophytic patterns and were rarely endophytic, which is consistent with our results [8,19]. Most GSTs in the high-risk group were of irregular morphology (78.6%). On the contrary, GSTs with regular morphology were seen more often in the low- and moderate-risk groups. Neill et al. [20] also showed that irregular morphology or lobulation was an independent risk factor for GST recurrence and metastasis, which is consistent with our study. A probable explanation for this result is that tumor cell heterogeneity increases concomitantly with increasing tumor aggressiveness, contributing to a faster growth rate in more aggressive tumor parts. Fat-positive signs around the lesion were more common in the high-risk group than in the other groups. Kim et al. [21] also found that GSTs with mesenteric fat infiltration were likely highly risky. This clinical outcome might be explained by the high ability of highly aggressive tumors to infiltrate the surrounding tissue. Alternatively, a larger tumor volume in the high-risk group might compress the surrounding blood vessels more easily, resulting in adipose tissue edema.

To the best of our knowledge, there are few nomogram models of CT features for predicting risk stratification for GSTs. In the present study, using the low-risk group as a reference, multivariate logistic regression analysis showed that the location, ulceration, longest diameter, and vascular-like enhancement were independent risk factors of high-risk GSTs. With the moderate-risk group as a reference, the morphology, necrosis, and feeding artery were independent predictors of high-risk GSTs. The AUC obtained from the internal validation using the bootstrap method was basically consistent with the results of the predicted model, which indicates the stability of the model. Two nomogram models were both successfully established to predict the high-risk GSTs and had good prediction efficiency. A logistic regression equation can graphically be present with a nomogram. It is convenient and straightforward to utilize a nomogram for risk of GSTs prediction through a simple addition operation, with practical value for the clinical evaluation of patients.

There were some limitations in the study. First, a retrospective study led to a selection bias. A possible non-uniformity in the CT scanner and the parameters, injection speed, and doses of contrast agent might also have impacted the results. Second, the study failed to perform a three-dimensional reconstruction of the CT images because of a lack of thin-slice CT images, which might also have impacted the results.

5. Conclusions

In summary, GSTs can be classified as high risk and non-high risk with MSCT features, such as the longest diameter, tumor location, morphology, necrosis, ulceration, feeding artery, and vascular-like enhancement. The nomogram model can better distinguish the risk classification of GSTs before surgery.

Author Contributions: S.W.: concept, design, definition of intellectual content, literature search, clinical studies, experimental studies, data acquisition, data analysis, manuscript preparation. P.D.: literature search, clinical studies, data acquisition. G.S.: concept, design, manuscript review. M.Z.: concept, design, manuscript review. M.W.: concept, design, definition of intellectual content, manuscript editing, and manuscript review. All authors have read and agreed to the published version of the manuscript.

Funding: This work was supported by the Affiliated TCM Hospital of Southwest Medical University Union Youth Nursery project of Natural Science (grant number 2018XYLH-035).

Institutional Review Board Statement: The study was performed in accordance with the ethical standards as laid out in the 1964 Declaration of Helsinki and its later amendments or comparable ethical standards and approved by the Institutional Review Board (protocol code YJ-KY2019068 and date of approval 30 October 2019).

Informed Consent Statement: The requirement of written informed consent was waived, because this was a retrospective study.

Data Availability Statement: All the data were collected from the Institutional Picture Archiving and Communication System (The Affiliated TCM Hospital of Southwest Medical University and Zhongshan Hospital, Fudan University).

Conflicts of Interest: The authors declare no conflict of interest.

Abbreviations

AFIP	Armed Forces Institute of Pathology
NIH	National Institutes of Health
GSTs	Gastric stromal tumors
GISTs	Gastrointestinal stromal tumors
MSCT	Multi-slice CT
AUC	Area under the receiver operating characteristic curve
TKI	Tyrosine kinase inhibitor
$\Delta CT_{arterial}$	CT value increment in arterial phase
ΔCT_{venous}	CT value increment in venous phase

References

1. Parab, T.M.; DeRogatis, M.J.; Boaz, A.M.; Grasso, S.A.; Issack, P.S.; Duarte, D.A.; Urayeneza, O.; Vahdat, S.; Qiao, J.-H.; Hinika, G.S. Gastrointestinal stromal tumors: A comprehensive review. *J. Gastrointest. Oncol.* **2019**, *10*, 144–154. [CrossRef]
2. Ao, W.; Cheng, G.; Lin, B.; Yang, R.; Liu, X.; Zhou, S.; Wang, W.; Fang, Z.; Tian, F.; Yang, G.; et al. A novel CT-based radiomic nomogram for predicting the recurrence and metastasis of gastric stromal tumors. *Am. J. Cancer Res.* **2021**, *11*, 3123–3134.

3. Chen, T.; Qiou, H.B.; Feng, X.Y.; Zhang, P.; Ye, L.Y.; Hu, Y.Y.; Liu, H.; Yu, J.; Tao, K.; Li, Y.; et al. Comparison of modified NIH and AFIP risk-stratification criteria for gastrointestinal stromal tumors:Amulticenter retrospective study. *Chin. J. Gastrointest. Surg.* **2017**, *20*, 845–851.
4. Chen, T.; Ye, L.-Y.; Feng, X.-Y.; Qiu, H.-B.; Zhang, P.; Luo, Y.-X.; Yuan, L.-Y.; Chen, X.-H.; Hu, Y.-F.; Liu, H.; et al. Performance of risk stratification systems for gastrointestinal stromal tumors: A multicenter study. *World J. Gastroenterol.* **2019**, *25*, 1238–1247. [CrossRef] [PubMed]
5. Belfiori, G.; Sartelli, M.; Cardinali, L.; Tranà, C.; Bracci, R.; Gesuita, R.; Marmorale, C. Risk stratification systems for surgically treated localized primary Gastrointestinal Stromal Tumors (GIST). Review of literature and comparison of the three prognostic criteria: MSKCC Nomogramm, NIH-Fletcher and AFIP-Miettinen. *Ann. Ital. Chir.* **2015**, *86*, 219–227. [PubMed]
6. Khoo, C.Y.; Chai, X.; Quek, R.; Teo, M.C.C.; Goh, B.K.P. Systematic review of current prognostication systems for primary gastrointestinal stromal tumors. *Eur. J. Surg. Oncol.* **2018**, *44*, 388–394. [CrossRef]
7. Miettinen, M.; Lasota, J. Gastrointestinal stromal tumors: Pathology and prognosis at different sites. *Semin. Diagn. Pathol.* **2006**, *23*, 70–83. [CrossRef]
8. Chen, T.; Xu, L.; Dong, X.; Li, Y.; Yu, J.; Xiong, W.; Li, G. The roles of CT and EUS in the preoperative evaluation of gastric gastrointestinal stromal tumors larger than 2 cm. *Eur. Radiol.* **2019**, *29*, 2481–2489. [CrossRef]
9. Maldonado, F.J.; Sheedy, S.P.; Iyer, V.R.; Hansel, S.L.; Bruining, D.H.; McCollough, C.H.; Harmsen, W.S.; Barlow, J.M.; Fletcher, J.G. Reproducible imaging features of biologically aggressive gastrointestinal stromal tumors of the small bowel. *Abdom. Radiol.* **2018**, *43*, 1567–1574. [CrossRef] [PubMed]
10. Iannicelli, E.; Carbonetti, F.; Federici, G.F.; Martini, I.; Caterino, S.; Pilozzi, E.; Panzuto, F.; Briani, C.; David, V. Evaluation of the Relationships Between Computed Tomography Features, Pathological Findings, and Prognostic Risk Assessment in Gastrointestinal Stromal Tumors. *J. Comput. Assist. Tomogr.* **2017**, *41*, 271–278. [CrossRef] [PubMed]
11. Grazzini, G.; Guerri, S.; Cozzi, D.; Danti, G.; Gasperoni, S.; Pradella, S.; Miele, V. Gastrointestinal stromal tumors: Relationship between preoperative CT features and pathologic risk stratification. *Tumori* **2021**, *107*, 556–563. [CrossRef]
12. Liu, M.; Liu, L.H.; Jin, E. Gastric sub-epithelial tumors: Identification of gastrointestinal stromal tumors using CT with a practical scoring method. *Gastric Cancer* **2019**, *22*, 769–777. [CrossRef] [PubMed]
13. Inoue, A.; Ota, S.; Nitta, N.; Murata, K.; Shimizu, T.; Sonoda, H.; Tani, M.; Ban, H.; Inatomi, O.; Ando, A.; et al. Difference of computed tomographic characteristic findings between gastric and intestinal gastrointestinal stromal tumors. *Jpn. J. Radiol.* **2020**, *38*, 771–781. [CrossRef]
14. Joensuu, H.; Hohenberger, P.; Corless, C.L. Gastrointestinal stromal tumour. *Lancet* **2013**, *382*, 973–983. [CrossRef]
15. Zhou, C.; Duan, X.H.; Zhang, X.; Hu, H.J.; Wang, D.; Shen, J. Predictive features of CT for risk stratifications in patients with primary gastrointestinal stromal tumour. *Eur. Radiol.* **2016**, *26*, 3086–3093. [CrossRef] [PubMed]
16. Xu, J.; Zhou, J.; Wang, X.; Fan, S.; Huang, X.; Xie, X.; Yu, R. A multi-class scoring system based on CT features for preoperative prediction in gastric gastrointestinal stromal tumors. *Am. J. Cancer Res.* **2020**, *10*, 3867–3881.
17. Su, Q.; Wang, Q.; Zhang, H.; Yu, D.; Wang, Y.; Liu, Z.; Zhang, X. Computed tomography findings of small bowel gastrointestinal stromal tumors with different histologic risks of progression. *Abdom. Radiol.* **2018**, *43*, 2651–2658. [CrossRef]
18. Jumniensuk, C.; Charoenpitakchai, M. Gastrointestinal stromal tumor: Clinicopathological characteristics and pathologic prognostic analysis. *World J. Surg. Oncol.* **2018**, *16*, 231. [CrossRef] [PubMed]
19. Li, H.; Ren, G.; Cai, R.; Chen, L.; Wu, X.R.; Zhao, J.X. A correlation research of Ki67 index, CT features, and risk stratification in gastrointestinal stromal tumor. *Cancer Med.* **2018**, *7*, 4467–4474. [CrossRef]
20. Neill, A.C.; Shinagare, A.B.; Kurra, V.; Tirumani, S.H.; Jagannathan, J.P.; Baheti, A.D.; Hornick, J.L.; George, S.; Ramaiya, N.H. Assessment of metastatic risk of gastric GIST based on treatment-naïve CT features. *Eur. J. Surg. Oncol.* **2016**, *42*, 1222–1228. [CrossRef] [PubMed]
21. Kim, H.C.; Lee, J.M.; Kim, K.W.; Park, S.H.; Kim, S.H.; Lee, J.Y.; Han, J.K.; Choi, B.I. Gastrointestinal stromal tumors of the stomach: CT findings and prediction of malignancy. *Am. J. Roentgenol.* **2004**, *183*, 893–898. [CrossRef] [PubMed]

Disclaimer/Publisher's Note: The statements, opinions and data contained in all publications are solely those of the individual author(s) and contributor(s) and not of MDPI and/or the editor(s). MDPI and/or the editor(s) disclaim responsibility for any injury to people or property resulting from any ideas, methods, instructions or products referred to in the content.

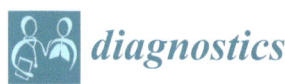

Article

Dynamic Contrast-Enhanced Magnetic Resonance Imaging for Measuring Perfusion in Pancreatic Ductal Adenocarcinoma and Different Tumor Grade: A Preliminary Single Center Study

Inga Zaborienė [1,*], Vestina Strakšytė [1], Povilas Ignatavičius [2], Giedrius Barauskas [2], Rūta Dambrauskienė [3] and Kristina Žvinienė [1]

1 Department of Radiology, Lithuanian University of Health Sciences, LT-50161 Kaunas, Lithuania
2 Department of Surgery, Lithuanian University of Health Sciences, LT-50161 Kaunas, Lithuania
3 Department of Oncology and Hematology, Lithuanian University of Health Sciences, LT-50161 Kaunas, Lithuania
* Correspondence: inga.zaboriene@lsmu.lt; Tel.: +370-326154

Abstract: Background: Dynamic contrast-enhanced magnetic resonance imaging is a noninvasive imaging modality that can supply information regarding the tumor anatomy and physiology. The aim of the study was to analyze DCE-MRI perfusion parameters in normal pancreatic parenchymal tissue and PDAC and to evaluate the efficacy of this diagnostic modality in determining the tumor grade. Methods: A single-center retrospective study was performed. A total of 28 patients with histologically proven PDAC underwent DCE-MRI; the control group enrolled 14 patients with normal pancreatic parenchymal tissue; the radiological findings were compared with histopathological data. The study patients were further grouped according to the differentiation grade (G value): well- and moderately differentiated and poorly differentiated PDAC. Results: The median values of K^{trans}, k_{ep} and iAUC were calculated lower in PDAC compared with the normal pancreatic parenchymal tissue ($p < 0.05$). The mean value of Ve was higher in PDAC, compared with the normal pancreatic tissue ($p < 0.05$). K^{trans}, k_{ep} and iAUC were lower in poorly differentiated PDAC, whereas Ve showed no differences between groups. Conclusions: Ve and iAUC DCE-MRI perfusion parameters are important as independent diagnostic criteria predicting the probability of PDAC; the Ktrans and iAUC DCE-MRI perfusion parameters may serve as effective independent prognosticators preoperatively identifying poorly differentiated PDAC.

Keywords: pancreatic adenocarcinoma; tumor grade; dynamic contrast-enhanced MRI

Citation: Zaborienė, I.; Strakšytė, V.; Ignatavičius, P.; Barauskas, G.; Dambrauskienė, R.; Žvinienė, K. Dynamic Contrast-Enhanced Magnetic Resonance Imaging for Measuring Perfusion in Pancreatic Ductal Adenocarcinoma and Different Tumor Grade: A Preliminary Single Center Study. *Diagnostics* **2023**, *13*, 521. https://doi.org/10.3390/diagnostics13030521

Academic Editors: Francescamaria Donati and Piero Boraschi

Received: 7 December 2022
Revised: 18 January 2023
Accepted: 24 January 2023
Published: 31 January 2023

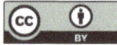

Copyright: © 2023 by the authors. Licensee MDPI, Basel, Switzerland. This article is an open access article distributed under the terms and conditions of the Creative Commons Attribution (CC BY) license (https://creativecommons.org/licenses/by/4.0/).

1. Introduction

Pathological grading of pancreatic ductal adenocarcinoma (PDAC) might be obtained preoperatively by fine needle biopsy (FNB). This way, some patients with a disease unsuitable for upfront surgery might be identified, even if considered resectable by high-quality imaging. However, FNB is associated with various complications and might postpone the treatment. Endoscopic ultrasonography-guided tissue acquisition (EUS-TA) represents the criterion standard for the diagnostic evaluation of pancreatic masses. However, the relatively high rate of false negatives still represents a common pitfall associated with this procedure [1]. If a poorly differentiated or anaplastic tumor is histologically confirmed, therapy might be started with a non-surgical approach. After neoadjuvant therapy, patients could undergo surgical exploration if the disease remains stable or in cases of downstaging. Therefore, noninvasive identification of tumor grade would be preferred in terms of improved patient selection. This is an interesting topic, as grading of the tumor is a significant prognostic factor in patients suffering from PDAC. Identifying new biomarkers is preferred to move toward an individual treatment of the patient, while unnecessary treatment could be prevented in others. Radiologists' knowledge of PDAC is based on morphological changes when performing imaging. Recently, minimal progress has been made in understanding the pathophysiology of PDAC via different imaging modalities, one of which is perfusion computed tomography (CT) [2–4].

Without the hazard of ionizing radiation, dynamic contrast-enhanced magnetic resonance imaging (DCE-MRI) is a noninvasive imaging modality that can provide anatomical and physiological information of the tumor [5–10]. Preliminary studies supported the importance of magnetic resonance (MR) perfusion in the evaluation of abdominal organs [5,11–14]. The aim of the study was to analyze DCE-MRI perfusion parameters in normal pancreatic parenchymal tissue and PDAC and to estimate the efficacy of this diagnostic modality in determining the tumor grade.

2. Materials and Methods

We performed a retrospective single-center study in the Department of Radiology at the Hospital of Lithuanian University of Health Sciences Kaunas Clinics. The Regional Biomedical Research Ethics Committee approved the study (protocol No. BE-2-22). All the patients gave informed consent. Forty-four (44) patients with histologically proven PDAC underwent DCE-MRI from September 2019 to January 2021. The inclusion criteria were as follows: histologically proven pancreatic head PDAC; tumor ≥ 2.0 cm in size; estimated glomerular filtration rate (eGFR) > 30 mL/min; absence of contraindications to MR examination. We included 28 subjects with pancreatic head PDAC. Perfusion qualitative and quantitative assessments were obtained in all cases. We excluded 16 patients who could not complete the examination because of pain or disagreed to participate in the study. The inclusion criteria for the control group patients were as follows: no history of abdominal disorders, no significant medical history of diabetes or other pancreatic disorders, no cystic or benign liver and cystic kidney lesions. In total, 14 patients with non-tumorous pancreatic tissue were included as controls. MRI was performed using a 1.5T MR system (Siemens Magnetom Avanto, Siemens Healthineers, Erlangen, Germany) in the supine position. Patients fasted for 6 to 8 h before the DCE-MRI scan. All DCE-MRI examinations were performed using an injection of 0.2 mL/kg Gd-based contrast media (Gadovist®, Bayer AG, Leverkusen, Germany), at a rate of 3.0 mL/s, followed by 20 mL of saline at the same injection rate. All the patients were instructed to breathe slowly during the examination. Two observers with 10 and 20 years of experience interpreting pancreatic MR images reviewed the original MR imaging data. A DCE-MRI postprocessing software program (Tissue 4D; Siemens Magnetom Avanto, Siemens Healthineers, Erlangen, Germany) was used to obtain both a time–signal–intensity curve (TSIC) and to generate perfusion maps for each healthy pancreatic parenchyma, tumor, and different tumor grade. Perfusion maps of the volume transfer coefficient (Ktrans), extracellular extravascular volume fraction (Ve), rate constant (K_{ep}), and initial area under the concentration curve in 60 s (iAUC) were generated. T1 mapping was computed from the T1-weighted acquisitions with different flip angles. The region of interest (ROI) was drawn on the abdominal aorta to obtain an arterial input function. The other three ROIs in the head of the pancreas were selected. The area of each ROI was 20 to 40 mm^2. The mean perfusion values of all the ROIs were calculated and used for further evaluation. The pancreatic duct, necrotic, or cystic areas of the tumor were avoided. The qualitative analysis was based on TSICs, which were classified based on their shape by two radiologists into different types. We selected types of curves from the study by Wanling Ma et al. as an example for further evaluation (Figure 1) [6].

The radiological findings were compared with histopathological data. Histopathological analysis was performed at the Department of Pathological Anatomy, Lithuanian University of Health Sciences. The study patients were further grouped according to the differentiation grade (G value): well- and moderately differentiated (G1 + G2) and poorly differentiated (G3) PDAC. Images of DCE-MRI of non-tumorous pancreatic tissue and PDAC are presented in Figures 2 and 3.

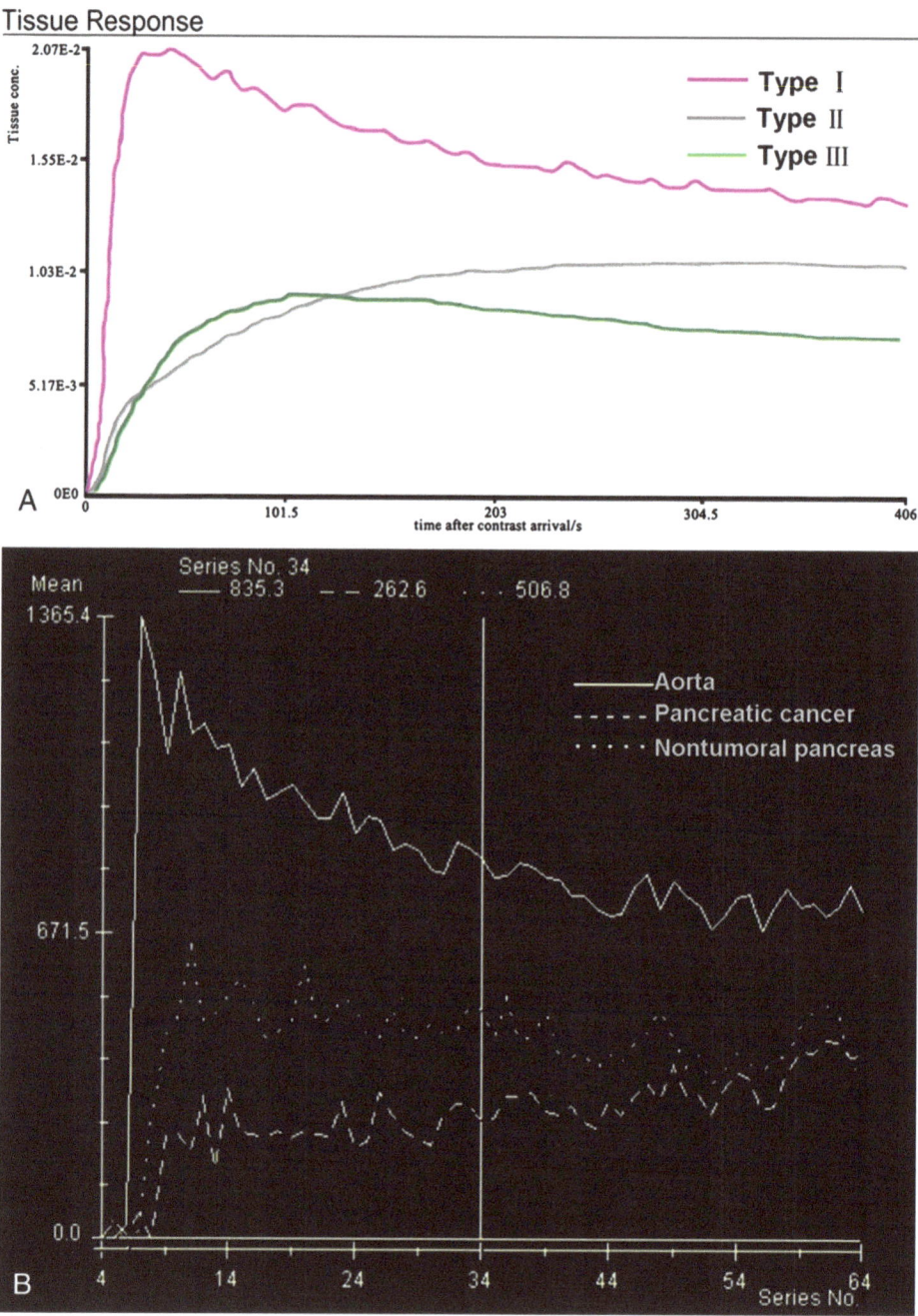

Figure 1. (**A**) SI-T curves of all nontumoral pancreatic tissue showed type I pattern enhancement. Pancreatic tumors showed type II or type III pattern enhancement; (**B**) Curve graph shows that pancreatic tumor enhances lesser than surrounding nontumoral pancreatic tissue. Time–signal–intensity curves selected for further data evaluation: type I, characterized by quick enhancement and quick washout; type II, with slow enhancement, which is followed by slow constant enhancement; type III, slow enhancement followed by slow washout [6].

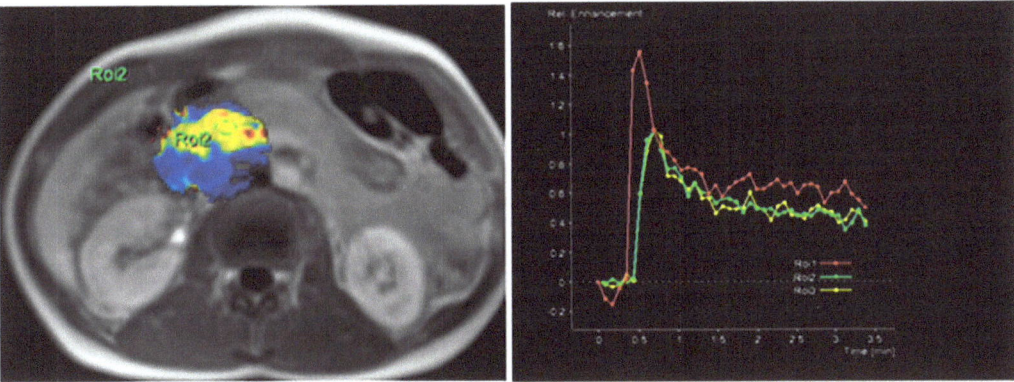

Figure 2. MRI perfusion images of non-tumorous pancreatic parenchymal tissue in the head of the pancreas with TSIC—Type I (characterized by fast enhancement and fast washout). Type I pattern enhancement was found in all tissues from control group patients.

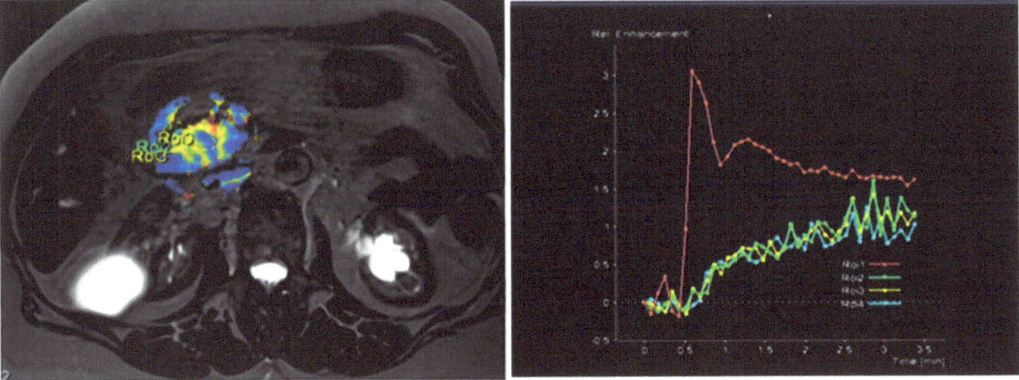

Figure 3. MRI perfusion images of G3 tumor in the head of the pancreas with TSIC—type II (slow enhancement and then continuous enhancement). The curve graph shows that pancreatic tumor enhances to a lesser extent than surrounding nontumoral pancreatic tissue. Most poorly differentiated (G3) tumors showed Type II pattern enhancement.

Statistical Analysis

We used the Kolmogorov–Smirnov and the Shapiro–Wilk tests to check data normality. Normally distributed data were expressed as mean values (SD—standard deviation), and abnormal distributed as medians. The Student's *t*-test and Mann–Whitney U-test were used for normally and non-normally distributed data, respectively. We used discriminant function analysis to determine the differences between groups and between well-/moderately and poorly differentiated PDAC.

We calculated cut-off points for best specificity, sensitivity, and accuracy, positive (PPV) and negative predictive values (NPV).

Statistical analysis was performed using ©SPSS for Windows 23.0 ™ software and ©Microsoft Excel 16™. Statistical significance was considered at *p*-value less than or equal to 0.05.

3. Results

3.1. General Patient's Characteristics

Radiological and histopathological data of 42 subjects were included. The control group enrolled 14 patients with normal pancreatic parenchymal tissue (Table 1). These patients underwent MRI due to other indications (IPMN—four subjects, benign liver lesions—seven subjects, cystic kidney lesions—three subjects). The mean age of patients was 60.64 (15.24) in this group. No difference in age or gender distribution between these groups was identified ($p = 0.209$ and $p = 0.306$, respectively, Table 1).

Table 1. The distribution between gender of PDAC and control group.

	Non-Tumorous Pancreatic Tissue ($n = 14$) Mean (SD) or N (%)	PDAC ($n = 28$) Mean (SD) or N (%)	p Value
Age	60.64 (15.24)	66.46 (15.24)	=0.209
Female	2 (14.3%)	8 (28.6%)	=0.306
Male	12 (85.7%)	20 (71.4%)	=0.306
Total	14 (100%)	28 (100%)	

Values are mean (standard deviation (SD)).

3.2. Normal Pancreatic Parenchyma vs. Pancreatic Ductal Adenocarcinoma (PDAC)

The median K^{trans}, k_{ep}, and iAUC values and the mean value (SD) of V_e for the normal pancreatic parenchymal tissue were 0.178 (min^{-1}), 0.861 (min^{-1}), 16.457 (mmol/s), and 0.196 (0.114), respectively. The median values of K^{trans}, k_{ep}, and Iauc for PDAC patients were 0.106 (min^{-1}), 0.406 (min^{-1}), and 9.045 (mmol/s), respectively; the mean value (SD) of V_e for PDAC was 0.313 (0.169).

The median values of K^{trans}, k_{ep}, and iAUC were calculated to be lower in PDAC compared with the normal pancreatic parenchymal tissue ($p < 0.05$). The mean value of Ve was higher in PDAC, compared with the normal pancreatic parenchymal tissue ($p < 0.05$). The data are presented in Table 2.

Table 2. DCE-MRI perfusion parameters in normal pancreatic parenchymal tissue and PDAC.

Parameters	Non-Tumorous Pancreatic Tissue Mean (SD) or Median * (q1–q3) Value	PDAC Mean (SD) or Median * (q1–q3) Value	p Value
K^{trans} * (min^{-1})	0.178 (0.0295–0.538)	0.106 (0.0298–0.538)	=0.033
k_{ep} * (min^{-1})	0.861 (0.519–3.035)	0.406 (0.199–1.054)	=0.006
V_e	0.196 (0.114)	0.313 (0.169)	=0.012
iAUC * (mmol/s)	16.457 (11.23–29.613)	9.045 (3.309–15.452)	=0.005

* Median in abnormal distribution of parameters. Abbreviations: SD—standard deviation; K^{trans}—volume transfer coefficient; Ve—extracellular extravascular volume fraction; K_{ep}—rate constant; iAUC—initial area under the concentration curve in 60 s.

We used the discriminant function analysis to determine differences between PDAC and the normal pancreatic parenchyma. All calculated MRI perfusion variables (Ktrans, Kep, Ve, and iAUC) were included to identify the most important ones. Cut-off points for all MRI perfusion parameters with their predictive values are presented in Table 3.

Table 3. Average of Ktrans, Kep, Ve, and iAUC in the presence of PDAC.

PDAC	K^{trans}	k_{ep}	V_e	iAUC
AUC	0.704	0.765	0.689	0.768
Cut-off point	<0.19	≤0.4	≥0.25	<15.75
Sensitivity	92.9	50.0	53.6	64.3
Specificity.	50.0	92.9	92.9	82.8
PPV	78.8	93.3	93.8	82.8
NPV	77.8	48.1	50.0	64.3

Abbreviations: PPV—positive predictive value; NPV—negative predictive value; ROC—receiver operating characteristic; K^{trans}—volume transfer coefficient; Ve—extracellular extravascular volume fraction; K_{ep}—rate constant; iAUC—initial area under the concentration curve in 60 s.

3.3. PDAC Independent Diagnostic Criteria

The logistic regression model was used to disclose the independent diagnostic MRI perfusion criteria of PDAC. Four main parameters—Ktrans, Kep, Ve, and iAUC—were included in the stepwise analysis to determine the most significant ones (Table 4 and Figure 4), disclosing iAUC and Ve as the most important independent discriminators.

Table 4. Logistic regression for disclosing the probability occurrence of PDAC.

	B	S.E.	*p* Value	Exp (B)	95% C.I. for EXP (B) Lower	95% C.I. for EXP (B) Upper
iAUC (mmol/s)	3.068	1.145	0.007	21.5	2.28	202.778
V_e	3.061	1.209	0.011	21.354	1.997	228.318

Abbreviations: Ve—extracellular extravascular volume fraction; iAUC—initial area under the concentration curve in 60 s.

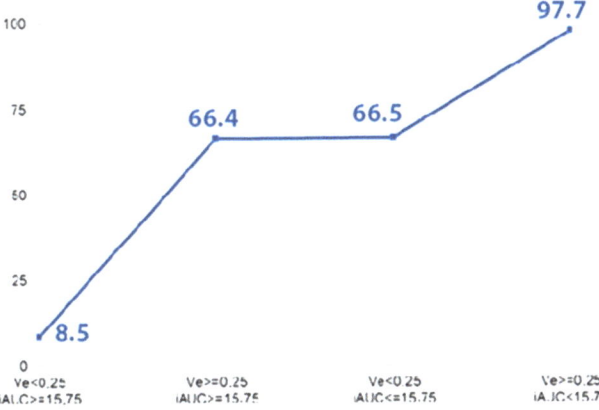

Figure 4. Disclosed probability for the PDAC. The graph shows the prognosticated probability of PDAC (%) (determined by logistic regression analysis) if the Ve and iAUC parameters or both of them exceed the defined cut-off value (Ve > 0.25, iAUC < 15.75). If both parameters are less than the determined cut-off point, the prognosticated probability for the presence of PDAC is 8.5%; if both values achieve the defined cut-off point, the estimated probability for the existence of PDAC is 97.7%.

3.4. Well-/Moderately Differentiated (G1/G2) PDAC vs. Poorly Differentiated (G3) PDAC

There were 10 (35.7%) subjects with well-/moderately (G1 + G2), and 18 (64.3%) with poorly differentiated (G3) tumors. Analysis revealed that K^{trans}, k_{ep}, and iAUC were lower in poorly differentiated PDAC, whereas Ve showed no differences in G1 + G2 and G3 PDAC. The distribution between perfusion parameters is presented in Table 5.

Table 5. DCE-MRI perfusion parameters in different grades of PDAC.

Parameters	Mean (SD) or Median * (q1–q3) Value (G1 + G2), (n = 10)	Mean (SD) or Median * (q1–q3) Value (G3), (n = 18)	p Value
K^{trans} * (min^{-1})	0.175 (0.132–0,182)	0.059 (0.034–0.106)	=0.020
k_{ep} * (min^{-1})	0.521 (0.369–1.091)	0.357 (0.165–0.623)	<0.001
V_e	0.335 (0.139)	0.300 (0.185)	=0.254
iAUC * (mmol/s)	15.600 (14.461–17.598)	5.202 (1.771–10.712)	=0.035

* Median in abnormal distribution of parameters; abbreviations: SD—standard deviation; K^{trans}—volume transfer coefficient; Ve—extracellular extravascular volume fraction; K_{ep}—rate constant; iAUC—initial area under the concentration curve in 60 s.

We performed discriminant function analysis to identify differences between well-/moderately and poorly differentiated PDAC. Four main MRI perfusion variables (Ktrans, Kep, Ve, and iAUC) were included to establish the most important ones.

The K^{trans} value less than 0.109 was concomitant to the presence of G3 PDAC with an 83.3% sensitivity and 90% specificity (AUC = 0.994); k_{ep} less than 0.344 was concomitant to the presence of PDAC with a 50% sensitivity and 90% specificity (AUC = 0.65); a higher than 0.272 Ve value was connected to the presence of G3 PDAC with a sensitivity of 44% and specificity of 30% (AUC = 0.428); an iAUC value less than 12.592 was concomitant to the presence of G3 PDAC with an 83.3% sensitivity and 90% specificity (AUC = 0.872). Cut-off points for all MRI perfusion parameters are presented in Table 6.

Table 6. Analysis of the poorly differentiated (G3) PDAC.

Poorly Differentiated (G3) PDAC	K^{trans}	k_{ep}	V_e	iAUC
AUC	0.994	0.65	0.428	0.872
Cut-off point	≤0.109	≤0.344	≥0.272	≤12.592
Sensitivity	83.3	50	44	83.3
Specificity.	90	90	30	90
PPV	94	90	53	94
NPV	75	50	23	75

Abbreviations: PPV—positive predictive value; NPV—negative predictive value; ROC—receiver operating characteristic; K^{trans}—volume transfer coefficient; Ve—extracellular extravascular volume fraction; K_{ep}—rate constant; iAUC—initial area under the concentration curve in 60 s.

3.5. Independent Diagnostic Criteria of Poorly Differentiated (G3) PDAC

The logistic regression model was chosen to disclose the independent diagnostic MRI perfusion criteria of poorly differentiated PDAC. Four main parameters—Ktrans, Kep, Ve, and iAUC—were included in the stepwise analysis to determine which of them were most important (Table 7 and Figure 5), identifying Ktrans and iAUC as significant independent discriminators.

Table 7. Logistic regression for estimating the probability occurrence of poorly differentiated (G3) PDAC.

	B	S.E.	p Value	Exp (B)	95% C.I. for EXP (B) Lower	95% C.I. for EXP (B) Upper
Ktrans	3.807	1.229	0.002	45	4.044	500.693
iAUC	3.281	1.462	0.025	26.599	1.516	466.594

Abbreviations: Ktrans—volume transfer coefficient; iAUC—initial area under the concentration curve in 60 s.

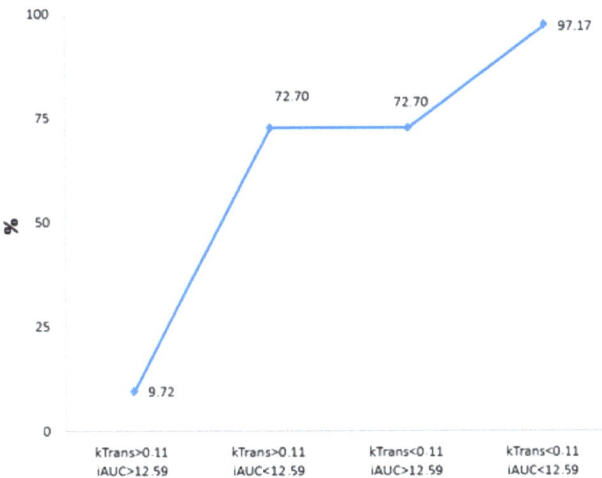

Figure 5. Calculated probability for the presence of poorly differentiated PDAC. The graph shows the prognosticated probability of G3 PDAC (%) if the Ktrans and iAUC parameters or both of them exceed the defined cut-off value (Ktrans < 0.11, iAUC < 12.59). If both parameters are less than the determined cut-off point, the prognosticated probability for the presence of G3 PDAC is 9.72%; if both values exceed the defined cut-off point, the estimated probability for the existence of PDAC is 97.17%.

4. Discussion

PDAC is a very heterogeneous tumor type; therefore, patients diagnosed with the same tumor stage often have markedly different clinical prognoses [15–17]. Diffusion-weighted imaging (DWI) with the apparent diffusion coefficient (ADC) predicts tumor grade and prognosis of various abdominal neoplasms, such as pancreatic neuroendocrine tumor, gastrointestinal tumors (GIST), rectal cancer, and hepatocellular carcinoma (HCC) [12,18–21].

The present study shows the significance of setting the role and value of the DCE-MRI analysis in diagnosing PDAC and evaluating the tumor grade without any ionizing radiation exposure for the patient. It is a noninvasive technique that can provide anatomical and physiological information about the tumor. DCE-MRI has been used to investigate microcirculation and microvasculature in different organs quantitatively. We analyzed the importance of MRI perfusion parameters in foreseeing PDAC and different tumor grades [4].

Another study of gallbladder cancer by Ji Hye Min et al. found the tumor ADC cut-off value to be an independent prognostic factor that ensures long-term disease-free survival (DFS) [16]. According to the literature, the differentiation grade of the tumor is a significant outcome prognosticator in PDAC patients [22]. Patients with low-grade (well-differentiated) PDAC have better survival rates than those with poorly differentiated PDAC [15,23–26]. Shibata K et al. reported that undifferentiated PDAC strongly predicts poor outcomes since it is related to hepatic metastases [15]. Tumor size and lymph node metastases influence survival less than tumor grade. Therefore, a noninvasive imaging modality able to predict a differentiation grade of PDAC before surgery would help to identify the aggressive prognosis of G3 tumors. This can allow optimizing therapeutic strategies and improve survival. Wasif N et al. in their study proposed the ability to include the tumor grade in PDAC staging—a novel TNMG staging system [10].

We agree with Facciorusso A et al., who recently confirmed contrast-enhanced harmonic endoscopic ultrasound (CH-EUS) as a helpful tool to identify the ideal target area for EUS-FNA avoiding the anechoic areas and vessels inside the tumor [27]. They also reported EUS-guided TA as a valuable tool in the diagnostic algorithm of pancreatic masses;

however, this method is still impaired by the relatively high rate of false negative results, mainly due to inadequate tissue samples. Most of these false negative cases are related to the presence of fibrosis and necrosis inside the tumor, thus usually requiring several needle passes to achieve adequate samples. Contrast enhancement was found to be able to properly characterize the areas of necrosis as well as the vessels. Therefore, this tool might help to identify the target area for FNA, thus decreasing the rate of false negative results by avoiding the areas rich in blood, necrosis, and fibrosis. Still, this method remains invasive.

Noninvasive preoperative identification of poorly differentiated PDAC may potentially define patients who may benefit from preoperative biopsy followed by neoadjuvant therapy for morphologically confirmed poorly differentiated PDAC or who may be enrolled in further clinical trials. In this way, patients might be eligible for individualized treatment.

In our previous study, we reported the significance of perfusion CT and MRI DWI in estimating poorly differentiated PDAC [13]. Still, one of the most significant disadvantages of perfusion CT remains a high radiation dose.

The qualitative assessment based on the signal intensity per time showed similar results to other studies reported in the literature [7,28–31]. All patients with non-tumorous pancreatic tissue showed a TSIC-shape 1. All PDAC patients showed a TSIC-shape 2, characterized by slow progressive enhancement. TSIC did not differ between different tumor grades because of overlap in the imaging features. The perfusion analysis showed a difference between Ktrans, Ve, Kep, and iAUC values obtained in non-tumorous pancreatic tissue, PDAC, and different tumor grade.

The K^{trans}, k_{ep}, and iAUC values of PDAC (0.106 min^{-1}, 0.406 min^{-1}, and 9.045 mmol/s, respectively) were lower than those of non-tumorous pancreatic tissue (0.178 min^{-1}, 0.861 min^{-1}, and 16.457 mmol/s, respectively). Moreover, all these perfusion values were significantly lower in G3 PDAC (0.059 min^{-1}, 0.357 min^{-1}, and 5.202 mmol/s, respectively). The Ktrans and Kep values reflect blood flow; thus, the described results agreed with the post-contrast behavior of the PDAC. According to Jin Xu et al., PDAC with poor blood supply had lower blood volume and blood flow when compared with normal pancreatic parenchyma. Therefore, more connective tissue and fibrous tissue proliferation in PDAC leads to the higher vascular pressure of EES, which further reduces the value of K^{trans} [32].

Jae Hyun Kim et al. [8] in their study also reported these values to be significantly lower in PDAC (0.042 min^{-1}, 0.761 min^{-1}, and 2.841 mmol/s) when compared with non-tumorous pancreatic tissue (0.387 min^{-1}, 6.376 min^{-1}, and 7.156 mmol/s). The authors assumed that these findings are predictable in regions where permeability is high compared with blood flow (in PDAC), and that Ktrans represents tissue blood flow as well as iAUC [8]. Significantly low Ktrans and iAUC values of PDAC correspond with the fact that pancreatic cancer is a hypovascular tumor [8]. Further, our results coincide with the results of pancreatic perfusion CT. We strongly believe that MRI perfusion parameters reflect the vascular physiology of solid hypovascular pancreatic tumors similar to perfusion CT parameters [2,13,32].

We also found a significant difference of Ktrans, Kep, and iAUC values between well-/moderately (G1/2) and poorly differentiated (G3) PDAC (0.175 min^{-1}, 0.521 min^{-1}, and 15.6 mmol/s and 0.059 min^{-1}, 0.357 min^{-1}, and 5.202 mmol/s respectively). These results are similar to the CT perfusion parameters calculated in our previous studies [2,13]. Ktrans and iAUC perfusion parameters were also significant independent discriminators for G3 PDAC. One of the strongest parts of our study is that none of the previously mentioned studies evaluated any MRI perfusion parameters for estimating poorly differentiated tumors. Only Wanling Ma reported some data about perfusion parameters and correlation with fibrotic tissue [6]. He found a negative correlation between K^{trans} of PDAC and fibrosis content and positive correlation of fibrosis to Ve. Yao X et al. also found statistically different values of K^{trans} between normal pancreatic tissue and PDAC. Calculations of perfusion parameters between different tumor grades were also not included [32].

Our study showed that there were significant differences in MRI perfusion parameters between non-tumorous pancreatic tissue and PDAC, as well as different tumor grades.

The differentiation between G1/2 and G3 PDAC during imaging is impossible. This confusion may lead to surgical treatment of G3 disease. Therefore, remarkably different perfusion parameters may provide helpful information for decision making. Our data demonstrate the potential role of DCE-MRI in the preoperative detection of high-grade tumors. Furthermore, the defined cut-off values of MRI perfusion parameters were found to be independent prognosticators for the presence of poorly differentiated PDAC.

If Ve and iAUC values exceeded the determined cut-off point, the estimated probability for the presence of PDAC reached almost 100% in this study. Therefore, estimated Ve and iAUC parameters may serve as promising independent diagnostic criteria predicting the probability of PDAC. Moreover, using the combination of Ktrans and iAUC values, the estimated probability for the presence of high-grade PDAC reached 97%.

Our study has some limitations. Firstly, a low number of patients were included in this retrospective study. Additionally, this was a single-center study performed with a specific MRI machine and software package for calculation of tissue perfusion parameters. To show the validity of our data, further standardized perfusion MRI protocols and multicenter studies are needed.

Finally, a control group of patients with a histologically proven diagnosis of chronic pancreatitis to evaluate the difference in DCE-MRI perfusion parameters would be of great value in establishing the reliability of DCE-MRI diagnosing PDAC.

5. Conclusions

- The estimated Ve and iAUC DCE-MRI perfusion parameters are important as independent diagnostic criteria predicting the probability of PDAC.
- If Ve and iAUC values are combined, the estimated probability for the presence of PDAC reaches almost 100%.
- The Ktrans and iAUC DCE-MRI perfusion parameters may be effective independent prognosticators preoperatively estimating poorly differentiated PDAC.
- If Ktrans and iAUC values are combined, the estimated probability for the presence of high-grade PDAC reaches 97%.

Author Contributions: Each named author has substantially contributed to conducting the underlying research and drafting this manuscript. Conception (constructing an idea or hypothesis for research)—G.B., K.Ž. and V.S.; design (planning methodology to reach the conclusions)—G.B., K.Ž. and P.I.; organizing and supervising the course of the article and taking responsibility—I.Z., V.S., R.D. and P.I.; materials and referred patients—K.Ž., R.D. and I.Z.; data collection and processing—I.Z.; analysis and interpretation—I.Z., G.B. and P.I.; literature review—I.Z., G.B. and V.S.; reviewing the article before submission for spelling and grammar and also for its intellectual content—G.B., V.S., K.Ž., R.D., I.Z. and P.I. All authors have read and agreed to the published version of the manuscript.

Funding: This research received no external funding.

Institutional Review Board Statement: The Regional Biomedical Research Ethics Committee approved the study, and all the patients gave their informed consent (study protocol No. BE-2-22, as of 13 May 2015).

Informed Consent Statement: Informed consent was obtained from all subjects involved in the study.

Data Availability Statement: Not applicable.

Conflicts of Interest: The authors declare no conflict of interest.

References

1. Gkolfakis, P.; Crinò, S.F.; Tziatzios, G.; Ramai, D.; Papaefthymiou, A.S.; Papanikolaou, I.; Triantafyllou, K.; Arvanitakis, M.; Lisotti, A.; Fusaroli, P.; et al. Comparative diagnostic performance of end-cutting fine-needle biopsy needles for EUS tissue sampling of solid pancreatic masses: A network meta-analysis. *Gastrointest. Endosc.* **2022**, *95*, 6. [CrossRef]
2. Zaborienė, I.; Barauskas, G.; Gulbinas, A.; Ignatavičius, P.; Lukoševičius, S.; Žvinienė, K. Dynamic perfusion CT—A promising tool to diagnose pancreatic ductal adenocarcinoma. *Open Med.* **2021**, *16*, 284–292. [CrossRef]

3. Yadav, A.K.; Sharma, R.; Kandasamy, D.; Pradhan, R.K.; Garg, P.K.; Bhalla, A.S.; Gamanagatti, S.; Srivastava, D.N.; Upadhyay, P.S.A.D. Perfusion CT—Can it resolve the pancreatic carcinoma versus mass forming chronic pancreatitis conundrum? *Pancreatology* **2016**, *16*, 979–987. [CrossRef]
4. Wang, L.; Zhu, H.Y.; Tian, J.M.; Huang, S.D.; Kong, L.S.; Lu, J.P. Magnetic resonance imaging in determination of myocardial ischemia and viability: Comparison with positron emission tomography and single-photon emission computed tomography in a porcine model. *Acta Radiol.* **2007**, *48*, 500–507. [CrossRef]
5. Kandel, S.; Kloeters, C.; Meyer, H.; Hein, P.; Hilbig, A.; Rogalla, P. Whole—organ perfusion of the pancreas using dynamic volume CT in patients with primary pancreas carcinoma: Acquisition technique, post-processing and initial results. *Eur. Radiol.* **2009**, *19*, 2641–2646. [CrossRef]
6. Ma, W.; Li, N.; Zhao, W.; Ren, J.; Wei, M.; Yang, Y.; Wang, Y.; Fu, X.; Zhang, Z.; Larson, A.C.; et al. Apparent Diffusion Coefficient and Dynamic Contrast-Enhanced Magnetic Resonance Imaging in Pancreatic Cancer: Characteristics and Correlation with Histopathologic Parameters. *Comput. Assist. Tomogr.* **2016**, *40*, 709–716. [CrossRef]
7. Huh, J.; Choi, Y.; Woo, D.C.; Seo, N.; Kim, B.; Lee, C.K.; Kim, I.S.; Nickel, D. Feasibility of test-bolus DCE-MRI using CAIPIRINHA-VIBE for the evaluation of pancreatic malignancies. *Eur. Radiol.* **2016**, *26*, 3949–3956. [CrossRef]
8. Kim, J.H.; Lee, J.M.; Park, J.H.; Kim, S.C.; Joo, I.; Han, J.K.; Choi, B.I. Solid pancreatic lesions: Characterization by using timing bolus dynamic contrast-enhanced MR imaging assessment—A preliminary study. *Radiology* **2013**, *266*, 185–196. [CrossRef]
9. Hu, R.; Yang, H.; Chen, Y.; Zhou, T.; Zhang, J.; Chen, T.W.; Zhang, X.M. Dynamic contrast-enhanced MRI for measuring pancreatic perfusion in acute pancreatitis: A. preliminary study. *Acad. Radiol.* **2019**, *26*, 1641–1649. [CrossRef]
10. Wasif, N.; Ko, C.Y.; Farrell, J.; Wainberg, Z.; Hines, O.J.; Reber, H.; Tomlinson, J.S. Impact of tumor grade on prognosis in pancreatic cancer: Should we include grade in AJCC staging? *Ann. Surg. Oncol.* **2010**, *17*, 2312–2320. [CrossRef]
11. Schraml, C.; Schwenzer, N.F.; Martirosian, P.; Claussen, C.D.; Schick, F. Perfudsion imaging of the pancreas using an arterial spin labeling technique. *J. Magn. Reson. Imaging* **2008**, *28*, 1459–1465. [CrossRef] [PubMed]
12. Shankar, S.; Kalra, N.; Bhatia, A.; Srinivasan, R.; Singh, P.; Radha, K.; Khandelwal, N.; Chawla, Y. Role of diffusion weighted imaging (DWI) for hepatocellular carcinoma (HCC) detection and its grading on 3T MRI: A prospective study. *J. Clin. Exp. Hepatol.* **2016**, *6*, 303–310. [CrossRef] [PubMed]
13. Zaboriene, I.; Zviniene, K.; Lukosevicius, S.; Ignatavicius, P.; Barauskas, G. Dynamic Perfusion Computed Tomography and Apparent Diffusion Coefficient as Potential Markers for Poorly Differentiated Pancreatic Adenocarcinoma. *Dig. Surg.* **2021**, *38*, 128–135. [CrossRef] [PubMed]
14. Tofts, P.S.; Brix, G.; Buckley, D.L.; Evelhoch, J.L.; Henderson, E.; Knopp, M.V.; Larsson, H.B.; Lee, T.-Y.; Mayr, N.A.; Parker, G.J.; et al. Estimating kinetic parameters from dynamic contrast enhanced T1-weighted MRI of a diffusible tracer: Standardized quantities and symbols. *J. Magn. Reson. Imaging* **1999**, *10*, 223–232. [CrossRef]
15. Shibata, K.; Matsumoto, T.; Yada, K.; Sasaki, A.; Ohta, M.; Kitano, S. Factors predicting recurrence after resection of pancreatic ductal carcinoma. *Pancreas* **2005**, *31*, 69–73. [CrossRef]
16. Min, J.H.; Kang, T.W.; Cha, D.I.; Kim, S.H.; Shin, K.S.; Lee, J.E.; Jang, K.-T.; Ahn, S.H. Apparent diffusion coefficient as a potential marker for tumour differentiation, staging and long-term outcomes in gallbladder cancer. *Eur. Radiol.* **2019**, *29*, 411–421. [CrossRef]
17. Alizadeh, A.A.; Aranda, V.; Bardelli, A.; Blanpain, C.; Bock, C.; Borowski, C.; Caldas, C.; Califano, A.; Doherty, M.; Elsner, M.; et al. Toward understanding and exploiting tumor heterogeneity. *Nat. Med.* **2015**, *21*, 846–853. [CrossRef]
18. Akashi, M.; Nakahusa, Y.; Yakabe, T.; Egashira, Y.; Koga, Y.; Sumi, K.; Noshiro, H.; Irie, H.; Tokunaga, O.; Miyazaki, K. Assessment of aggressiveness of rectal cancer using 3-T MRI:correlation between the apparent diffusion coefficient as a potential imaging biomarker and histologic prognostic factors. *Acta Radiol.* **2014**, *55*, 524–531. [CrossRef]
19. Jang, K.M.; Kim, S.H.; Lee, S.J.; Choi, D. The value of gadoxetic acid-enhanced and DWI MRI for prediction of grading of pancreatic neuroendocrine tumors. *Acta Radiol.* **2014**, *55*, 140–148. [CrossRef]
20. Kang, T.W.; Kim, S.H.; Jang, K.M.; Choi, D.; Ha, S.Y.; Kim, K.M.; Kang, W.K.; Kim, M.J. Gastrointestinal stromal tumors: Correlation of modified NIH risk stratification with diffusion weighted MR imaging as an imaging biomarker. *Eur. J. Radiol.* **2015**, *84*, 33–40. [CrossRef]
21. Kim, M.; Kang, T.W.; Kim, Y.K.; Kim, S.H.; Kwon, W.; Ha, S.Y.; Ji, S.A. Pancreatic neuroendocrine tumor: Correlation of apparent diffusion coefficient or WHO classification with recurrence-free survival. *Eur. J. Radiol.* **2016**, *85*, 680–687. [CrossRef] [PubMed]
22. Lee, N.K.; Kim, S.; Moon, J.I.; Shin, N.; Kim, D.U.; Seo, H.I.; Kim, H.S.; Han, G.J.; Kim, J.Y.; Lee, J.W. Diffusion-weighted magnetic resonance imaging of gallbladder adenocarcinoma: Analysis with emphasis on histologic grade. *Clin. Imaging* **2016**, *40*, 345–351. [CrossRef] [PubMed]
23. Dallongeville, A.; Corno, L.; Silvera, S.; Boulay-Coletta, I.; Zins, M. Initial Diagnosis and Staging of Pancreatic Cancer Including Main Differentials. *Semin. Ultrasound CT MR* **2019**, *40*, 436–468. [CrossRef] [PubMed]
24. De Castro, S.M.; Kuhlmann, K.F.; van Heek, N.T.; Busch, O.R.C.; Offerhaus, G.J.; van Gulik, T.M.; Obertop, H.; Gouma, D.J. Recurrent disease after microscopically radical (R0) resection of periampullary adenocarcinoma in patients without adjuvant therapy. *J. Gastrointest. Surg.* **2004**, *8*, 775–784. [CrossRef]
25. Kremer, B.; Vogel, I.; Luttges, J.; Klöppel, G.; Henne-Bruns, D. Surgical possibilities for pancreatic cancer: Extended resection. *Ann. Oncol.* **1999**, *10*, 252–256. [CrossRef]

26. Park, J.Y.; King, J.; Reber, H.; Hines, O.J.; Mederos, M.A.; Wang, H.L.; Dawson, D.; Wainberg, Z.; Donahue, T.; Girgis, M. Poorly differentiated histologic grade correlates with worse survival in SMAD4 negative pancreatic adenocarcinoma patients. *J. Surg. Oncol.* **2021**, *123*, 389–398. [CrossRef]
27. Facciorusso, A.; Mohan, B.P.; Crinò, S.F.; Ofosu, A.; Ramai, D.; Lisotti, A.; Chandan, S.; Fusaroli, P. Contrast-enhanced harmonic endoscopic ultrasound-guided fine-needle aspiration versus standard fine-needle aspiration in pancreatic masses: A meta-analysis. *Exper. Revies. Gastroenterol. Hepatol.* **2021**, *15*, 821–828. [CrossRef]
28. Kim, H.; Keene, K.S.; Sarver, D.B.; Lee, S.K.; Beasley, T.M.; Morgan, D.E.; Posey, J.A., III. Quantitative perfusion and diffusion-weighted magnetic resonance imaging of gastrointestinal cancers treated with multikinase inhibitors: A pilot study. *Gastrointest. Cancer Res.* **2014**, *7*, 75–81.
29. Xu, J.; Liang, Z.; Hao, S.; Zhu, L.; Ashish, M.; Jin, C.; Fu, D.; Ni, Q. Pancreatic adenocarcinoma: Dynamic 64-slice helical CT with perfusion imaging. *Abdom Imaging* **2009**, *34*, 759–766. [CrossRef]
30. Tofts, P.S. Modeling tracer kinetics in dynamic Gd-DTPA MR imaging. *J. Magn. Reson. Imaging* **1997**, *7*, 91–101. [CrossRef]
31. Donati, F.; Boraschi, P.; Cervelli, R.; Pacciardi, F.; Lombardo, C.; Boggi, U.; Falaschi, F.; Caramella, D. 3T MR perfusion of solid pancreatic lesions using dynamic contrast-enhanced DISCO sequence: Usefulness of qualitative and quantitative analyses in a pilot study. *Magn. Reson. Imaging* **2019**, *59*, 105–113. [CrossRef]
32. Yao, X.; Zeng, M.; Wang, H.; Sun, F.; Rao, S.; Ji, Y. Evaluation of pancreatic cancer by multiple breath-hold dynamic contrast-enhanced magnetic resonance imaging at 3.0T. *Eur. J. Radiol.* **2012**, *81*, e917–e922. [CrossRef]

Disclaimer/Publisher's Note: The statements, opinions and data contained in all publications are solely those of the individual author(s) and contributor(s) and not of MDPI and/or the editor(s). MDPI and/or the editor(s) disclaim responsibility for any injury to people or property resulting from any ideas, methods, instructions or products referred to in the content.

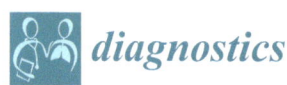

Review

Intraductal Papillary Mucinous Neoplasm of the Pancreas: A Challenging Diagnosis

Charikleia Triantopoulou [1,*], Sofia Gourtsoyianni [2], Dimitrios Karakaxas [3] and Spiros Delis [3]

1. Department of Radiology, Konstantopouleio General Hospital, 14233 Athens, Greece
2. 1st Department of Radiology, School of Medicine, National and Kapodistrian University of Athens, Areteion Hospital, 11528 Athens, Greece; sgty76@gmail.com
3. Department of Surgery, Konstantopouleio General Hospital, 14233 Athens, Greece; dimitrios.karakaksas@gmail.com (D.K.); sdelis55@hotmail.com (S.D.)
* Correspondence: ctriantopoulou@gmail.com

Abstract: Intraductal papillary mucinous neoplasm of the pancreas (IPMN) was classified as a distinct entity from mucinous cystic neoplasm by the WHO in 1995. It represents a mucin-producing tumor that originates from the ductal epithelium and can evolve from slight dysplasia to invasive carcinoma. In addition, different aspects of tumor progression may be seen in the same lesion. Three types are recognized, the branch duct variant, the main duct variant, which shows a much higher prevalence for malignancy, and the mixed-type variant, which combines branch and main duct characteristics. Advances in cross-sectional imaging have led to an increased rate of IPMN detection. The main imaging characteristic of IPMN is the dilatation of the pancreatic duct without the presence of an obstructing lesion. The diagnosis of a branch duct IPMN is based on the proof of its communication with the main pancreatic duct on MRI-MRCP examination. Early identification by imaging of the so-called worrisome features or predictors for malignancy is an important and challenging task. In this review, we will present recent imaging advances in the diagnosis and characterization of different types of IPMNs, as well as imaging tools available for early recognition of worrisome features for malignancy. A critical appraisal of current IPMN management guidelines from both a radiologist's and surgeon's perspective will be made. Special mention is made of complications that might arise during the course of IPMNs as well as concomitant pancreatic neoplasms including pancreatic adenocarcinoma and pancreatic endocrine neoplasms. Finally, recent research on prognostic and predictive biomarkers including radiomics will be discussed.

Keywords: intraductal papillary mucinous tumor; pancreas; CT; MRI; PETA; EUS

Citation: Triantopoulou, C.; Gourtsoyianni, S.; Karakaxas, D.; Delis, S. Intraductal Papillary Mucinous Neoplasm of the Pancreas: A Challenging Diagnosis. *Diagnostics* **2023**, *13*, 2015. https://doi.org/10.3390/diagnostics13122015

Academic Editors: Francescamaria Donati and Piero Boraschi

Received: 23 April 2023
Revised: 31 May 2023
Accepted: 4 June 2023
Published: 9 June 2023

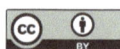

Copyright: © 2023 by the authors. Licensee MDPI, Basel, Switzerland. This article is an open access article distributed under the terms and conditions of the Creative Commons Attribution (CC BY) license (https://creativecommons.org/licenses/by/4.0/).

1. Introduction

With the advances in multidetector computed tomography (MDCT) imaging and the continuing increase in overall cross-sectional imaging, pancreatic cystic lesions are more and more commonly encountered including intraductal papillary mucinous neoplasms (IPMNs) of the pancreas. The crude prevalence rate of pancreatic cystic lesions and IPMNs is 2.1% and was found to increase significantly with age in a large-scale, single-center cohort study of 21,745 asymptomatic healthy individuals [1]. In the same study, IPMNs were found to comprise 82% of incidental pancreatic cystic lesions demonstrated on CT examinations.

IPMNs arise from the epithelial lining of the pancreatic ducts. Different patterns of progression may be seen in the histopathology, from hyperplasia to invasive carcinoma [2]. They affect men and females equally and are identified usually in the 6th-7th decade [3]. Three main types may be identified: branch duct (BD) type, main duct type, subdivided into the segmental main duct (SMD) and diffuse main duct (DMD) subtypes, and mixed type (MT), combining both main types.

Imaging aims not only at the accurate diagnosis of an IPMN but also to provide information on the so-called worrisome features for malignancy. Taking into consideration the heterogenous group of lesions that this entity represents, it is of utmost importance to have in place clear diagnostic protocols and follow dedicated guidelines. The literature is extensive and, in some points, controversial concerning surgical indications, as well as the length of imaging follow-up.

Recent research in radiomics using computed tomography (CT) and magnetic resonance imaging (MRI) has shown promise in developing prognostic and predictive biomarkers in an effort to personalize IPMN patient management.

In this review, our aim is to focus on the challenges that IPMNs pose to the reporting radiologists, who should recognize them, as they have a pivotal role in patient management, including early implementation of appropriate therapy, namely surgical removal, allowing for cure.

2. Imaging Findings

A branch duct IPMN is easily recognized as a cystic dilatation of the pancreatic duct side branches. Grape-like clusters of cysts may be also seen communicating with the main pancreatic duct that is not dilated (Figure 1). A BD-type IPMN may be identified in any part of the pancreas. In diffuse main duct IPMNs, a uniform dilatation is noticed throughout the main pancreatic duct, while a patulous ampulla of Vater may be also identified. Segmental main duct IPMNs appear as a focal dilatation of the main pancreatic duct (Figure 2). Mixed IPMNs involve both the main pancreatic duct and side branches (Figure 3).

The main imaging characteristic of a main duct IPMN is the dilatation of the main pancreatic duct, without the presence of an obstructing lesion (Figure 4). If the diameter of the main pancreatic duct exceeds 10 mm, it is considered a high-risk stigma [4]. Cross-sectional imaging, whether MDCT or MRI, reveals the exact location of the cystic lesion, stratifies the type of IPMN, and allows for accurate measurement of the extent of the lesion. This is particularly important as the IPMN could be multifocal (Figure 5), while different types may co-exist in the same patient (Figure 6).

The duct/cyst content is hypodense in both unenhanced and after-iv-contrast-administration CT images, with fluid attenuation; while it is of high signal intensity in T2-weighted images and low signal intensity in T1-weighted images. Intraductal calcifications are rare, but when present are associated with malignant transformation [5]. Papillary growth is best appreciated after intravenous contrast administration [2] (Figure 7). Thick walls and the presence of mural nodules contribute to the irregular ductal margins in such cases. In addition to intravenous contrast enhancement, other available contrast mechanisms when performing MRI/MRCP examination of the pancreas, such as Diffusion Weighted Imaging (DWI), allow the identification of worrisome features such as enhancing mural nodule > 5 mm or thickened/enhancing cyst wall as per the international consensus guidelines for the management of IPMN published in 2017 [4]. However, the diagnosis/characterization of a mural nodule might not always be easy and endoscopic ultrasound (EUS) is recommended to simultaneously evaluate the architecture of the cyst and obtain a biopsy.

Several studies challenge the cutoff value of main pancreatic duct (MPD) $\geq$ 10 mm as a high-risk stigma, while a recent study investigated whether there is a different threshold of the MPD corresponding to malignancy of IPMNs according to the tumor location (head–neck versus body–tail) [6]. Different cutoff values of MPD based on CT and MRI measurements were associated with malignancy. For IPMNs involving the MPD, the threshold was found to be 8.2 mm for lesions located in the pancreatic head and neck, while for lesions in the body and tail of the pancreas, the proposed threshold was 7.7 mm.

Regarding BD type, the diagnosis and differentiation from other pancreatic cystic lesions are based on the proof of communication of the cystic lesion with the main pancreatic duct, best identified via MRI-MRCP examination. The branch duct type may be solitary or in the form of multiple cystic lesions. Solitary branch duct IPMNs are located mainly in the uncinate process and have a grape-like microcystic or a unilocular or multilocular macrocystic appearance [2] on MRCP images. Compared with 2D MRCP examination, 3D

MRCP has been shown to provide better image quality, providing an improved evaluation of the pancreatic duct and morphological aspects of IPMN, being more helpful in identifying the communicating duct, in addition to being preferred for surgical planning [7].

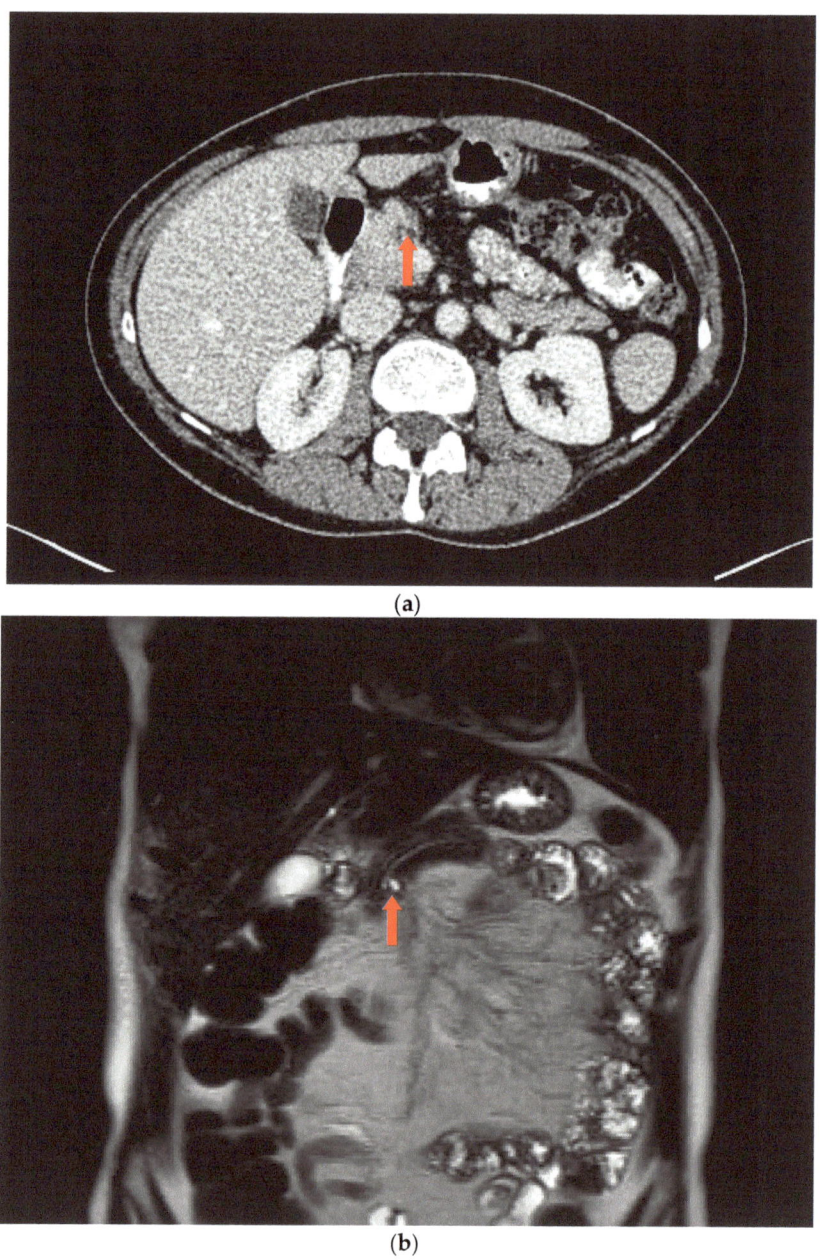

Figure 1. Contrast-enhanced CT image (**a**) and coronal T2-w MR image (**b**), show a small branch duct IPMN (arrow) communicating with the main duct. The IPMN is more easily seen on the MR image.

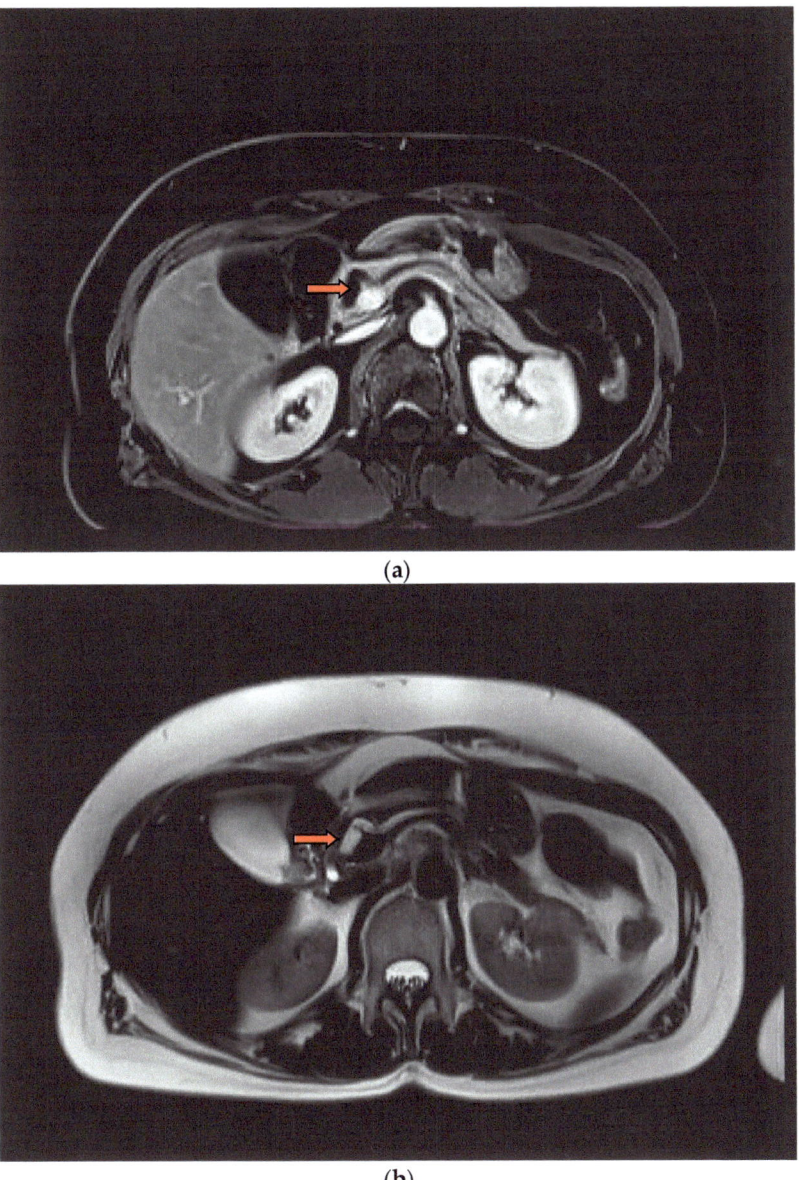

Figure 2. Contrast-enhanced T1-w MR image (**a**) and T2-w MR image (**b**), demonstrate a marked dilatation of the main pancreatic duct in the head and neck of the pancreas, consistent with a segmental main duct IPMN (arrow).

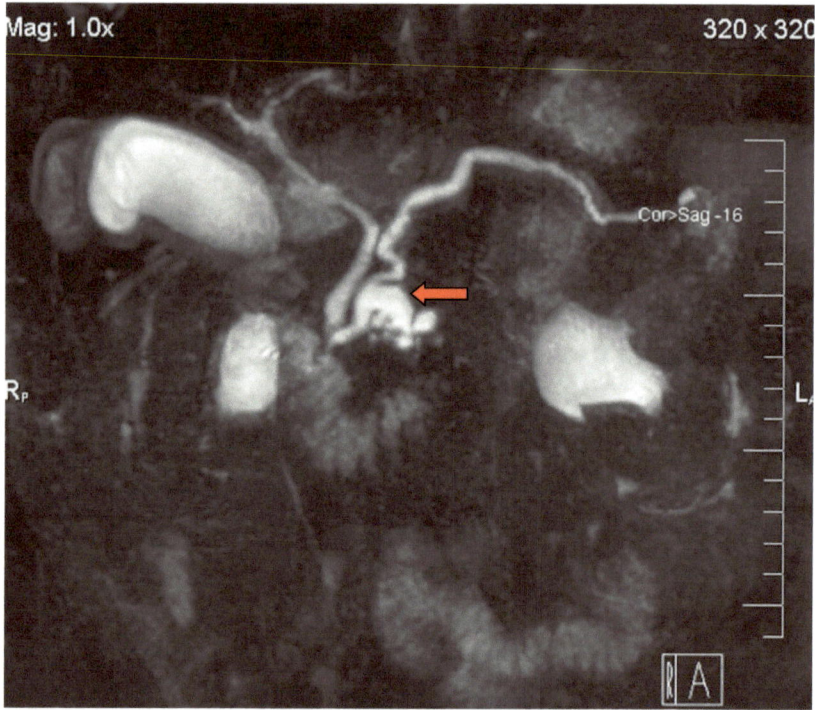

Figure 3. A mixed-type IPMN (arrow) is seen in the pancreatic head on this MRCP image.

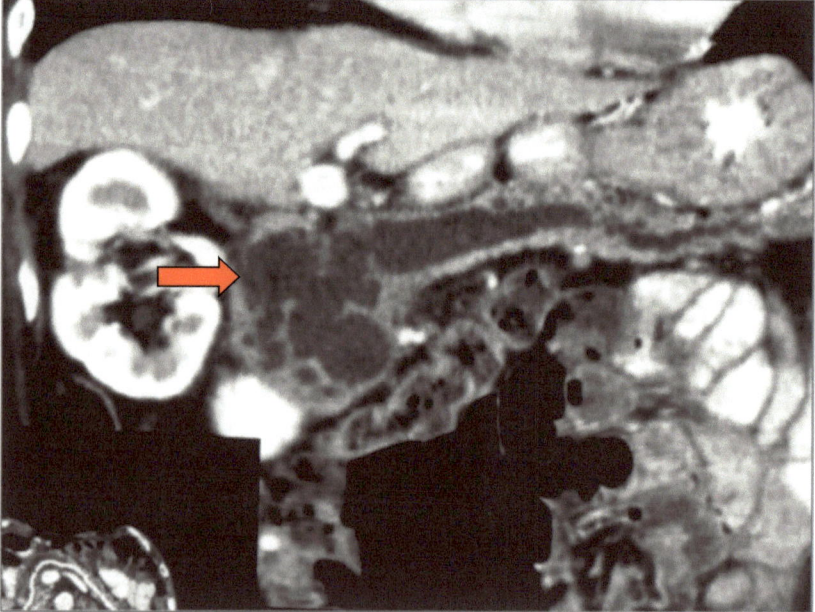

Figure 4. Curved reconstructed CT image in the course of the dilated pancreatic duct shows a typical case of main duct IPMN (arrow).

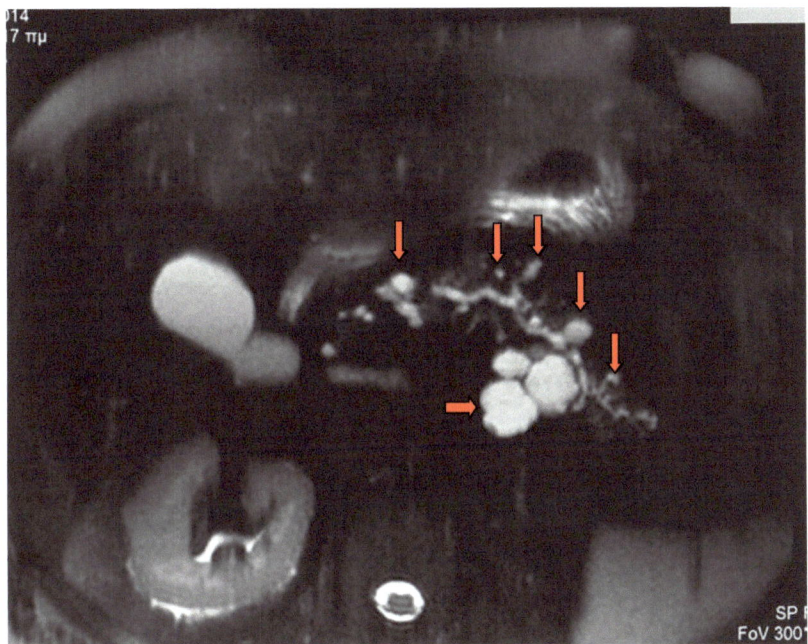

Figure 5. T2-w fs MR image shows many IPMNs of different sizes and morphology throughout the pancreas (arrows).

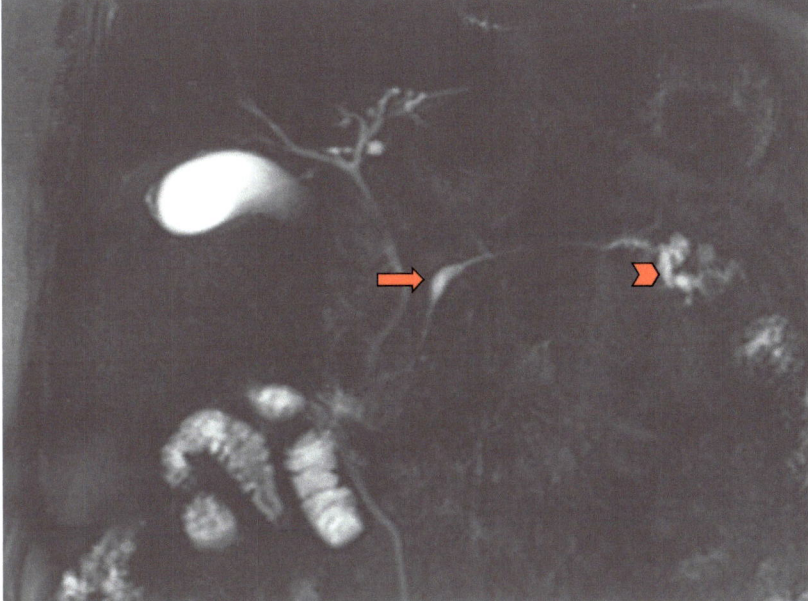

Figure 6. MRCP image shows a segmental main duct IPMN in the body (arrow) and a branch duct IPMN in the tail of the pancreas (arrowhead).

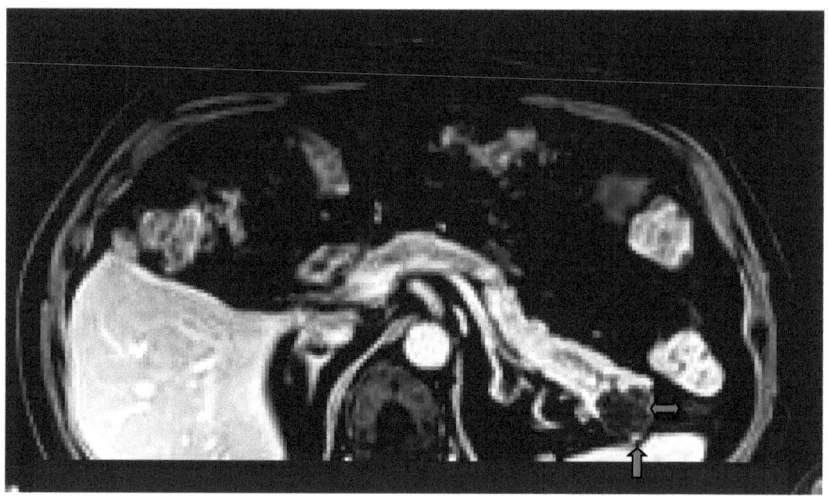

Figure 7. IPMN in the pancreatic tail, presenting as a cystic lesion on contrast-enhanced T1-w MR image. Enhancing mural nodules are obvious (arrows).

The exploitation of the quantitative parameter of diffusion-weighted imaging (DWI) might prove to be helpful in differential diagnosis between mucinous and serous cystic tumors and in IPMN characterization (benign vs malignant). For this purpose, a spin-echo echo-planar DWI sequence with multiple b values (0, 150, 500, 1000, and 1500 s/mm^2) was studied at 3T MRI, and different ADC values were proposed [8].

A different quantitative MRI measurement that might prove to be helpful is proton density fat fraction (PDFF [%]) calculated in a multi-echo 3D DIXON sequence obtained at 3T MRI, which has been found to be significantly higher in pancreatic parenchyma of patients with intraductal papillary mucinous neoplasm with a concomitant invasive carcinoma (IPMN-IC) (Figure 8) compared to a normal pancreas group and an IPMN group without invasive carcinoma, thus serving as a potential biomarker for the malignant development of IPMN [9].

Conversely, Yamada et al. [10] demonstrated that parenchymal fatty infiltration, expressed by a lower CT density of the pancreas in patients with IPMN, may serve as an early imaging biomarker for developing malignancy in the pancreas, for both high-grade dysplasia/derived pancreatic ductal adenocarcinoma (PDAC) and for concomitant PDAC. For this purpose, the authors utilized the pancreatic index (PI) measured on CT images calculated by dividing the CT density of the pancreas by that of the spleen.

In the retrospective study of Lee et al. [11] comparing the diagnostic performance and intermodality agreement between contrast-enhanced CT and MRI for prediction of malignancy, enhancing mural nodule of ≥5 mm, abrupt main pancreatic duct caliber change, lymphadenopathy, larger main pancreatic duct size, and faster cyst growth rate were found to be more common in malignant than benign IPMNs. The diagnostic performance of contrast-enhanced CT and MRI were comparable, with good intermodality agreement. In a later study by Min et al. [12], it was shown that MRI is superior to CT for identifying IPMN-associated mural nodules. Nevertheless, diagnostic performance for differentiating malignant from benign IPMNs was found to be similar between CT and MRI.

Many studies have evaluated the usefulness of 18-fluorodeoxyglucose positron emission tomography/computed tomography (18-FDG PET/CT) in the characterization of IPMN of the pancreas. In 2019, Yamashita et al. [13] showed that 18-FDG PET accumulation was significantly related to malignancy in IPMN with a sensitivity of 0.82 and specificity of 0.71. In another systematic review [14], it was shown that 18-FDG PET/CT imaging had a very high positive and negative predictive value, as well as a specificity and accuracy of

95% and 91%, respectively in identifying malignancy (either high-grade dysplasia and/or invasive) in IPMNs.

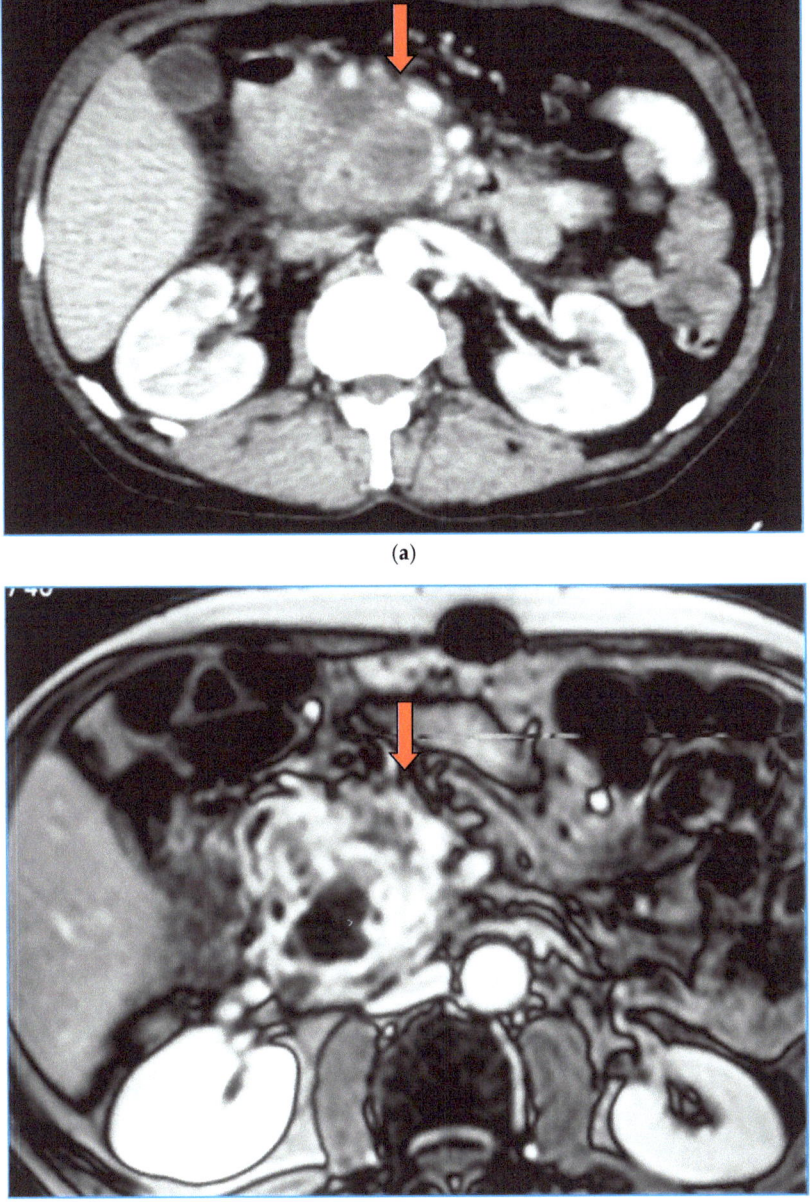

(a)

(b)

Figure 8. Contrast-enhanced CT image (**a**) and T1-w MR image post iv contrast administration (**b**), show an IPMN with invasive carcinoma (arrow) in the pancreatic head infiltrating the superior mesenteric vein.

Finally, a recent meta-analysis [15] evaluating the role of all imaging modalities in the differentiation of benign and malignant IPMNs concluded that PET/CT showed the highest AUC. MRI/MRCP and PET/CT can be used interchangeably as a first-line examination based on the overall diagnostic accuracy in the diagnosis of malignant IPMN. A negative PET/CT examination in a patient with a suspicion of a malignant IPMN on CT and/or MRI permits a safe follow-up plan and may help to avoid unnecessary surgery.

In conclusion, CT is mandatory for staging and resectability evaluation. MRI offers the advantage of a better depiction of cystic lesions and their communication with the pancreatic duct by means of MRCP imaging. Furthermore, MRI is advantageous when equivocal liver lesions need to be characterized. At the same time, PET/CT has an additional role in indeterminate IPMNs, concerning the possibility of malignant transformation, and is used in selected cases.

3. IPMN-Related Complications

IPMNs are frequently asymptomatic, but in some cases, epigastric pain is reported. Fistulas may develop between IPMNs and various organs [16,17]. Their presence is usually related to invasive carcinoma and may involve the duodenum (64%), the common bile duct (56%), or the stomach (17%). The hypothesized mechanism for the formation of pancreaticogastric and pancreaticoduodenal fistulas is by contiguous invasion [18]. In cases of benign IPMNs, the mechanism differs and is associated with the increase of the intraductal pressure due to the presence of dense mucin causing ductal dilatation and wall disruption. Chronic inflammatory infiltration of the pancreatic tissue has been described as another possible mechanism in these cases [19].

Another rare complication that has been reported is pseudomyxoma peritonei caused by a ruptured pancreatic duct and mucin spread in the peritoneum [20]. The duct rupture and the subsequent mucin spread is a serious event as it is related to tumor seeding. Intraductal hemorrhage has also been reported in some cases, detected as high attenuation content on unenhanced CT images or as high signal intensity on fat-suppressed T1-weighted MR images. Intraductal hemorrhage may also lead to perforation and fistula formation [21].

Acute pancreatitis (AP) may also complicate an IPMN with a rate that varies from 12 to 67% [22]. The rate of AP does not seem to differ among benign and malignant IPMNs. Patients with IPMN are more prone to develop acute pancreatitis than patients with pancreatic adenocarcinoma because of the obstruction of the main duct by thick, abundant mucin and marked ductal dilatation. It is important to recognize an IPMN in cases of repeated episodes of AP, as these patients require surgery. The differential diagnosis between IPMN and AP-related pseudocysts is often challenging.

In patients with no high-risk stigmata who develop recurrent acute pancreatitis, endoscopic sphincterotomy could be offered as a minimally invasive technique to reduce the rate of these episodes. In selected patients, it can be a safe and effective treatment, without obviating the need for follow-up.

IPMNs are considered one of the main precursor lesions of pancreatic ductal adenocarcinoma (PDAC) following the tumoral intraepithelial neoplasm pathway. When an IPMN progresses to an invasive PDAC, it is referred to as an "IPMN with an invasive carcinoma" or "intraductal papillary mucinous carcinoma" (IPMC). IPMCs have distinct molecular, biological, and prognostic characteristics and account for about 10% of resected pancreatic cancers of ductal origin [23]. It is of utmost importance to differentiate IPMN-associated adenocarcinomas from other pseudo-IPMN lesions that can be secondary duct ectasias, retention cysts, large-duct-type PDACs, pseudocysts, cystic tumor necrosis, simple mucinous cysts, groove pancreatitis-associated paraduodenal wall cysts, or congenital cysts [24].

4. IPMN Management Guidelines

Currently, three primary guidelines exist regarding the management of the continuously increasing number of diagnosed IPMN cases. All three try to answer the critical question of "to operate or to follow up", as this poses a critical dilemma faced by involved clinicians. The guidelines are based on objective imaging, laboratory, and clinical findings to reduce the number of unnecessary pancreatic operations and their associated morbidity and mortality rates.

These are the International Association of Pancreatology Guidelines first published in 2006 and revised in 2012 and 2017, the European evidence-based Guidelines published in 2013 and updated in 2018, and the American Gastroenterology Association Guidelines published in 2015. All agree on the main surgical intervention indications categorized as "Worrisome Features-Relative Indications" or "High Risk Stigmata-Absolute Indications" of a branch duct IPMN [4,25,26] (Table 1).

Table 1. Surgical intervention indications.

High-Risk Stigmata
enhancing solid component ≥ 5 mm
main pancreatic duct ≥ 10 mm
obstructive jaundice
Worrisome Features
thickened and enhancing cyst wall
enhancing mural nodule < 5 mm
main pancreatic duct 5–9 mm
cyst ≥ 3 cm
lymphadenopathy
abrupt change in caliber of the pancreatic duct with distal pancreatic atrophy
cyst growth rate ≥ 5 mm in two years
elevated CA 19-9

Worrisome features or relative indications according to the International Association of Pancreatology and European guidelines, respectively, cannot be solely used to predict the malignant course of an IPMN neoplasia. Patients with worrisome features had a significantly better 5-year disease-specific survival compared with those with high-risk stigmata (96% vs. 60%, respectively). The surgical intervention indications also differ between the guidelines, as the European guidelines warrant surgical resection in cases where there is one relative indication in surgically fit patients. In contrast, the International Association of Pancreatology guidelines require the presence of at least one worrisome feature leading to further diagnostic evaluation with EUS to better assess the risk of malignancy. The American Gastroenterology Association guidelines recommend surgery for cases presenting with an MPD ≥ 5 mm and the presence of a solid component or cytology positive for malignancy [4,25,26].

"Worrisome features" on imaging include a cyst of 3 cm, an enhancing mural nodule < 5 mm, thickened enhancing cyst walls, main pancreatic duct dilatation with a diameter 5–9 mm, abrupt change in the caliber of the main pancreatic duct with distal pancreatic atrophy, lymphadenopathy, an elevated serum level of carbohydrate antigen (CA)19-9, and a rapid rate of cyst growth > 5 mm/2 years. The evaluation of these patients by endoscopic ultrasonography (EUS) using techniques such as Doppler EUS or contrast-enhanced harmonic EUS is mandatory. The presence of blood supply in a mural nodule can further stratify the lesion and it is important for patient management [4].

Conversely, the presence of "High-risk Stigmata" on CT, MRI, or EUS (i.e., obstructive jaundice in a patient with a cystic lesion of the pancreatic head, enhancing mural nodule of 5 mm, or main pancreatic duct diameter of 10 mm) is a clear indication for lesion resection in surgically fit patients without further testing. This is based on the high frequency of invasive carcinoma and high-grade dysplasia in MD-IPMN, which is 61.6% (range, 36–100%), while the mean frequency of invasive IPMN is 43.1% (range, 11–81%). Precursor lesions of pancreatic cancer such as IPMNs with HGD, pancreatic intraepithelial neoplasia 3 (PanIN 3), and mucinous cystic neoplasia (MCN) with HGD should be resected as this is the only chance for patient cure [4].

Given the higher malignant potential of main duct and mixed-type IPMNs, an early surgical excision decision in surgically fit patients can be justified [27,28]. All patients with cysts of 3 cm in size without "Worrisome Features" should undergo surveillance according to size stratification [4]. Additionally, the Shin score published in 2010 is a complimentary tool that comprises five variables, namely, age, history of pancreatitis, CA19-9 level, pancreatic duct diameter, and mural nodules. Patients with a Shin score of <1 warrant surveillance, while those with a score of >4 should undergo surgery. There are no clear guidelines for the treatment of patients with Shin scores of 2 or 3, which should be individualized [29].

Given the growing number of incidentally diagnosed cases in asymptomatic patients, a dilemma will frequently arise regarding therapeutic handling. Symptomatic patients may have a higher likelihood of malignancy or complications. Surgical intervention is often recommended, especially if the IPMN has high-risk features such as large size, main pancreatic duct involvement, or worrisome imaging findings. However, symptomatic patients may "deserve" more conservative management, especially in cases when there is a lack of high-risk features. Surveillance and regular imaging follow-up are usually recommended. This allows for the detection of any changes in the IPMN that may warrant intervention. In the presence of high-risk features, though, surgical intervention may still be considered. Eventually, the decision of how to proceed has to be, as much as possible, individualized and be taken in the context of a multidisciplinary team discussion.

In conclusion, following the initial evaluation with detailed patient history, physical examination, and laboratory tests, imaging studies should assess the size, location, and morphology of the IPMN and identify any high-risk or worrisome features. A multidisciplinary team will then evaluate the patient's symptoms and overall health and discuss the patient's clinical situation, risk factors, and potential management options. According to the aforementioned guidelines, asymptomatic, low-risk IPMN cases should be followed-up every 6–12 months, asymptomatic, high-risk IPMN cases should be considered for surgical intervention after evaluating the patient's overall health and risk-benefit analysis, and symptomatic IPMN cases should be offered a surgical intervention, especially if high-risk features are present. When resection takes place, the pathology report will direct the further type and timeframe of the follow-up plan.

5. EUS-FNA Added Value for IPMN Stratification

The added value of EUS-FNA and cytological interpretation is well recognized, especially for the evaluation of a small BD-IPMN without worrisome features. The recognition of a high-grade epithelial atypia, although insufficient for a malignant interpretation, represents a more sensitive predictor of invasive carcinoma or HGD than positive cytology [4,26]. The presence of cellular atypia in epithelial cells in the cyst fluid shows an 80% accuracy in the prediction of invasive carcinoma and HGD in a mucinous cyst, while more cancers can be detected in small IPMNs than the use of "worrisome features". Concerning molecular analysis of the cyst fluid, although still evolving, it is crucial for the recognition of a mucinous cyst. There is evidence that the detection of KRAS mutations supports accurately the diagnosis of a mucinous, but not necessarily malignant, cyst. Recent studies have evaluated the role of GNAS mutations, showing that this may help in distinguishing mucinous cysts from benign cysts [30,31]. Patients with positive fluid obtained cytology should be considered for surgery [32].

6. Surgical Considerations Regarding IPMN Management

Referral to a high-volume center for IPMN cases is without any doubt the cornerstone of their management, given the high level of complexity and experience required for their correct diagnosis and follow-up, or even more important, the technical difficulty and postoperative management of the required surgical operations and different types of resections [33–35].

IPMNs are considered in most cases as pre-malignant neoplasms and their resection must follow standard oncological principles such as a negative pathology report of the resection margin and proper lymphadenectomy [36]. Moreover, IPMNs can be characterized as the result of a pancreatic "field defect" because there is a possibility that all pancreatic ductal epithelial cells are at risk of dysplastic change [37].

Carbohydrate antigen (CA) 19-9 is a tumor biomarker related to pancreatic adenocarcinoma. When elevated in cases of IPMN, it is considered a worrisome feature in current guidelines and a relative criterion for resection. This biomarker has a prognostic value as CA 19-9 levels > 37 U/mL are associated not only with an increased likelihood of invasive carcinoma but also with worse overall and disease-free survival.

There are only three types of pancreatic resection that can assure the best oncological postoperative outcomes. These are pancreatoduodenectomy, distal pancreatectomy, and total pancreatectomy. Limited resections are considered only in a case-by-case setting and for a small minority of cases and they can be performed as focal non-anatomic excision or enucleation [38]. Cases of BD-IPMN without clinical, radiologic, cytopathologic, or serologic suspicion of invasive carcinoma may be treated in such a way. They are associated sometimes with leakage of mucin followed by pseudomyxoma peritonei and present with a higher rate of pancreatic fistulae and higher recurrence percentages from potential residual neoplasm [39–41].

Pancreatoduodenectomy is indicated in cases of dilatation of the main pancreatic duct in the head of the pancreas or the uncinate process, while lesions in the body and tail of the organ are treated with distal pancreatectomy with or without splenic preservation. Total pancreatectomy is the treatment of choice for diffuse multifocal disease, familial history of pancreatic adenocarcinoma, and failure to achieve a negative resection margin due to high-grade dysplasia in repeated intraoperative frozen sections. Total pancreatectomy postoperative sequelae are considered much more acceptable than the high risk of carcinoma development. However, due to long-term postoperative outcomes, total pancreatectomy cannot be advocated for all IPMNs even if multiple, and should only be offered in younger patients who can better handle the consequences of diabetes and exocrine insufficiency [42,43].

The intraoperative frozen section of the resection margin is a prerequisite for a safe oncologic outcome in cases when a partial pancreatectomy is attempted. The extent of the resection is based solely on its findings. High-grade dysplasia and carcinoma warrant extension of the resection or even total excision of the organ, but low-grade dysplasia is a finding that does not need any further modification of the procedure [44].

Moreover, it is interesting and at the same time important from an oncological outcome perspective, that T1a invasive intraductal papillary mucinous carcinoma has an excellent postoperative survival course, in cases with no lymphatic involvement, compared to pancreatic ductal adenocarcinoma, probably because of the more indolent behavior of this type of neoplasia [45].

7. Histopathological Correlation

IPMNs are characterized by abundant mucinous production and proliferation of mucinous epithelial cells resulting in papillary epithelial growth. Intraductal oncocytic papillary neoplasms (IOPNs), and intraductal tubulopapillary neoplasms (ITPNs) were considered variants of IPMN. In the 5th edition of the World Health Organization (WHO) Report, published in 2019, IOPNs and ITPNs are classified as distinctive neoplasms.

A combination of differentiations can be displayed in IPMNs using immunolabeling. The main differentiations are related to the neoplastic epithelium, which can be gastric-foveolar, intestinal, and pancreatobiliary. Gastric–foveolar differentiation is the most common type and is mainly seen in BD-IPMNs. Intestinal differentiation is the second most common type and is characterized by the presence of long finger-like (villous) papillae. Intestinal-type IPMN is the precursor of all colloid carcinomas of the pancreas.

The identification of the various types of differentiation in IPMNs is important but not as clinically significant as the degree of dysplasia assigned to them [46]. The grading system is simplified in low- vs. high-grade. Grading of dysplasia has clinical importance as high-grade neoplasms are more likely to have an associated invasive carcinoma. The presence of high-grade dysplasia in resected neoplasms has a major prognostic and predictive value as it is associated with a higher risk of progression in the remnant pancreas after surgery [47,48].

8. Concomitant Pancreatic Neoplasms

Patients with IPMN are at a well-recognized risk of developing concomitant pancreatic adenocarcinoma (PDAC) [49]. The term concomitant PDAC with IPMN refers to a PDAC that is separated from the IPMN by an uninvolved segment of the pancreatic duct and with no clearly visible areas of transition in between.

There are many retrospective studies reporting cases of patients with IPMN developing adenocarcinoma in areas not related to pancreatic cysts, with incidences of between 4% and 11% [50–57]. Adenocarcinoma may develop many years after the diagnosis of IPMN. In a prospective study, which followed 89 patients with IPMN over a 17-year period, four developed concomitant pancreatic adenocarcinoma [58]. This fact supports the role of long-term follow-up in patients with IPMNs.

It is quite difficult to differentiate pancreatic adenocarcinoma from malignant IPMN as they share almost the same imaging characteristics. The only criterion that may be used for the differential diagnosis is that in cases of pancreatic adenocarcinoma with obstruction of the pancreatic duct, there is upstream ductal dilatation and atrophy of the parenchyma. Conversely, in cases of IPMN, the duct is dilated but there is no parenchymal atrophy. As both cases need surgery, accurate differential diagnosis is not mandatory, and the radiologist should focus on resectability evaluation using the same criteria as for pancreatic cancer.

Identical genetic alterations can well explain the co-existence of IPMN with PDAC. Somatic-activating mutations in the KRAS and GNAS genes have been described in both diseases and are the most common alterations. There is increasing evidence that PDACs in the vicinity of IPMN lesions are often significantly smaller and have a different biological behavior compared to PDACs with no associated IPMN, being less aggressive and associated with longer survival [59].

Another important observation supported by the literature is that the occurrence of IPMNs in association with pancreatic neuroendocrine tumors (PNETs) is more frequent than expected [60]. Patients with concomitant IPMN and PNET have been reported in many studies at a rate of 2.8% and 4.6% of all cases [61–63]. Goh et al. [61] hypothesized that this association could be related to the existence of common underlying risk factors and genetic alterations.

There are two proposed hypotheses for the tumorigenesis of concomitant PNET and IPMN published: (1) one cell type in a unique tumor could transdifferentiate into another cell type; and (2) two cell types could arise from a common neoplastic progenitor; the latter hypothesis being supported by many investigators.

Terada et al. [64] suggested that IPMN has the potential for endocrine differentiation. They found that argentaffin-serotonin- and gastrin-secreting cells were present in IPMN but not in normal pancreatic ductal cells. However, Hashimoto et al. [65] studied a case of mixed PNET and IPMN and found positivity for exocrine markers expressed on some endocrine tumor cells, supporting the contention that the endocrine tumor cells might transdifferentiate to ductal tumor cells.

Some reports suggest that there is a lack of awareness of the potential for the concomitance of PNET and IPMN, thus leading to the poor examination of specimens and a high rate of underreported or undetected cases [66]. Therefore, it is important that radiologists and pathologists are aware of the possibility of concomitant IPMN with PNET in order to recognize these neoplasms early, as this may certainly affect patient management and prognosis.

9. Advanced Endoscopic Procedures

EUS-guided needle confocal laser endomicroscopy (nCLE) is a novel technique that permits real-time microscopic imaging of intra-cystic epithelium allowing in vivo pathological analysis of pancreatic cystic lesions (PCLs). Characteristic features of IPMNs have been well established in recent literature.

In a recent meta-analysis (7 studies and 324 patients), this technique was evaluated for the differential diagnosis between mucinous and non-mucinous cystic pancreatic lesions. The sensitivity, specificity, and accuracy were 85% (95%CI: 71–93%), 99% (95%CI: 90–100%), and 99% (95%CI: 98–100%), respectively, while the risk of post-procedure acute pancreatitis was only 1% [67].

The INDEX study was designed as a post hoc analysis to identify multiple nCLE imaging variables that would detect advanced neoplasia in IPMNs [68]. The variables with the highest inter-observer agreement according to this study were papillary epithelial thickness and darkness. Specifically, papillary epithelial thickness visualized by nCLE (width ≥ 50 μm) had a specificity of 100% (95%CI: 69–100%) for the detection of advanced neoplasia. Additionally, estimation of the papillary epithelial darkness (cut-off ≤ 90 pixel intensity) revealed a specificity of 100% (95%CI: 69–100%), while the sensitivity and AUC were reported to be 87.5% (95%CI: 62–99%) and 0.90, respectively [68].

However, we should mention the potential limitations of nCLE. Manually evaluation of papillary epithelial thickness and darkness may lead to differences in the inter-observer interpretation of images. The development of an artificial intelligence model has partially solved these issues and identified advanced neoplasia in IPMNs with a sensitivity of 83% and specificity of 88%, which are above the minimum levels of the Fukuoka or AGA guidelines [69].

There is clear evidence that nCLE is an important diagnostic technique. Despite this, its incorporation into the diagnostic clinical routine is still lacking. High equipment costs are the main limitation, while continuous training in image acquisition and interpretation is definitely needed. Complications such as acute pancreatitis are still slightly higher than the standard EUS-FNA examination and care should be taken for their prevention.

10. Molecular Biomarkers

The introduction of next-generation sequencing (NGS) offers a new possibility in the accurate diagnosis and classification of pancreatic cystic lesions (PCLs). Small gene panels or whole exome NGS can be used. By these methods, the evaluation of intact cell and cell-free nucleic acid is allowed, as these can be found in the cyst fluid. The presence of DNA mutations (KRAS, CDKN2A, SMAD4, PTEN, PIK3CA, and TP53) can be associated not only with pancreatic adenocarcinoma but also with mucinous cystic lesions and IPMNs.

Molecular analysis of cyst fluid is of utmost importance as it can contribute to the risk estimation of IPMNs. In a large meta-analysis based on six studies, McCarty et al. [70] reported that the presence of KRAS and GNAS mutations succeeded in the detection of mucinous PCLs with a very high specificity of 99% (95%CI: 67–100%), and also a high diagnostic accuracy of 97% (95%CI: 95–98%). Additionally, dual KRAS/GNAS mutation had 94% sensitivity, 91% specificity, and 97% accuracy for diagnosing IPMNs. Recently, Ren et al. found that uncommon BRAF mutations are characteristics of a significant subset of IPMNs that lack KRAS mutations. These observations indicate that RAS-MAPK dysregulation is often found in these tumor types [71].

Risk stratification of IPMNs is quite challenging. Singhi et al. [72] used next-generation sequencing in order to evaluate DNA mutations in IPMNs that were associated with advanced neoplasia. They analyzed 102 patients with a proven diagnosis by histopathology. The presence of TP53, PIK3CA, and/or PTEN mutations was evaluated. Ultimately, they reported 88% sensitivity and 95% specificity in the diagnosis of IPMN-related advanced neoplasia.

Cyst fluid molecular analysis by next-generation sequencing presents many advantages compared to measuring cyst CEA levels, which is the standard technique, with better accuracy, and furthermore, offers the possibility of providing risk estimation for IPMNs. However, it is not readily available and the high cost represents a financial barrier to universal adaptation. These advanced techniques should be used in centers with high expertise in the management of cystic pancreatic lesions.

11. Radiomics–Future Directions

Despite improvements in imaging, the morphologic features of IPMNs on CT and/or MRI are still not clear enough to assess dysplasia. This is the reason why even the most recently revised guidelines may lead to unnecessary pancreatic surgery in benign cases. Lekkerkerker et al. conducted a very important study in an effort to compare the ICGs (2012) with the European (2013) and American guidelines (2015) and evaluated their performance on 75 patients with histopathologically proven IPMNs. It was shown that surgery was justified in only half of the cases (54%, 53%, and 59% of the patients, respectively) [73].

There is obviously a need to develop new biomarkers that could non-invasively assess the risk of malignancy with greater accuracy in the heterogenous group of IPMNs. Radiomics is based on data mining from medical images in order to combine qualitative and quantitative information [74]. It is based on the computerized extraction of quantifiable data from radiological images from different sources. Through this extraction, mineable databases are created that can be used for diagnosis assessment, prognosis estimation, and prediction evaluation.

Three are not many studies that have evaluated the role of radiomics in differentiating IPMNs with high-grade dysplasia (HGD) or advanced neoplasia from indolent lesions with low-grade dysplasia (LGD) [75–78]. In most of these studies, CT scans were used and patients with confirmed surgical histopathology were included. A recent multicenter study by Cui et al. [79], presents a radiomic nomogram based on MRI to predict high-grade dysplasia or adenocarcinoma in branch duct IPMNs. Clinical variables were combined with a radiomic signature that incorporated nine features. Their results were promising as the predictive nomogram they created diagnosed advanced neoplasia with AUC values of 0.903 (in the training cohort; with a sensitivity of 95% and a specificity of 73%), and 0.884 (in one of two external validation cohorts; with a sensitivity of 79% and a specificity of 90%) [79].

In a more recent study, the authors used contrast-enhanced CT-based radiomics to differentiate between LGD, HGD, and invasive IPMN. A large retrospective series of 408 consecutive patients with histologically proven IPMN after resection was used [80]. They showed many, and significant, differences in the training cohort between patients with benign and malignant IPMNs (in 85/107 radiomic features). The results were really promising considering that the multivariate model differentiated benign from malignant tumors in the training cohort with an area under the ROC curve (AUC) of 0.84, a sensitivity of 0.82, and a specificity of 0.74, while in an external validation cohort, the scores were an AUC of 0.71, a sensitivity of 0.69, and a specificity of 0.57. Thus, preoperative CT-based radiomic analysis has the potential to differentiate benign from malignant IPMNs.

There is no doubt that radiomics represent a promising non-invasive tool for the accurate classification and risk estimation of pancreatic cystic lesions and, specifically, IPMNs and will impact proper patient management. Radiomics has so far demonstrated a great potential for diagnosis, prognosis, and risk evaluation in pancreatic neoplastic cysts, providing prognostic and predictive biomarkers. However, it is still a novel technique and has been used to date mainly for clinical trials in academic centers. Protocol standardization is challenging as it may affect all steps of image analysis [81].

12. Conclusions

IPMNs are classified into three subtypes MD-IPMN, BD-IPMN, and mixed-type. Each subtype has different clinical/imaging presentation and management strategies, which further adds to the diagnostic complexity. The management of IPMN is dependent on risk stratification based on various factors including size, extension, and the presence of dysplasia. Imaging ambiguity remains a challenge in both diagnosis and further stratification of this entity. Advances in radiomics are expected to provide tumor-specific treatment strategies and optimize patient management in the future.

It is of utmost importance for radiologists to be familiar with current guidelines and to participate in multidisciplinary meetings, as each case requires a tailored approach and personalized treatment might be offered. There is a great need to reduce the rate of futile surgeries without missing the therapeutic window in selected cases. Radiologists will have an increasing role in the chain of patient management and should adapt new techniques in their daily clinical practice. Precise diagnosis should also contain detailed information including proposing prognostic and predictive imaging biomarkers and providing guidance for the best patient treatment.

Author Contributions: Conceptualization, C.T. and S.G.; methodology, C.T., S.G., D.K. and S.D.; literature research, S.G. and D.K.; resources, C.T.; writing—original draft preparation, C.T., S.G. and D.K.; writing—review and editing, C.T., S.G., D.K. and S.D.; supervision, C.T. and S.D. All authors have read and agreed to the published version of the manuscript.

Funding: This research received no external funding.

Institutional Review Board Statement: Ethical review and approval were waived for this study due to the study type (review).

Informed Consent Statement: Not applicable (review).

Data Availability Statement: No new data were created or analyzed in this study. Data sharing is not applicable to this review article.

Conflicts of Interest: The authors declare no conflict of interest.

References

1. Chang, Y.R.; Park, J.K.; Jang, J.Y.; Kwon, W.; Yoon, J.H.; Kim, S.W. Incidental pancreatic cystic neoplasms in an asymptomatic healthy population of 21,745 individuals: Large-scale, single-center cohort study. *Medicine* **2016**, *95*, e5535. [CrossRef]
2. Matos, C.; Baleato, S. Ducts. In *Clinical MRI of the Abdomen Why, How, When*; Gourtsoyiannis, N., Ed.; Springer: Berlin, Germany, 2011.
3. Fasanella, K.E.; McGrath, K. Cystic lesions and intraductal neoplasms of the pancreas. *Best Pract. Res. Clin. Gastroenterol.* **2009**, *23*, 35–48. [CrossRef]
4. Tanaka, M.; Fernández-Del Castillo, C.; Kamisawa, T.; Jang, J.Y.; Levy, P.; Ohtsuka, T.; Salvia, R.; Shimizu, Y.; Tada, M.; Wolfgang, C.L. Revisions of international consensus Fukuoka guidelines for the management of IPMN of the pancreas. *Pancreatology* **2017**, *17*, 738–753. [CrossRef] [PubMed]
5. Taouli, B.; Vilgrain, V.; Vullierme, M.-P.; Terris, B.; Denys, A.; Sauvanet, A.; Hammel, P.; Menu, Y. Intraductal papillary mucinous tumors of the pancreas: Helical CT with histopathologic correlation. *Radiology* **2000**, *217*, 757–764. [CrossRef] [PubMed]
6. Zhou, H.; Li, X.; Wang, Y.; Wang, Z.; Zhu, J.; Wang, Z.; Chen, X. Threshold of main pancreatic duct for malignancy in intraductal papillary mucinous neoplasm at head-neck and body-tail. *BMC Gastroenterol.* **2022**, *22*, 473. [CrossRef] [PubMed]
7. Yoon, L.S.; Catalano, O.A.; Fritz, S.; Ferrone, C.R.; Hahn, P.F.; Sahani, D.V. Another dimension in magnetic resonance cholangiopancreatography: Comparison of 2- and 3-dimensional magnetic resonance cholangiopancreatography for the evaluation of intraductal papillary mucinous neoplasm of the pancreas. *J. Comput. Assist. Tomogr.* **2009**, *33*, 363–368. [CrossRef]
8. Boraschi, P.; Scalise, P.; Casotti, M.T.; Kauffmann, E.F.; Boggi, U.; Donati, F. Cystic Lesions of the Pancreas: Is Apparent Diffusion Coefficient Value Useful at 3 T Magnetic Resonance Imaging? *J. Comput. Assist. Tomogr.* **2022**, *46*, 363–370. [CrossRef]
9. Sotozono, H.; Kanki, A.; Yasokawa, K.; Yamamoto, A.; Sanai, H.; Moriya, K.; Tamada, T. Value of 3-T MR imaging in intraductal papillary mucinous neoplasm with a concomitant invasive carcinoma. *Eur. Radiol.* **2022**, *32*, 8276–8284. [CrossRef]
10. Yamada, D.; Kobayashi, S.; Takahashi, H.; Yoshioka, T.; Iwagami, Y.; Tomimaru, Y.; Shigekawa, M.; Akita, H.; Noda, T.; Asaoka, T.; et al. Pancreatic CT density is an optimal imaging biomarker for earlier detection of malignancy in the pancreas with intraductal papillary mucinous neoplasm. *Pancreatology* **2022**, *22*, 488–496. [CrossRef]
11. Lee, J.E.; Choi, S.-Y.; Min, J.H.; Yi, B.H.; Lee, M.H.; Kim, S.S.; Hwang, J.A.; Kim, J.H. Determining Malignant Potential of Intraductal Papillary Mucinous Neoplasm of the Pancreas: CT versus MRI by Using Revised 2017 International Consensus Guidelines. *Radiology* **2019**, *293*, 134–143. [CrossRef]
12. Min, J.H.; Kim, Y.K.; Kim, S.K.; Kim, H.; Ahn, S. Intraductal papillary mucinous neoplasm of the pancreas: Diagnostic performance of the 2017 international consensus guidelines using CT and MRI. *Eur. Radiol.* **2021**, *31*, 4774–4784. [CrossRef] [PubMed]
13. Yamashita, Y.I.; Okabe, H.; Hayashi, H.; Imai, K.; Nakagawa, S.; Nakao, Y.; Yusa, T.; Itoyama, R.; Yama, T.; Umesaki, N.; et al. Usefulness of 18-FDG PET/CT in Detecting Malignancy in Intraductal Papillary Mucinous Neoplasms of the Pancreas. *Anticancer Res.* **2019**, *39*, 2493–2499. [CrossRef] [PubMed]

14. Srinivasan, N.; Koh, Y.X.; Goh, B.K. Systematic review of the utility of 18-FDG PET in the preoperative evaluation of IPMNs and cystic lesions of the pancreas. *Surgery* **2019**, *165*, 929–937. [CrossRef] [PubMed]
15. Liu, H.; Cui, Y.; Shao, J.; Shao, Z.; Su, F.; Li, Y. The diagnostic role of CT, MRI/MRCP, PET/CT, EUS and DWI in the differentiation of benign and malignant IPMN: A meta-analysis. *Clin. Imaging* **2021**, *72*, 183–193. [CrossRef]
16. Koizumi, M.; Sata, N.; Yoshizawa, K.; Tsukahara, M.; Kurihara, K.; Yasuda, Y.; Nagai, H. PostERCP pancreatogastric fistula associated with an intraductal papillary-mucinous neoplasm of the pancreas—A case report and literature review. *World J. Surg. Oncol.* **2005**, *3*, 70. [CrossRef]
17. Okada, K.-I.; Furuuchi, T.; Tamada, T.; Sasaki, T.; Suwa, T.; Shatari, T.; Takenaka, Y.; Hori, M.; Sakuma, M. Pancreatobiliary fistula associated with an intraductal papillary-mucinous pancreatic neoplasm manifesting as obstructive jaundice: Report of a case. *Surg. Today* **2008**, *38*, 371–376. [CrossRef]
18. Jung, I.S.; Shim, C.S.; Cheon, Y.K.; Bhandari, S.; Cha, S.W.; Moon, J.H.; Cho, Y.D.; Kim, J.H.; Kim, Y.S.; Lee, M.S.; et al. Invasive intraductal papillary mucinous tumor of the pancreas with simultaneous invasion of the stomach and duodenum. *Endoscopy* **2004**, *36*, 186–189. [CrossRef]
19. Jausset, M.F.; Delvaux, D.; Dumitriu, A.; Bressenot, O.; Bruot, J.; Mathias, D.; Regent, V.; Laurent, V. Benign Intraductal Papillary-MucinousNeoplasm of the Pancreas Associated with Spontaneous Pancreaticogastric and Pancreaticoduodenal Fistulas. *Digestion* **2010**, *82*, 42–46. [CrossRef]
20. Rosenberger, L.H.; Stein, L.; Witkiewicz, A.K.; Kennedy, E.P.; Yeo, C.J. Intraductal papillary mucinous neoplasm (IPMN) with extra-pancreatic mucin: A case series and review of the literature. *J. Gastrointest. Surg.* **2012**, *16*, 762–770. [CrossRef]
21. Yamada, Y.; Mori, H.; Hijiya, N.; Matsumoto, S.; Takaji, R.; Ohta, M.; Kitano, S.; Moriyama, M. Intraductal papillary mucinous neoplasms of the pancreas complicated with intraductal hemorrhage, perforation, and fistula formation: CT and MR imaging findings with pathologic correlation. *Abdom. Imaging* **2012**, *37*, 100–109. [CrossRef]
22. Venkatesh, P.G.; Navaneethan, U.; Vege, S.S. Intraductal papillary mucinous neoplasm and acute pancreatitis. *J. Clin. Gastroenterol.* **2011**, *45*, 755–758. [CrossRef] [PubMed]
23. Poultsides, G.A.; Reddy, S.; Cameron, J.L.; Hruban, R.H.; Pawlik, T.M.; Ahuja, N.; Jain, A.; Edil, B.H.; Iacobuzio-Donahue, C.A.; Schulick, R.D.; et al. Histopathologic basis for the favorable survival afterresection of intraductal papillary mucinous neoplasm-associated invasive adenocarcinoma of the pancreas. *Ann. Surg.* **2010**, *251*, 470–476. [CrossRef] [PubMed]
24. Muraki, T.; Jang, K.T.; Reid, M.D.; Pehlivanoglu, B.; Memis, B.; Basturk, O.; Mittal, P.; Kooby, D.; Maithel, S.K.; Sarmiento, J.M.; et al. Pancreatic ductal adenocarcinomas associated with intraductalpapillary mucinous neoplasms (IPMNs) versus pseudo-IPMNs:relative frequency, clinicopathologic characteristics anddifferential diagnosis. *Mod. Pathol.* **2022**, *35*, 96–105. [CrossRef]
25. European Study Group on Cystic Tumors of the Pancreas. European evidence-based guidelines on pancreatic cystic neoplasms. *Gut* **2018**, *67*, 789–804. [CrossRef]
26. Vege, S.S.; Ziring, B.; Jain, R.; Moayyedi, P.; Adams, M.A.; Dorn, S.D.; Dudley-Brown, S.L.; Flamm, S.L.; Gellad, Z.F.; Gruss, C.B.; et al. American gastroenterological association institute guideline on the diagnosis and management of asymptomatic neoplastic pancreatic cysts. *Gastroenterology* **2015**, *148*, 819–822. [CrossRef] [PubMed]
27. Sahora, K.; Mino-Kenudson, M.; Brugge, W.; Thayer, S.P.; Ferrone, C.R.; Sahani, D.; Pitman, M.B.; Warshaw, A.L.; Lillemoe, K.D.; Fernandez-del Castillo, C.F. Branch duct intraductal papillary mucinous neoplasms: Does cyst size change the tip of the scale? A critical analysis of the revised international consensus guidelines in a large single-institutional series. *Ann. Surg.* **2013**, *258*, 466–475. [CrossRef]
28. Sahora, K.; Fernández-del Castillo, C.; Dong, F.; Marchegiani, G.; Thayer, S.P.; Ferrone, C.R.; Sahani, D.V.; Brugge, W.R.; Warshaw, A.L.; Lillemoe, K.D.; et al. Not all mixed-type intraductal papillary mucinous neoplasms behave like main-duct lesions: Implications of minimal involvement of the main pancreatic duct. *Surgery* **2014**, *156*, 611–621. [CrossRef]
29. Shin, S.H.; Han, D.J.; Park, K.T.; Kim, Y.H.; Park, J.B.; Kim, S.C. Validating a simple scoring system to predict malignancy and invasiveness of intraductal papillary mucinous neoplasms of the pancreas. *World J. Surg.* **2010**, *34*, 776–783. [CrossRef]
30. Wu, J.; Matthaei, H.; Maitra, A.; Dal Molin, M.; Wood, L.D.; Eshleman, J.R.; Goggins, M.; Canto, M.I.; Schulick, R.D.; Edil, B.H.; et al. Recurrent GNAS mutations define an unexpected pathway for pancreatic cyst development. *Sci. Transl. Med.* **2011**, *3*, 92ra66. [CrossRef]
31. Singhi, A.D.; Nikiforova, M.N.; Fasanella, K.E.; McGrath, K.M.; Pai, R.K.; Ohori, N.P.; Bartholow, T.L.; Brand, R.E.; Chennat, J.S.; Lu, X.; et al. Preoperative GNAS and KRAS testing in the diagnosis of pancreatic mucinous cysts. *Clin. Cancer Res.* **2014**, *20*, 4381–4389. [CrossRef]
32. Genevay, M.; Mino-Kenudson, M.; Yaeger, K.; Konstantinidis, I.T.; Ferrone, C.R.; Thayer, S.; Castillo, C.F.-D.; Sahani, D.; Bounds, B.; Forcione, D.; et al. Cytology adds value to imaging studies for risk assessment of malignancy in pancreatic mucinous cysts. *Ann. Surg.* **2011**, *254*, 977–983. [CrossRef] [PubMed]
33. Pulvirenti, A.; Pea, A.; Rezaee, N.; Gasparini, C.; Malleo, G.; Weiss, M.J.; Cameron, J.L.; Wolfgang, C.L.; He, J.; Salvia, R. Perioperative outcomes and long-term quality of life after total pancreatectomy. *J. Br. Surg.* **2019**, *106*, 1819–1828. [CrossRef] [PubMed]
34. Seiko Hirono and Hiroki Yamaue. Surgical strategy for intraductal papillary mucinous neoplasms of the pancreas. *Surg. Today* **2020**, *50*, 50–55. [CrossRef] [PubMed]

35. Stoop, T.F.; Ateeb, Z.; Ghorbani, P.; Scholten, L.; Arnelo, U.; Besselink, M.G.; Del Chiaro, M. Surgical outcomes after total pancreatectomy:a high-volume center experience. *Ann. Surg. Oncol.* **2021**, *28*, 1543–1551. [CrossRef]
36. Pollini, T.; Andrianello, S.; Caravati, A.; Perri, G.; Malleo, G.; Paiella, S.; Marchegiani, G.; Salvia, R. The management of intraductal papillary mucinous neoplasms of the pancreas. *Minerva Chir.* **2019**, *74*, 414–421. [CrossRef]
37. Remotti, H.E.; Winner, M.; Saif, M.W. Intraductal papillary mucinous neoplasms of the pancreas: Clinical surveillance and malignant progression, multifocality and implications of a Field-Defect. *JOP J. Pancreas* **2012**, *13*, 135–138.
38. Kaiser, J.; Fritz, S.; Klauss, M.; Bergmann, F.; Hinz, U.; Strobel, O.; Schneider, L.; Büchler, M.W.; Hackert, T. Enucleation: A treatment alternative for branch duct intraductal papillary mucinous neoplasms. *Surgery* **2017**, *161*, 602–610. [CrossRef]
39. Avula, L.R.; Hagerty, B.; Alewine, C. Molecular mediators of peritoneal metastasis in pancreatic cancer. *Cancer Metastasis Rev.* **2020**, *39*, 1223–1243. [CrossRef]
40. Choi, S.H.; Park, S.H.; Kim, K.W.; Lee, J.Y.; Lee, S.S. Progression of unresected intraductal papillary mucinous neoplasms of the pancreas to cancer: A systematic review and meta-analysis. *Clin. Gastroenterol. Hepatol.* **2017**, *15*, 1509–1520. [CrossRef]
41. Imaoka, H.; Yamao, K.; Hijioka, S.; Hara, K.; Mizuno, N.; Tanaka, T.; Kondo, S.; Tajika, M.; Shimizu, Y.; Niwa, Y. Pseudomyxoma peritonei arising from intraductal papillary neoplasm after surgical pancreatectomy: Report of 2 cases and review of the literature. *Clin. J. Gastroenterol.* **2012**, *5*, 15–19. [CrossRef]
42. Stoop, T.F.; Ateeb, Z.; Ghorbani, P.; Scholten, L.; Arnelo, U.; Besselink, M.G.; Del Chiaro, M. Impact of endocrine and exocrine insufficiency on quality of life after total pancreatectomy. *Ann. Surg. Oncol.* **2020**, *27*, 587–596. [CrossRef] [PubMed]
43. Scholten, L.; Latenstein, A.E.; van Eijck, C.; Erdmann, J.; van der Harst, E.; Mieog, J.S.D.; Molenaar, I.Q.; van Santvoort, H.C.; DeVries, J.H.; Besselink, M.G.; et al. Outcome and long-term quality of life aftertotal pancreatectomy (PANORAMA): A nationwide cohort study. *Surgery* **2019**, *166*, 1017–1026. [CrossRef] [PubMed]
44. Nara, S.; Shimada, K.; Sakamoto, Y.; Esaki, M.; Kosuge, T.; Hiraoka, N. Clinical significance of frozen section analysis duringresection of intraductal papillary mucinous neoplasm: Should a positive pancreatic margin for adenoma or borderline lesion be resected additionally? *J. Am. Coll. Surg.* **2009**, *209*, 614–621. [CrossRef] [PubMed]
45. Takeda, Y.; Imamura, H.; Yoshimoto, J.; Fukumura, Y.; Yoshioka, R.; Mise, Y.; Kawasaki, S.; Saiura, A. Survival comparison of invasive intraductal papillary mucinous neoplasm versus pancreatic ductal adenocarcinoma. *Surgery* **2022**, *172*, 336–342. [CrossRef] [PubMed]
46. Assarzadegan, N.; Babaniamansour, S.; Shi, J. Updates in the Diagnosis of Intraductal Neoplasms of the Pancreas. *Front. Physiol.* **2022**, *13*, 856803. [CrossRef] [PubMed]
47. Amini, N.; Habib, J.R.; Blair, A.; Rezaee, N.; Kinny-Köster, B.; Cameron, J.L.; Hruban, R.H.; Weiss, M.J.; Fishman, E.K.; Lafaro, K.J.; et al. Invasive and non-invasive progression after resection of non-invasive intraductal papillary mucinous neoplasms. *Ann. Surg.* **2022**, *272*, 370–377. [CrossRef] [PubMed]
48. Rezaee, N.; Barbon, C.; Zaki, A.; He, J.; Salman, B.; Hruban, R.H.; Cameron, J.L.; Herman, J.M.; Ahuja, N.; Lennon, A.M.; et al. Intraductal papillary mucinous neoplasm (IPMN) with high-grade dysplasia is a risk factor for the subsequent development of pancreatic ductal adenocarcinoma. *HPB* **2016**, *18*, 236–246. [CrossRef]
49. Law, J.K.; Wolfgang, C.L.; Weiss, M.J.; Lennon, A.M. Concomitant pancreatic adenocarcinoma in a patient with branch-duct intraductal papillary mucinous neoplasm. *World J. Gastroenterol.* **2014**, *20*, 9200–9204.
50. Kamisawa, T.; Tu, Y.; Egawa, N.; Nakajima, H.; Tsuruta, K.; Okamoto, A. Malignancies associated with intraductal papillary mucinous neoplasm of the pancreas. *World J. Gastroenterol.* **2005**, *11*, 5688–5690. [CrossRef]
51. Yamaguchi, K.; Kanemitsu, S.; Hatori, T.; Maguchi, H.; Shimizu, Y.; Tada, M.; Nakagohri, T.; Hanada, K.; Osanai, M.; Noda, Y.; et al. Pancreatic ductal adenocarcinoma derived from IPMN and pancreatic ductal adenocarcinoma concomitant with IPMN. *Pancreas* **2011**, *40*, 571–580. [CrossRef]
52. Yamaguchi, K.; Ohuchida, J.; Ohtsuka, T.; Nakano, K.; Tanaka, M. Intraductal papillary-mucinous tumor of the pancreas concomitant with ductal carcinoma of the pancreas. *Pancreatology* **2002**, *2*, 484–490. [CrossRef] [PubMed]
53. Tamura, K.; Ohtsuka, T.; Ideno, N.; Aso, T.; Kono, H.; Nagayoshi, Y.; Shindo, K.; Ushijima, Y.; Ueda, J.; Takahata, S.; et al. Unresectable pancreatic ductal adenocarcinoma in the remnant pancreas diagnosed during every-6-month surveillance after resection of branch duct intraductal papillary mucinous neoplasm: A case report. *JOP J. Pancreas* **2013**, *14*, 450–453.
54. Sawai, Y.; Yamao, K.; Bhatia, V.; Chiba, T.; Mizuno, N.; Sawaki, A.; Takahashi, K.; Tajika, M.; Shimizu, Y.; Yatabe, Y.; et al. Development of pancreatic cancers during long-term follow-up of side-branch intraductal papillary mucinous neoplasms. *Endoscopy* **2010**, *42*, 1077–1084. [CrossRef] [PubMed]
55. Tada, M.; Kawabe, T.; Arizumi, M.; Togawa, O.; Matsubara, S.; Yamamoto, N.; Nakai, Y.; Sasahira, N.; Hirano, K.; Tsujino, T.; et al. Pancreatic cancer in patients with pancreatic cystic lesions: A prospective study in 197 patients. *Clin. Gastroenterol. Hepatol.* **2006**, *4*, 1265–1270. [CrossRef]
56. Yamaguchi, K.; Nakamura, K.; Yokohata, K.; Shimizu, S.; Chijiiwa, K.; Tanaka, M. Pancreatic cyst as a sentinel of in situ carcinoma of the pancreas. Report of two cases. *Int. J. Pancreatol.* **1997**, *22*, 227–231. [CrossRef]
57. Uehara, H.; Nakaizumi, A.; Ishikawa, O.; Iishi, H.; Tatsumi, K.; Takakura, R.; Ishida, T.; Takano, Y.; Tanaka, S.; Takenaka, A. Development of ductal carcinoma of the pancreas during follow-up of branch duct intraductal papillary mucinous neoplasm of the pancreas. *Gut* **2008**, *57*, 1561–1565. [CrossRef]

58. Tanno, S.; Nakano, Y.; Koizumi, K.; Sugiyama, Y.; Nakamura, K.; Sasajima, J.; Nishikawa, T.; Mizukami, Y.; Yanagawa, N.; Fujii, T.; et al. Pancreatic ductal adenocarcinomas in long-term follow-up patients with branch duct intraductal papillary mucinous neoplasms. *Pancreas* 2010, *39*, 36–40. [CrossRef]
59. Tanaka, M. International consensus on the management of intraductal papillary mucinous neoplasm of the pancreas. *Ann. Transl. Med.* 2015, *3*, 286.
60. Larghi, A.; Stobinski, M.; Galasso, D.; Lecca, P.G.; Costamagna, G. Concomitant intraductal papillary mucinous neoplasm and pancreatic endocrine tumour: Report of two cases and review of the literature. *Dig. Liver Dis.* 2009, *41*, 759–761. [CrossRef]
61. Goh, B.K.; Ooi, L.L.; Kumarasinghe, M.P.; Tan, Y.M.; Peng-Cheow, C.; Chow, P.K.; Chung, F.Y.A.; Wai-Wong, K. Clinicopathological features of patients with concomitant intraductal papillary mucinous neoplasm of the pancreas and pancreatic endocrine neoplasm. *Pancreatology* 2006, *6*, 520–526. [CrossRef]
62. Zhao, X.; Stabile, B.E.; Mo, J.; Wang, J.; French, S.W. Nesidioblastosis coexisting with islet cell tumor and intraductal papillary mucinous hyperplasia. *Arch. Pathol. Lab. Med.* 2001, *125*, 1344–1347. [CrossRef]
63. Marrache, F.; Cazals-Hatem, D.; Kianmanesh, R.; Palazzo, L.; Couveland, A.; O'Toole, D.; Maire, F.; Hammel, P.; Levy, P.; Sauvanet, A.; et al. Endocrine tumor and intraductal papillary mucinous neoplasm of the pancreas: A fortuitous association? *Pancreas* 2005, *31*, 79–83. [CrossRef] [PubMed]
64. Terada, T.; Ohta, T.; Kitamura, Y.; Ashida, K.; Matsunaga, Y.; Kato, M. Endocrine cells in intraductal papillary-mucinous neoplasms of the pancreas. A histochemical and immunohistochemical study. *Virchows Arch.* 1997, *431*, 31–36. [CrossRef] [PubMed]
65. Hashimoto, Y.; Murakami, Y.; Uemura, K.; Hayashidani, Y.; Sudo, T.; Ohge, H.; Sueda, T.; Shimamoto, F.; Hiyama, E. Mixed ductal-endocrine carcinoma derived from intraductal papillary mucinous neoplasm (IPMN) of the pancreas identified by human telomerase reverse transcriptase (hTERT) expression. *J. Surg. Oncol.* 2008, *97*, 469–475. [CrossRef] [PubMed]
66. Kadota, Y.; Shinoda, M.; Tanabe, M.; Tsujikawa, H.; Ueno, A.; Masugi, Y.; Oshima, G.; Nishiyama, R.; Tanaka, M.; Mihara, K.; et al. Concomitant pancreatic endocrine neoplasm and intraductal papillary mucinous neoplasm: A case report and literature review. *World J. Surg. Oncol.* 2013, *11*, 75. [CrossRef]
67. Konjeti, V.R.; McCarty, T.R.; Rustagi, T. Needle-based Confocal Laser Endomicroscopy (nCLE) for Evaluation of Pancreatic Cystic Lesions: A Systematic Review and Meta-analysis. *J. Clin. Gastroenterol.* 2020, *56*, 72–80. [CrossRef] [PubMed]
68. Krishna, S.G.; Hart, P.A.; DeWitt, J.M.; DiMaio, C.J.; Kongkam, P.; Napoleon, B.; Othman, M.O.; Yew Tan, D.M.; Strobel, S.G.; Stanich, P.P.; et al. EUS-guided confocal laserendomicroscopy: Prediction of dysplasia in intraductal papillary mucinous neoplasms (with video). *Gastrointest. Endosc.* 2020, *91*, 551–563. [CrossRef] [PubMed]
69. Machicado, J.D.; Chao, W.-L.; Carlyn, D.E.; Pan, T.-Y.; Poland, S.; Alexander, V.L.; Maloof, T.G.; Dubay, K.; Ueltschi, O.; Middendorf, D.M.; et al. High performance in risk stratification of intraductal papillary mucinous neoplasms by confocal laser endomicroscopy image analysis with convolutional neural networks (with video). *Gastrointest. Endosc.* 2021, *94*, 78–87. [CrossRef]
70. McCarty, T.R.; Paleti, S.; Rustagi, T. Molecular analysis of EUS-acquired pancreatic cyst fluid for KRAS and GNAS mutations for diagnosis of intraductal papillary mucinous neoplasia and mucinous cystic lesions: A systematic review and meta-analysis. *Gastrointest. Endosc.* 2021, *93*, 1019–1033. [CrossRef]
71. Ren, R.; Krishna, S.G.; Chen, W.; Frankel, W.L.; Shen, R.; Zhao, W.; Avenarius, M.R.; Garee, J.; Caruthers, S.; Jones, D. Activation of the RAS pathway through uncommon BRAF mutations in mucinous pancreatic cysts without KRAS mutation. *Mod. Pathol.* 2021, *34*, 438–444. [CrossRef]
72. Singhi, A.D.; McGrath, K.; Brand, R.E.; Khalid, A.; Zeh, H.J.; Chennat, J.S.; Fasanella, K.E.; Papachristou, G.I.; Slivka, A.; Bartlett, D.L.; et al. Preoperative next-generation sequencing of pancreatic cyst fluid is highly accurate in cyst classification and detection of advanced neoplasia. *Gut* 2018, *67*, 2131–2141. [CrossRef]
73. Lekkerkerker, S.J.; Besselink, M.G.; Busch, O.R.; Verheij, J.; Engelbrecht, M.R.; Rauws, E.A.; Fockens, P.; van Hooft, J.E. Comparing 3 guidelines on the management of surgically removed pancreatic cysts with regard to pathological outcome. *Gastrointest. Endosc.* 2017, *85*, 1025–1031. [CrossRef]
74. Gillies, R.J.; Kinahan, P.E.; Hricak, H. Radiomics: Images Are More than Pictures, They Are Data. *Radiology* 2016, *278*, 563–577. [CrossRef] [PubMed]
75. Hanania, A.N.; Bantis, L.E.; Feng, Z.; Wang, H.; Tamm, E.P.; Katz, M.H.; Maitra, A.; Koay, E.J. Quantitative imaging to evaluate malignant potential of IPMNs. *Oncotarget* 2016, *7*, 85776–85784. [CrossRef] [PubMed]
76. Permuth, J.B.; Choi, J.; Balarunathan, Y.; Kim, J.; Chen, D.T.; Chen, L.; Orcutt, S.; Doepker, M.P.; Gage, K.; Zhang, G.; et al. Combining radiomic features with a miRNA classifier may improve prediction of malignant pathology for pancreatic intraductal papillary mucinous neoplasms. *Oncotarget* 2016, *7*, 85785–85797. [CrossRef]
77. Attiyeh, M.A.; Chakraborty, J.; Gazit, L.; Langdon-Embry, L.; Gonen, M.; Balachandran, V.P.; D'Angelica, M.I.; DeMatteo, R.P.; Jarnagin, W.R.; Kingham, T.P.; et al. Preoperative risk prediction for intraductal papillary mucinous neoplasms by quantitative CT image analysis. *HPB* 2019, *21*, 212–218. [CrossRef] [PubMed]
78. Hoffman, D.H.; Ream, J.M.; Hajdu, C.H.; Rosenkrantz, A.B. Utility of whole-lesion ADC histogram metrics for assessing the malignant potential of pancreatic intraductal papillary mucinous neoplasms (IPMNs). *Abdom. Radiol.* 2017, *42*, 1222–1228. [CrossRef]
79. Cui, S.; Tang, T.; Su, Q.; Wang, Y.; Shu, Z.; Yang, W.; Gong, X. Radiomic nomogram based on MRI to predict grade of branching type intraductal papillary mucinous neoplasms of the pancreas: A multicenter study. *Cancer Imaging* 2021, *21*, 26. [CrossRef]

80. Tobaly, D.; Santinha, J.; Sartoris, R.; Dioguardi Burgio, M.; Matos, C.; Cros, J.; Couvelard, A.; Rebours, V.; Sauvanet, A.; Ronot, M.; et al. CT-Based Radiomics Analysis to Predict Malignancyin Patients with Intraductal Papillary MucinousNeoplasm (IPMN) of the Pancreas. *Cancers* **2020**, *12*, 3089. [CrossRef] [PubMed]
81. Cheng, S.; Shi, H.; Lu, M.; Wang, C.; Duan, S.; Xu, Q.; Shi, H. Radiomics Analysis for PredictingMalignant Potential of IntraductalPapillary Mucinous Neoplasms of thePancreas: Comparison of CT and MRI. *Acad. Radiol* **2022**, *29*, 367–375. [CrossRef]

Disclaimer/Publisher's Note: The statements, opinions and data contained in all publications are solely those of the individual author(s) and contributor(s) and not of MDPI and/or the editor(s). MDPI and/or the editor(s) disclaim responsibility for any injury to people or property resulting from any ideas, methods, instructions or products referred to in the content.

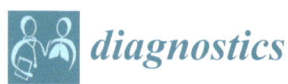

Review

Rare Solid Pancreatic Lesions on Cross-Sectional Imaging

Ana Veron Sanchez [1,*], Nuria Santamaria Guinea [2], Silvia Cayon Somacarrera [3], Ilias Bennouna [1], Martina Pezzullo [4] and Maria Antonietta Bali [1]

[1] Hôpital Universitaire de Bruxelles, Institut Jules Bordet, 1070 Brussels, Belgium; ilias.bennouna@hubruxelles.be (I.B.)
[2] Clatterbridge Cancer Centre, Liverpool L7 8YA, UK
[3] Hospital Universitario Marques de Valdecilla, 39008 Santander, Spain
[4] Hôpital Universitaire de Bruxelles, Hôpital Erasme, 1070 Brussels, Belgium
* Correspondence: ana.veron@hubruxelles.be

Abstract: Several solid lesions can be found within the pancreas mainly arising from the exocrine and endocrine pancreatic tissue. Among all pancreatic malignancies, the most common subtype is pancreatic ductal adenocarcinoma (PDAC), to a point that pancreatic cancer and PDAC are used interchangeably. But, in addition to PDAC, and to the other most common and well-known solid lesions, either related to benign conditions, such as pancreatitis, or not so benign, such as pancreatic neuroendocrine neoplasms (pNENs), there are solid pancreatic lesions considered rare due to their low incidence. These lesions may originate from a cell line with a differentiation other than exocrine/endocrine, such as from the nerve sheath as for pancreatic schwannoma or from mesenchymal cells as for solitary fibrous tumour. These rare solid pancreatic lesions may show a behaviour that ranges in a benign to highly aggressive malignant spectrum. This review includes cases of an intrapancreatic accessory spleen, pancreatic tuberculosis, solid serous cystadenoma, solid pseudopapillary tumour, pancreatic schwannoma, purely intraductal neuroendocrine tumour, pancreatic fibrous solitary tumour, acinar cell carcinoma, undifferentiated carcinoma with osteoclastic-like giant cells, adenosquamous carcinoma, colloid carcinoma of the pancreas, primary leiomyosarcoma of the pancreas, primary and secondary pancreatic lymphoma and metastases within the pancreas. Therefore, it is important to determine the correct diagnosis to ensure optimal patient management. Because of their rarity, their existence is less well known and, when depicted, in most cases incidentally, the correct diagnosis remains challenging. However, there are some typical imaging features present on cross-sectional imaging modalities that, taken into account with the clinical and biological context, contribute substantially to achieve the correct diagnosis.

Keywords: pancreas; solid; rare

1. Introduction

In addition to the most common solid pancreatic lesions related to benign conditions, such as chronic pancreatitis, or to malignancy mainly represented by PDAC and pNENs, there are several rare pancreatic solid lesions that can be very challenging to correctly diagnose due to knowledge scarcity secondary to their very low incidence.

A variety of epithelial tumours may arise within the pancreas, with ductal, acinar and neuroendocrine differentiation. In addition, most of the mesenchymal tumours found in extrapancreatic locations may also arise within the pancreas. However, in cases such as the solid pseudopapillary neoplasm, there is no defined cell lineage identified.

These lesions can present a benign, potentially malignant and malignant behaviour and may show typical and atypical imaging features on cross-sectional imaging modalities. Combining these imaging findings with epidemiological, clinical and biological data may contribute to achieving the correct diagnosis.

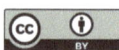

Table 1 reports the rare solid pancreatic lesions classified in three sections based on their behaviour: benign, potentially malignant and malignant.

Table 1. Classification of rare solid pancreatic lesions.

Benign	Potentially Malignant	Malignant
Intrapancreatic splenic tissue	Solid pseudopapillary tumour	Acinar cell carcinoma
Tuberculosis	Schwannoma	Undifferentiated carcinoma with osteoclastic-like giant cells.
Solid serous cystadenoma	Purely intraductal neuroendocrine tumour	Adenosquamous carcinoma
	Fibrous solitary tumour	Colloid carcinoma
		Primary leiomyosarcoma
		Lymphoma (primary and secondary)
		Metastases

Due to their rarity, statistical data regarding the incidence and prevalence are not easy to find and published literature about these pancreatic lesions mainly consists of case reports or series. Table 2 reports incidence/prevalence data of these rare solid pancreatic lesions. Therefore, the aim of this pictorial review is to gather rare solid lesions that can be encountered in the pancreas and describe the cross-sectional imaging features, highlighting their respective hallmarks, with a focus on differential diagnosis and on patient management.

Table 2. No. of cases/incidence/prevalence of rare solid pancreatic lesions depicted.

Rare Solid Pancreatic Lesions	No. of Cases/Incidence/Prevalence
Intrapancreatic splenic tissue	61 cases/3000 autopsies
Tuberculosis	116 cases
Solid serous cystadenoma	22 cases
Solid pseudopapillary tumour	2% of all exocrine pancreatic neoplasms
Schwannoma	<80 cases reported
Purely intraductal neuroendocrine tumour	7 cases reported
Fibrous solitary tumour	29 cases reported
Acinar cell carcinoma	<2% of all primary pancreatic neoplasms
Undifferentiated carcinoma with osteoclasic-like giant cells	<1% of all malignant pancreatic neoplasms
Adenosquamous carcinoma	0.38–10% prevalence
Colloid carcinoma	1% of all pancreatic tumours
Primary leiomyosarcoma	0.1% of malignant pancreatic neoplasms
Primary lymphoma	<0.5% of all primary pancreatic neoplasms, 1% of all extranodal lymphomas
Secondary lymphoma	30% cases of extranodal lymphoma
Metastases	2–5% of pancreatic malignancies

Concerning image acquisition, it is crucial to note the importance of including a pancreatic parenchymal phase, obtained 35–40 s after intravenous contrast administration, as it ensures a relatively increased enhancement of the pancreatic parenchyma and shows higher differences in attenuation between normal parenchyma and hypovascular tumours, as well as allowing assessment of arteries [1]. This parenchymal phase is followed by a portal venous phase, obtained at 70 s, to assess the veins, as venous flow artifacts observed in the pancreatic phase will be avoided [1]. In addition, hepatic enhancement will be increased and metastases will be detected more easily. Dynamic study finishes with a delayed venous phase, at 180 s.

2. Benign Lesions (Table S1)

2.1. Intrapancreatic Splenic Tissue (Figure 1)

Intrapancreatic splenic tissue (IPST) may occur under the form of accessory spleen or splenosis. Accessory spleens are congenital abnormalities, in which the earliest forms of spleen fail to fuse during the fifth week of embryonic life [2] and are usually located next to their embryonic origin or along their migration path [3]. Splenosis, though, is an acquired condition, in which a heterotopic transplantation of splenic tissue takes place [4], frequently after spleen surgery or trauma. It can be found anywhere throughout the abdomen, the pelvis and even the chest [5], although it occurs most frequently in the liver [6] and is rare within the pancreas [7]. Sixty-one accessory spleens were found within the pancreatic tail in a 3000-patient autopsy study [8].

The pancreatic tail is a preferred IPST location, either in the form of IPAS or splenosis [9] and it has been described as the second most common site of accessory spleen [10].

IPST commonly appears incidentally on cross-sectional techniques as a well-defined nodule, presenting clear demarcated borders with the adjacent parenchyma. It shows the same signal intensity as the spleen, with the same behaviour following intravenous contrast administration, heterogeneously enhancing in a zebra-pattern, during the arterial phase [11] due to different flow rate of contrast through the red and white pulp [12], and becoming homogeneous during the portal phase. However, this heterogeneous enhancement may be missing, especially in small lesions [11]. An elevated signal intensity in diffusion-weighted images (DWIs) using a high b-value is also suggestive of IPST [13]. IPST may grow and potentially mimic malignancy [14].

Spleen surgery or trauma history may be very helpful to achieve a correct diagnosis that is crucial to avoid unnecessary surgery or biopsy.

IPST should be included in the differential diagnosis of pancreatic hypervascular lesions, namely pNENs, solid pseudopapillary tumour (SPT) and pancreatic metastasis (PM) from renal clear cell carcinoma (RCC). Epidermoid cyst and inflammatory pseudotumour have been described as associated with IST [15–17], and the diagnosis under these circumstances may be challenging.

Tc-99m-labelled heat-denatured red blood cells (Tc-99m-DRBCs) are currently the gold standard technique to specifically prove the diagnosis of IST [18], as Tc-99m-DRBCs are trapped by reticuloendothelial cells.

2.2. Pancreatic Tuberculosis (Figure 2)

Pancreatic tuberculosis (PT) occurs very rarely, predominantly during a multiorgan abdominal spread of the infection [19]. Only 116 cases have been reported in the literature [20]. When isolated, its diagnosis is not suspected and is frequently achieved after histologic examination, following resection [21]. It has been theorised that pancreatic enzymes serve as shields against *Mycobacterium tuberculosis* [22].

In the western world, PT occurs mainly in immunocompromised patients [21,23]. It seems to be more frequent between the fourth and fifth decades of life [24,25]. Gender association is not clear [26,27].

The most frequent clinical presentations are vague non-specific symptoms (fatigue, fever, weight loss, nausea and vomiting) [28] or a history of acute or chronic pancreatitis [21]. Less frequently, it can also present as obstructive jaundice or gastrointestinal bleeding [29].

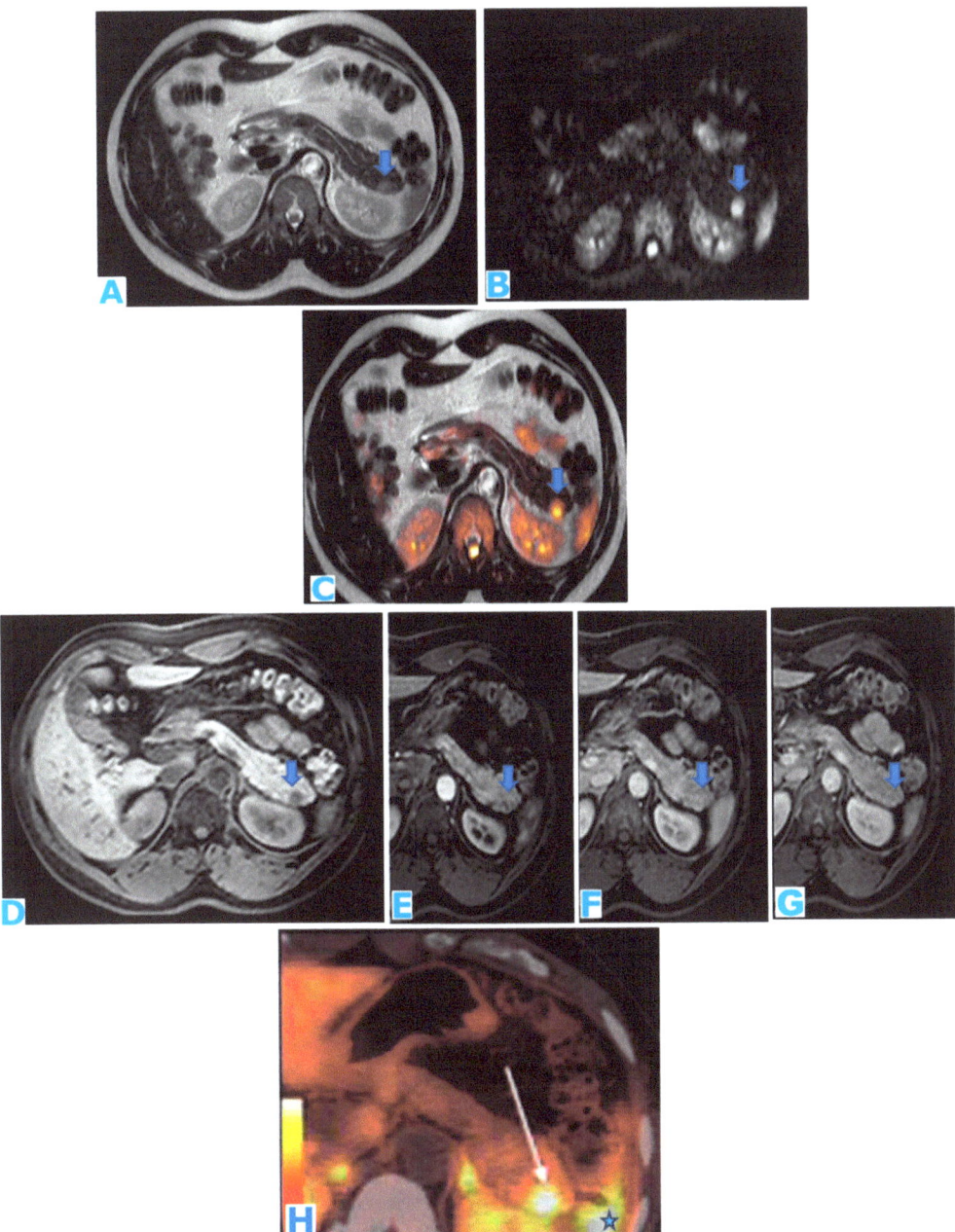

Figure 1. (**A**): axial T2-weighted images (T2WIs), (**B**): DWI, (**C**): axial T2WI-DWI fused images, (**D**): non-contrast-enhanced (NCE) fat-saturated (FS) T1-weighted images (T1WI), (**E**–**G**): axial contrast-enhanced (CE) dynamic FST1WI, (**E**): pancreatic parenchymal phase, (**F**): portal venous phase, (**G**): delayed venous phase, (**H**): Ga-68-DOTATOC PET-CT. Incidentally discovered IPAS in a 56 year-old patient, during check-up examination for elevation of pancreatic enzymes. Note a slightly hyperintense

lesion within the pancreatic tail in T2WI (arrow in (**A**)), with diffusion restriction (arrow in (**B**,**C**)), conspicuous in the unenhanced phase (arrow in (**D**)) but not so much following intravenous contrast administration (arrow in (**E**–**G**)). Endoscopic ultrasound-guided fine-needle aspiration (EUS-FNA) obtained small epithelioid cells, with antichromogranin- and synaptophysin-positive immunostaining and concluded a pNEN grade II (Ki 67 = 5%). However, in the PET-CT, the lesion (arrow in (**H**)) showed the same uptake as the spleen (* in (**H**)) and no non-physiological uptake was found, so an IPAS was suspected on imaging. The FNA result was a false positive for NEN secondary to contamination of normal neuroendocrine pancreatic tissue as the patient underwent a left-sided pancreatectomy with spleen preservation and the histological examination concluded IPAS.

The body of the pancreas seems to be the favoured location, closely followed by the head [25,30].

Presentation patterns are focal masses [31], multiple small nodules [23] and, less frequently, a diffuse involvement, mimicking an acute pancreatitis [32], with increased signal intensity in T2-weighted images (T2WIs) [21].

Focal pattern PT may appear as a well-defined cystic–solid mass, with varying aspects depending on the proportion of cystic and solid components [23]: hypodense on CT, hypo- or isointense in T1-weighted images (T1WIs) and heterogeneous in T2WIs. After intravenous contrast administration, peripheral enhancement with central necrosis or enhancing solid components may be depicted [25]. When predominantly cystic, PT may be misdiagnosed as a cystic tumour, such as a cystadenoma, a pseudocyst in the setting of chronic pancreatitis or an infected abscess. If, on the other hand, PT consists of a mainly solid lesion associated with biliary or main pancreatic duct (MPD) dilatation, it may be indistinguishable from PDAC (especially if accompanied by peripancreatic lymph nodes and signs of vascular invasion), lymphoma and metastasis [33].

Calcifications are frequently encountered [34]. Dilatation of the bile and pancreatic ducts may occur, though infrequently, despite the mass effect on the ducts [28]. Displacement and stenosis of an otherwise normal MPD are frequent features, without much prestenotic dilatation [34]. Vascular invasion has been described [25,35].

As lymph nodes are the most common tuberculosis site within the abdomen, accompanying peripancreatic lymphadenopathy is frequently found [36], mostly showing peripheral enhancement with central low attenuation, corresponding to granulation tissue encircling central caseous necrosis [37]. This appearance, although highly suggestive, is not pathognomonic of PT.

Both cytology and histological examination following imaging-guided fine-needle aspiration (FNA) or biopsy (FNB), respectively, are the gold standard diagnosing techniques. PT can be effectively treated with antituberculous therapy [38].

2.3. Solid Serous Cystadenoma (Figure 3)

Solid serous cystadenoma (SSCA) is the rarest variant of pancreatic serous cystadenoma, accounting for only 3% of all cases [39], and with only 22 cases reported in the literature [40]. Serous cystadenomas are benign tumours, usually composed of cysts that can measure up to 2 cm, with a typical honeycomb appearance. A central scar, often calcified, is frequently identified [41].

The solid variant is frequently misdiagnosed, because cystic spaces are either absent or scarce and too tiny [42]. In addition, serous cystadenomas may contain intratumoral haemorrhage, which adds to the high density of these lesions, contributing to the solid appearance. It occurs most commonly in elderly women, as an incidental finding, with no site of preference [40]. If symptomatic, the presentation is usually non-specific, with abdominal pain, abdominal mass and, rarely, jaundice [43].

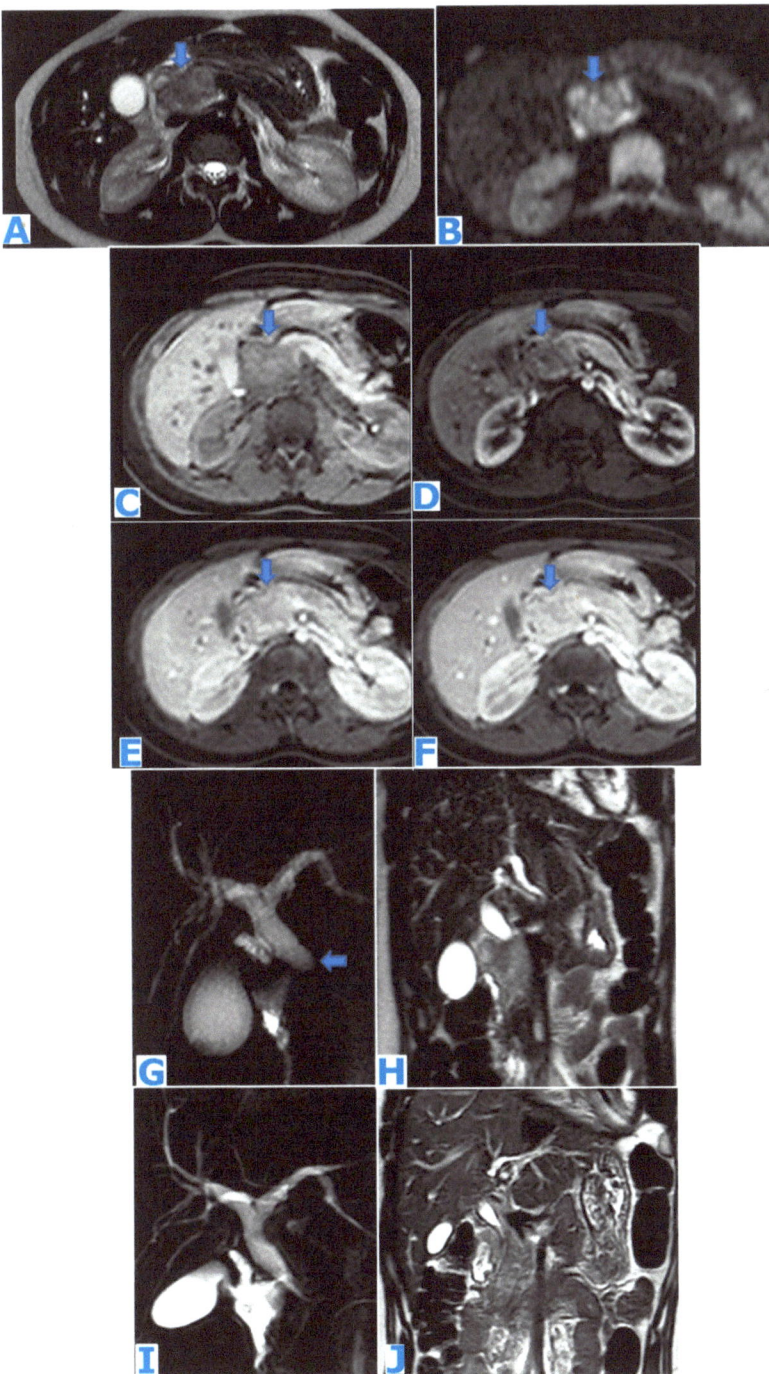

Figure 2. (**A**): axial T2WI, (**B**): DWI, (**C**): NCE FST1WI, (**D**–**F**): axial CE dynamic FST1WI (**D**): pancreatic parenchymal phase, (**E**): portal venous phase, (**F**): delayed venous phase, (**G**): MCRP, (**H**): coronal

T2WI, (**I**): posttreatment MCRP, (**J**): posttreatment coronal T2WI. Primary pancreatic tuberculosis in a 15-year-old patient from Burundi presenting with abdominal pain and anicteric cholestasis. Note in the T2WI a hyperintense mass in the head of the pancreas (arrow in (**A**)) causing an abrupt biliary duct cutoff (arrow in (**G**)) and upstream dilatation. The mass shows diffusion restriction (arrow in (**B**)) and progressive enhancement in the dynamic sequences (arrows in (**C–F**)). EUS-guided FNA revealed necrosis, Langhans giant cells, lymphocytes and macrophages organised in granulomas. Thoracic radiography (not shown) was normal, and diagnosis was primary pancreatic tuberculosis. Both the lesion and mass effect on the common bile duct completely resolved after treatment (**I,J**).

As the remaining serous cystadenomas, SSCAs are well-delimited lesions, hypointense in T1WIs and hyperintense in T2WIs [44]. Its most salient feature is an early rapid enhancement followed by isointensity in the portal phase, a fact that frequently leads to a misdiagnosis of pNEN [40,45,46]. T2WIs and especially MR cholangiopancreatography (MRCP), a heavily T2WI sequence with an echo time 10 times longer than that of regular T2WIs, help diagnose the hyperintense cyst [47]. A mild dilatation of the pancreatic duct may happen, due to compression.

Preoperative diagnosis is challenging, and aside from pNEN, it is also commonly mistaken for SPT, PM and even PDAC [47].

Once the diagnosis is suspected at cross-sectional imaging, a confirmation by EUS-FNA is achieved in only half of patients [42], as SSCA's nature may cause the sample to lack the epithelial tissue required for diagnosis.

As in typical serous cystadenomas, surgery is only recommended when causing symptoms, due to compression of neighbouring organs [48] or if diagnosis remains uncertain after workup [43].

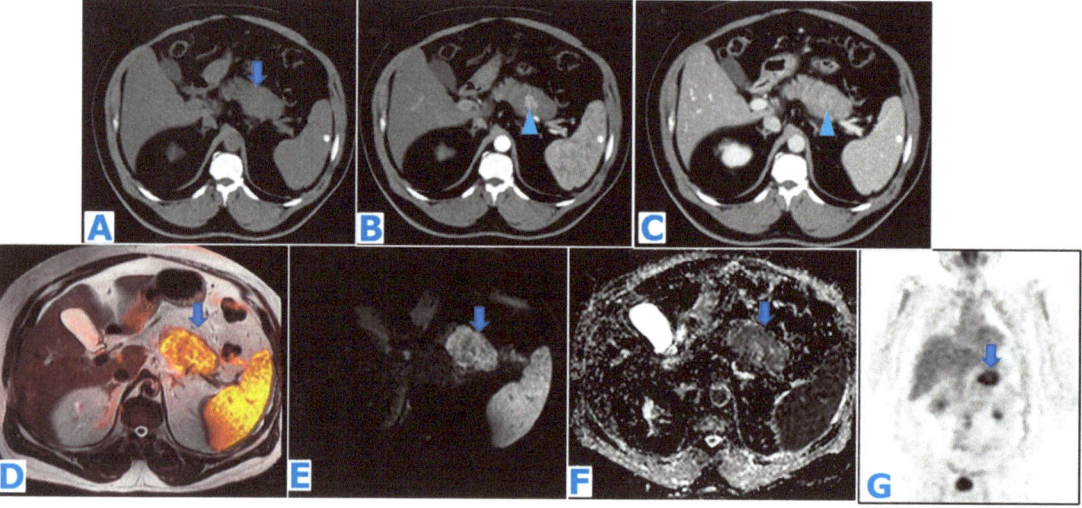

Figure 3. (**A**): axial NCE-CT, (**B**): axial CE pancreatic parenchymal phase CT, (**C**): axial CE portal venous phase CT, (**D**): axial T2WI-DWI fusion, (**E**): DWI, (**F**): ADC, (**G**): coronal FDG-PET. Solid serous cystadenoma. A 67-year-old patient with fatigue and abdominal pain, referred from another institution with the diagnosis of pancreatic neoplasm. CA 19.9 within normal limits. CT shows a solid lesion in the body of the pancreas (arrow in (**A**)), with central enhancement in the arterial phase (arrowhead in (**B**)), which persists during portal phase (arrowhead in (**C**)). There is no downstream MPD dilatation. Note the diffusion restriction (arrow in (**D–F**)) and the peripheral hypermetabolic uptake on the PET-CT (arrow in (**G**)). EUS-guided FNB only obtained inflammatory cells, with no evidence of malignancy. The lesion remained suspicious, and the patient underwent a left pancreatectomy. Histological examination revealed a SSCA.

3. Potentially Malignant Lesions (Table S2)

3.1. Solid Pseudopapillary Tumour (Figures 4 and 5)

SPT is a rare pancreatic neoplasm accounting for 2% of all exocrine pancreatic neoplasms [49]. It is an epithelial tumour, but its pathogenesis remains unclear as its cells of origin are unlike any other cell found within the embryonic or adult pancreas [50]. It has been hypothesised that it arises from pluripotential embryonic stem cells [51].

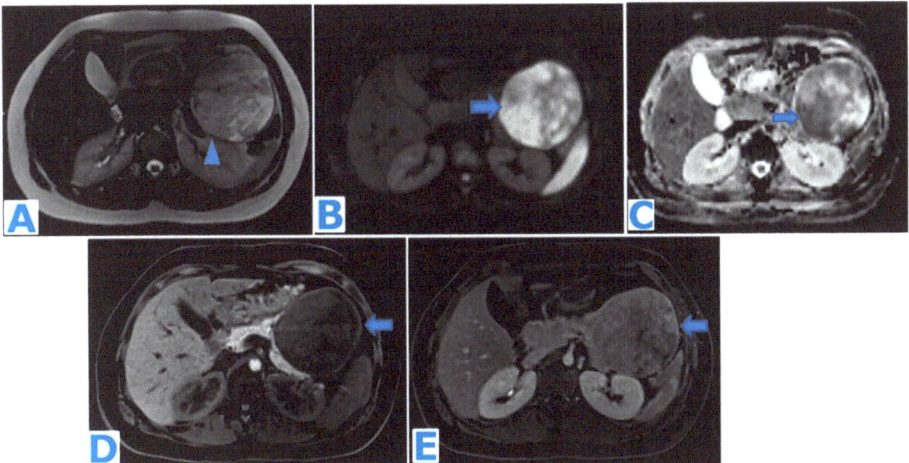

Figure 4. (**A**): axial T2WI, (**B**): DWI, (**C**): ADC, (**D**): axial NE FST1WI, (**E**): axial CE portal venous phase FST1WI. Pancreatic solid pseudopapillary tumour in a 20-year-old woman as an incidental finding during a pregnancy check-up. A 10 cm pancreatic mass was found, with a fibrous capsule (arrowhead in (**A**)), diffusion restriction (arrows in (**B**,**C**)) and heterogeneous enhancement (arrow in (**D**,**E**)). Imaging findings were compatible with a pancreatic SPT, and it was histologically proven following distal pancreatectomy.

SPT occurs tenfold more frequently in women than in men and this has given origin to a hypothesis linking the tumour to female sex hormones [51,52] or pointing to genital ridges close to the pancreatic anlage during organogenesis as a possible origin [53]. Published cases occurring in men report usually an older age and curiously an aggressive behaviour [54]. Its target populations are women younger than 40 years old [55].

There is no association with a functional endocrine syndrome [56] or with any laboratory finding [57].

This tumour grows at a slow rate, thus it does not cause symptoms and it is incidentally discovered in about 15% of patients [55,56]. When present, symptoms are non-specific [50,55,58]. Jaundice happens very rarely [55]. Hemoperitoneum secondary to tumour rupture, either spontaneous or traumatic [59,60], has been described as a rare presentation.

As a result of its slow growth rate and soft nature, SPT usually presents with a large size at diagnosis (mean size 5 cm) [61].

The tail of the pancreas is a favoured location [50]. An extrapancreatic site of origin is possible, though rare [62–66].

MPD or biliary dilatation almost never occurs [67].

Distant metastases, usually present at the time of diagnosis, occur in about 15% of patients [68] and are predominantly hepatic, peritoneal or lymphatic [68–70].

SPT is depicted in cross-sectional images as a homogeneous solid lesion that, as it becomes larger, outgrows the blood supply and suffers degenerative changes. Formation of pseudopapillae occurs as loss of tissue takes place. The stalks of these pseudopapillae contain fragile blood vessels and, as a result, intralesional haemorrhage happens frequently [71–73]. All these events contribute to a heterogeneous appearance with variable solid and cystic components and intralesional haemorrhagic and necrotic parts [50]. Intralesional haemorrhagic traces are considered to be pathognomonic findings [74,75]. Internal fluid–fluid levels may also be identified [76]. The different components will be better depicted on MR thanks to its high contrast resolution. A pseudocapsule, reflecting the tumour slow growth, is almost always depictable in tumours larger than 3 cm, granting well-delineated borders. True to its fibrous nature, it is typically hypointense in both T1- and T2WIs and enhances moderately after intravenous contrast injection [76]. Dystrophic calcifications are found in up to 30% of cases [59], with a variety of patterns [77], and occur more frequently in larger tumours [50], as necrotic components fail to reabsorb. Following intravenous contrast administration, SPT shows a heterogeneous nature in the arterial phase, even when small in size, followed by a progressive enhancement in the portal venous phase [78].

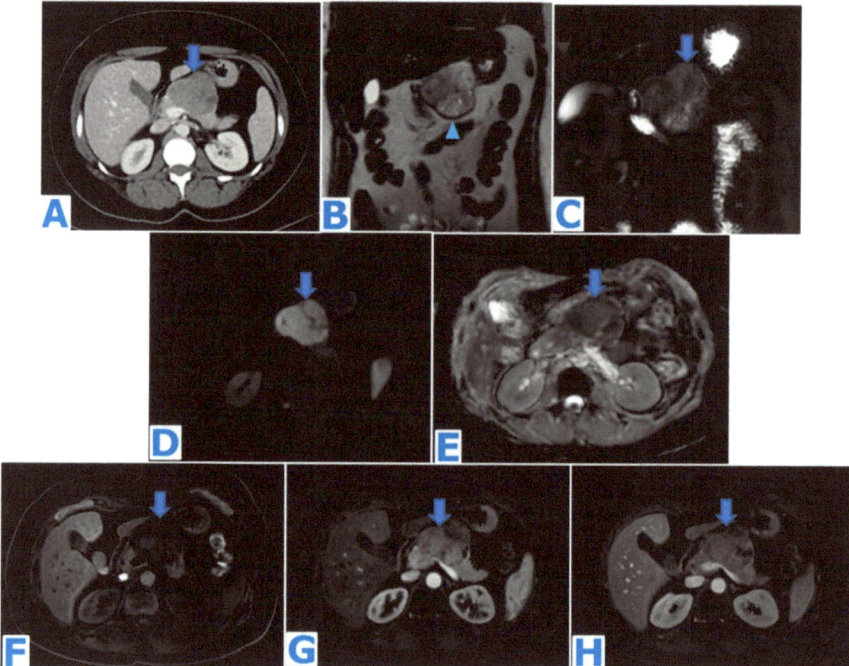

Figure 5. (**A**): axial CE portal venous phase CT, (**B**): coronal T2WI, (**C**): MRCP, (**D**): DWI, (**E**): ADC, (**F**): axial NCE FST1WI, (**G**): axial CE pancreatic parenchymal phase FST1WI, (**H**): axial CE portal venous phase FST1WI. Pancreatic solid pseudopapillary tumour in a 30-year-old woman as an incidental finding during a CT scan for abdominal pain. CT showed a mass within the body of the pancreas (arrow in (**A**)). The lesion was well defined by a fibrous capsule (arrowhead in (**B**)). MPD was displaced, with normal caliber (arrow in (**C**)). The lesion showed diffusion restriction (arrow in (**D**,**E**)) and progressive heterogeneous enhancement (arrow in (**F**–**H**)). Due to the microcystic appearance in T2WIs, the lesion was initially thought to be a microcystic serous cystadenoma, even if it lacked some characteristic features. Nevertheless, given its size and presence of symptoms, it was removed. Histological examination revealed a SPT.

Surgical resection may be considered without prior biopsy if the presentation is classic. In atypical presentations, diagnosis is achieved through histological examination following biopsy.

Tumour resection is the treatment with curative intent, with a success rate close to 90% [79]. SPTs usually have a benign behaviour but malignancy has been reported in 10–15% [49,68,70]. Even if metastatic, the prognosis is good, as long an R0 resection is achieved [80]. The only significant proven malignancy predictors are pancreatic duct dilatation, vessel encasement and the presence of metastases [81]. It is extremely important to continue surveillance in the long term, as SPTs are prone to recur and develop metastases as a late event, even years after surgery [82].

3.2. Pancreatic Schwannoma (Figure 6)

Pancreatic schwannoma (PS) is a rare tumour that arises from Schwann cells found in the sheath of vagus nerve branches on their course through the pancreas [83].

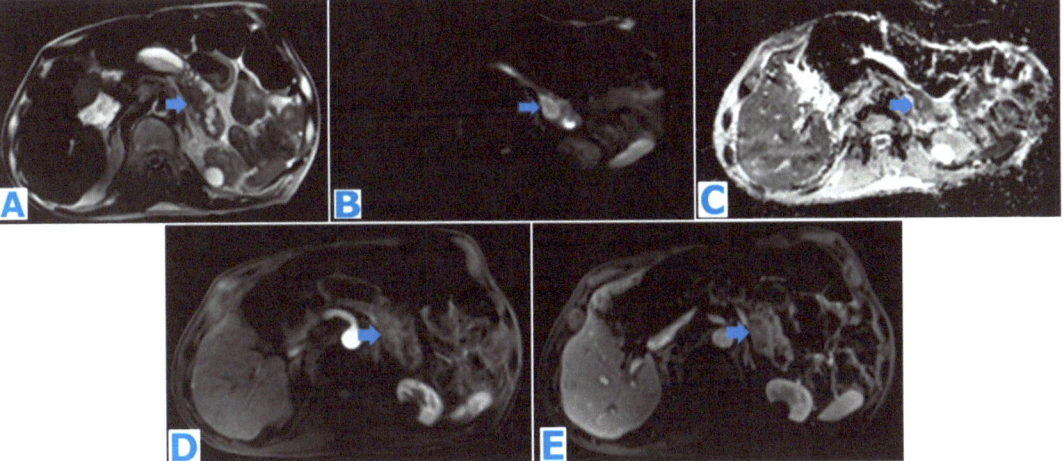

Figure 6. (**A**): axial T2WI, (**B**): DWI, (**C**): ADC, (**D**): axial CE early arterial phase FST1WI, (**E**): axial CE pancreatic parenchymal phase FST1WI. Pancreatic schwannoma in a 70-year-old male patient during follow-up for a duodenal gastrointestinal stromal tumour (GIST), removed five years prior through cephalic duodenopancreatectomy. A pancreatic lesion is noted within the pancreatic tail (arrow in (**A**)). Observe MPD dilatation unrelated to the lesion, due to surgical procedure. The lesion showed diffusion restriction (arrow in (**B**,**C**)) and progressive heterogeneous enhancement following intravenous contrast administration (arrow in (**D**,**E**)). EUS-guided FNA obtained fragments of mesenchymal tissue with minimal nuclear atypia and positive immunostaining for anti-S-100, and cytological report concluded schwannoma. Tumour board decided conservative management and the lesion is currently under surveillance.

Only 10% of cases are associated with genetic disorders, such as neurofibromatosis type 2 (NF2), multiple meningiomas and schwannomatosis, and, rarely, with neurofibromatosis type 1 (NF1), with an increased risk of malignant transformation [84].

There are less than 80 reported cases in the literature, with most of the cases occurring in adults (average age 55 years), with a slightly higher incidence in women [85].

Patients mostly present with non-specific abdominal complaints [86], although the prevalence of symptoms suspicious for a PDAC (such as weight loss, palpable mass and jaundice) is not neglectable [85].

Levels of CA 19-9 and carcinoembryonic antigen (CEA) are usually within normal values. Most tumours have been found within the head [87].

Tumour size varies greatly and, with increasing size, there is also proportionate likelihood of degeneration occurring. Microscopically, two distinct areas are found within the tumour: Antoni A, solid, with a compact cellular organisation and a well-developed vascular net, and Antoni B, hypocellular with loose myxoid stroma, less vascularity and degenerative alterations (haemorrhage, calcification, cyst formation, hyalinisation and xanthoma infiltration) [88,89]. The tumour's appearance is determined by the proportion of Antoni A and B areas; thus, the imaging features are non-specific and preoperative diagnosis is challenging [90].

On CT, benign schwannomas are usually depicted as encapsulated round masses with a variable proportion of avidly enhancing (Antoni A areas) and non-enhancing (Antoni B areas) components, following intravenous contrast administration [91]. On MR, hypointense signal in T1WIs and heterogeneously hyperintense signal in T2WIs are commonly found [92], in addition to progressive enhancement in T1WIs [93].

Suspicious signs of malignancy are rapid growth, invasion of neighbouring structures, a solid inhomogeneous and irregular mass with avid contrast enhancement and associated thrombosis [94].

PS is usually associated with a hypermetabolic appearance on FDG-PET, even if benign [95].

Differential diagnosis should include SPT, pNEN and pancreatic cystadenoma. The diagnosis of PS should be considered when a well-circumscribed lesion with or without a cystic component is encountered, showing increased FDG uptake on PET-CT [95].

Diagnosis is achieved after histological examination following EUS-guided biopsy.

If asymptomatic, a conservative management may be considered, given its benign nature and stable size or slow growth rate [96]. On the other hand, if symptomatic, resection should be considered. Follow-up after surgery should be carried on, as the risk of recurrence remains unknown [97].

3.3. Purely Intraductal Pancreatic Neuroendocrine Tumour (Figure 7)

Intraductal growth of a pNEN is encountered in two different scenarios. Most frequently, it is found in the form of a parenchymal lesion that extends into the pancreatic duct and grows along its extent. This presentation is very rare and very few cases have been published [98–104]. The other, and even rarer, setting is a true intraductal origin, where a NEN arises within the main pancreatic duct as a polypoid mass that grows along the duct [98,105,106] but it is not connected to a parenchymal lesion [107]. Only seven cases of purely intraductal pNENs have been reported in the literature [107]. Purely intraductal pNEN has been hypothesised to rise from totipotential stem cells located within the epithelium of the main duct [108]. As the tumour grows, the tumour may block the duct lumen and, as a result, it can cause pancreatitis. In fact, these tumours frequently present as a chronic pancreatitis. This exclusively intraductal lesion is not conspicuous on CT, and it may be obscured by the pancreatitis signs, so it is most frequently diagnosed after surgery. MRCP proves to be very useful as it can depict the intraductal tumour as a filling defect. Intraductal pNEN may also be identified following intravenous contrast administration as an avidly enhancing lesion in the arterial phase. This type of presentation occurs mostly associated with non-functioning pNENs [107]. An inflammatory stricture in the setting of chronic pancreatitis constitutes the other differential diagnosis possibility. There are so few cases in the literature that no data can be extrapolated.

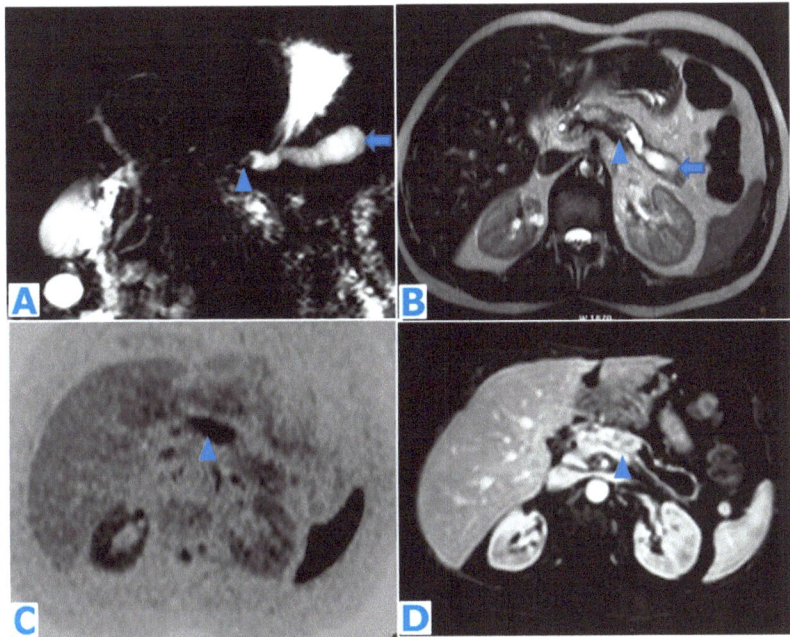

Figure 7. (**A**): MRCP, (**B**): axial T2WI, (**C**): DWI, (**D**): axial CE arterial phase FST1WI. Intraductal pancreatic NEN in a 55-year-old patient with a known history of a testicular tumour, admitted for acute pancreatitis, with no risk factors. Note the marked dilatation of the distal MPD (arrows in (**A**,**B**)) with a proximal filling defect (arrowheads in (**A**,**B**)) which corresponds to the intraductal tumour. The intraductal mass shows diffusion restriction (arrowhead in (**C**)) and intense enhancement following intravenous contrast administration (arrowhead in (**D**)). A total pancreatectomy was decided by the MDT and histological examination concluded grade 2 intraductal pNEN.

3.4. Pancreatic Solitary Fibrous Tumour (Figure 8)

This type of extrapleural solitary fibrous tumour is a fibroblastic mesenchymal tumour, previously known as haemangiopericytoma. It was first described in the pleura in 1931 [109], derived from mesenchymal cells from pleural connective tissue, but since then, it has been documented in almost every anatomic site, including the retroperitoneum [110].

Pancreatic solitary fibrous tumour (PSFT) is a rare neoplasm, with only 29 cases reported [111]. It shows no gender preference, and the median age reported at diagnosis is 53 years [112]. The main symptoms reported at presentation are abdominal pain and jaundice, though most frequently tumours are incidental findings [113].

Patients may present with refractory and recurrent hypoglucemia as a paraneoplastic syndrome (Doege–Potter syndrome), caused by an increased production of insulin-like growth factor II [113]. Being a mesenchymal tumour, there is no association with tumour markers.

PSFT arises most commonly within the pancreatic head [111].

It shows a true capsule and well-defined margins, and it does not tend to invade the surrounding parenchyma [114]. Its most salient feature is its hypervascularity, and it usually enhances homogeneously and progressively in the arterial and portal phase [115]. In larger tumours, central necrosis occurs, and it has been described that a malignant type may present a heterogeneous appearance with haemorrhage, necrosis and calcifications [115].

Dilatation of the main pancreatic duct has been observed in some cases, as well as biliary dilatation in tumours located within the head [116], but these findings are not a constant, despite the large size of tumours. Lymphadenopathies are not frequently associated [111].

FDG-PET has not been shown to be useful in distinguishing indolent from aggressive PSFT [117], contrary to previous hypotheses.

The main differential diagnosis based on imaging findings is pNEN [118]. Other options should include leiomyosarcoma, GIST, perivascular epithelioid cell tumour (PEComa) and SPT in younger patients.

Definite diagnosis is achieved by EUS-guided biopsy. Curative treatment is complete surgical resection [119], with good results, since most of the published cases were disease free after surgery [115]. Adjuvant radio- or chemotherapy treatments have not achieved successful results [120]. Negative margins have proved to decrease the rate of local recurrence and to improve survival [120]. Follow-up is recommended, as about 12–22% of all solitary fibrous tumours are aggressive, with local recurrence and metastases [121].

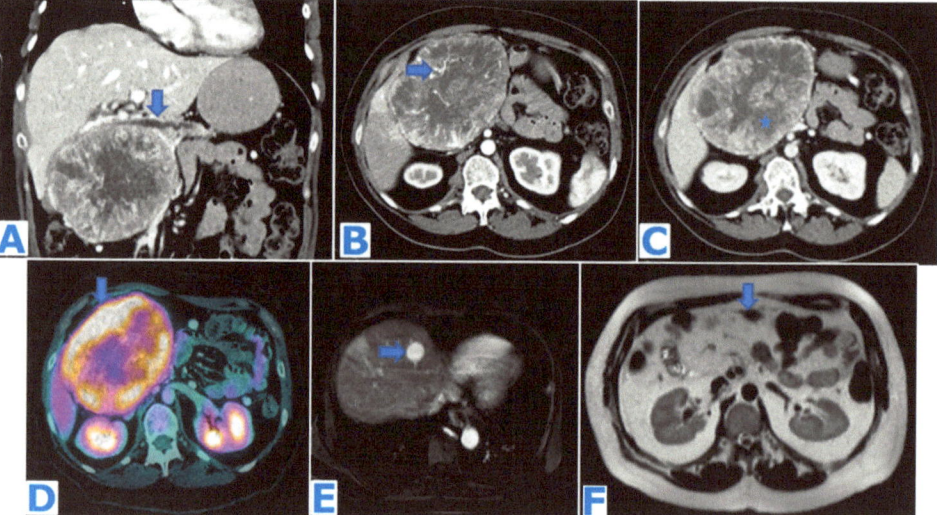

Figure 8. (**A**): CE-CT portal phase coronal MPR, (**B**): axial CE arterial phase CT, (**C**): axial CE portal venous phase CT, (**D**): FDG-PET CT. Follow-up images (**E**): axial CE arterial phase FST1WI, (**F**): axial T2WI. Malignant pancreatic solitary fibrous tumour in a 47-year-old patient who presented with a palpable mass within the right hypochondrium. She had a history of a nasal fibrous solitary tumour 10 years prior. CT showed an enormous solid mass in the head of the pancreas, causing mild dilatation of the pancreatic duct (arrow in (**A**)). Note the central necrosis (* in (**C**)) and the hypervascularity of the non-necrotic periphery (arrow in (**B**)), which is highly metabolic on the FDG-PET (arrow in (**D**)). The patient underwent a total pancreatectomy and the histological examination concluded PSFT. It turned out to have a malignant outcome and the patient developed liver (arrow in (**E**)) and omental (arrow in (**F**)) metastases within the year following the surgery.

4. Malignant Lesions (Table S3)

4.1. Acinar Cell Carcinoma (Figures 9 and 10)

Acinar cell carcinoma is a rare epithelial malignant primary pancreatic tumour, named after the acinar differentiation of its cells. Even though acinar cells constitute most of the pancreatic parenchyma, acinar cell carcinoma (ACC) paradoxically represents less than 2% of primary pancreatic neoplasms [122].

ACC occurs mostly in men (men to women ratio of 3.6) with a bimodal presentation, with two incidence peaks at 8–15 and 60 years [123–125].

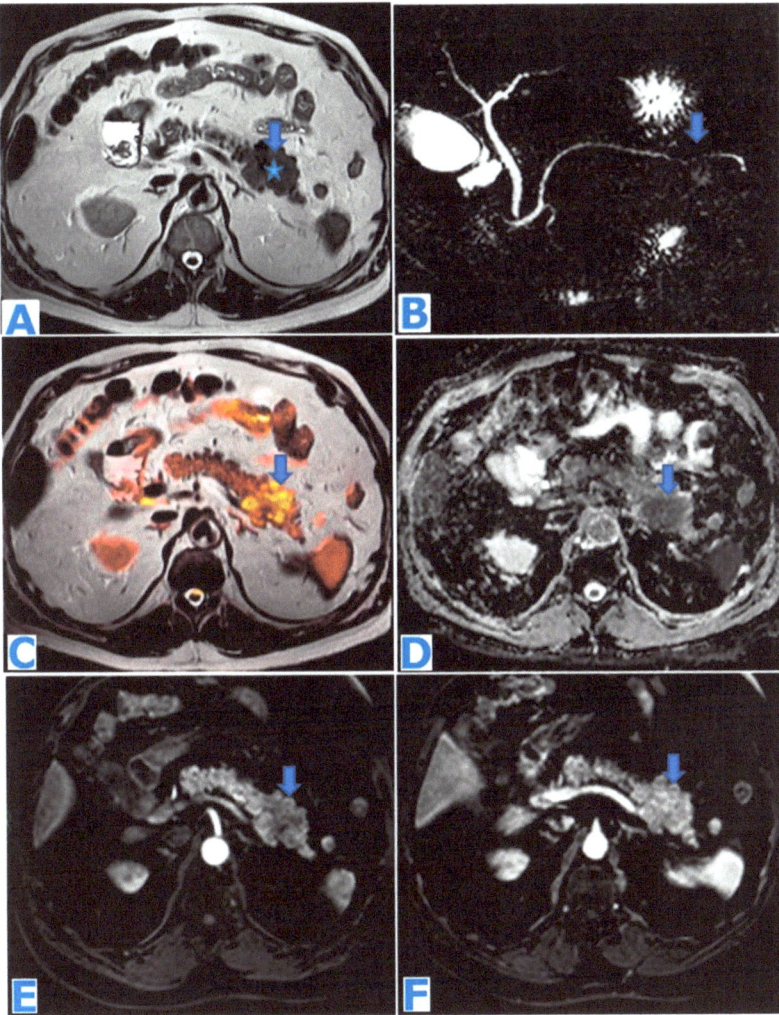

Figure 9. (**A**): axial T2WI, (**B**): MRCP following secretin injection, (**C**): axial T2 DWI fusion, (**D**): ADC, (**E**): axial CE pancreatic parenchymal phase FST1WI, (**F**): axial CE portal venous phase FST1WI. Acinar cell adenocarcinoma in a 79-year-old patient with previous episodes of pancreatitis of unknown cause and elevated lipase in current laboratory results. A solid well-defined mass (arrow in (**A**)) with lobulated contours and minimal MPD stenosis (* in (**A**)) is found in the distal pancreas. It shows diffusion restriction (arrows in (**C**,**D**)). Note the duct penetrating sign following secretin injection (arrow in (**B**)). It is hypoenhancing in the early arterial phase (arrow in (**E**)) with progressive enhancement during pancreatic parenchymal phase (arrow in (**F**)). No adenopathies are found. Findings were non-specific and did not fulfill the diagnosis criteria for PDAC. Diagnosis was achieved at histological examination following EUS-guided FNB.

It arises throughout the pancreas, with no favoured location.

Presenting symptoms are non-specific, with abdominal pain and weight loss being the most common. Pancreatitis and obstructive jaundice are rare [126,127] as, despite their large size, ACCs do not tend to cause ductal obstruction [128,129].

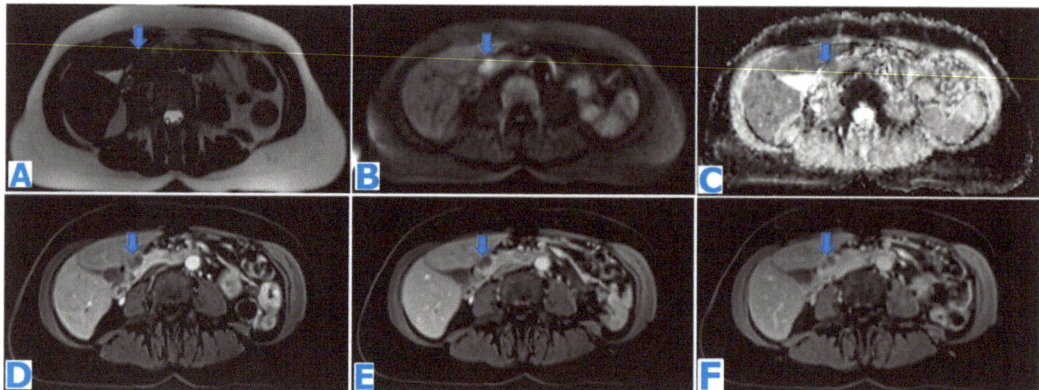

Figure 10. (**A**): axial T2WI, (**B**): DWI, (**C**): ADC, (**D**): CE pancreatic parenchymal phase FST1WI, (**E**): axial CE portal venous phase FST1WI, (**F**): axial CE delayed venous phase FST1WI. Acinar cell adenocarcinoma incidentally discovered in a 70-year-old female patient during a routine echography. Note the lesion within the head of the pancreas, rather exophytic and heterogeneous (arrow in (**A**)), with diffusion restriction (arrows in (**B**,**C**)). During the dynamic sequences following intravenous contrast administration (arrows in (**D**–**F**)), the lesion shows capsular enhancement while the center remains hypointense, due to necrosis/cystic changes. Due to its exophytic appearance, the lesion was thought to be within the pancreaticoduodenal groove and, hence, was diagnosed as a GIST. Histopathological examination following EUS-guided FNB revealed an ACC.

Elevated lipase, secreted by the tumour, may be the presenting sign of ACC and may be used as a tumour marker [130]. As a result, fat necrosis may be triggered, either subcutaneously, presenting as nodules, or within the cancellous bone, causing polyarthralgia [131,132]. These symptoms, together with peripheral eosinophilia, constitute a paraneoplastic syndrome [133] that may occur after tumour recurrence. An elevated alpha-fetoprotein may sometimes be found [134]. Levels of CA 19-9 and carcinoembryonic antigen (CEA) are usually within normal values.

At the time of presentation, almost half of patients present with hepatic and lymph node metastases [135].

On cross-sectional imaging, ACC usually appears as a large (average size at diagnosis of 10cm [136–138]), well-defined and oval or round exophytic mass (it may even be found attached to the surface of the pancreas on the histological examination [130]). Calcifications are found in one third of patients [136,137,139]. It usually shows a solid appearance, but internal haemorrhage, necrosis and cystic changes are common in larger lesions [136]. On unenhanced CT, it is usually iso-hypodense to the pancreatic parenchyma, and it shows a hypovascular nature, hypoenhancing in the arterial phase and becoming more enhancing than the pancreatic parenchyma in the portal venous phase [140]. An enhancing capsule may also be identified.

Concerning the cross-sectional imaging test of choice, the combination of CT and MR works well in depicting the imaging features. MR outperforms CT in describing tumour limits, intratumoral bleeding, local invasion and ductal dilatation, whereas CT is better at detecting calcification [141].

Differential diagnosis should include PDAC, pNENs, SPT and, in children, also pancreatoblastoma. PDAC usually shows a smaller size with no calcification or cystic changes [142]. Its margins are not well delineated, and invasion of neighbouring structures is one of its hallmarks. ACCs are often mistaken for large pNENs, as they may show heterogeneous density/SI due to haemorrhage, necrosis, cystic changes and calcifications, but ACCs are mainly hypovascular. SPTs may also mimic ACCs, but the target population is the key: they occur almost exclusively in young women, in which ACCs rarely occur [143]. Pancreatoblastoma may cause a differential diagnosis issue, as it usually occurs in infants and children [144]. Its frequently also presents with liver metastases, but it is more aggressive than ACC.

Even if almost half of patients present at diagnosis with hepatic and regional lymph nodes metastases [135,145], ACC shows a better prognosis than PDAC, with a 5-year survival rate of 50% [146,147]. However, ACC has a higher rate of recurrence [141].

Surgical resection with negative margins is the only therapeutic approach that improves long-term survival. Recent studies suggest that the outcome of combining surgery and chemotherapy is more favourable than that of only surgery [148].

4.2. Undifferentiated Carcinoma with Osteoclastic-like Giant Cells (Figure 11)

Undifferentiated carcinoma with osteoclastic-like giant cells (UCOGC) is an extremely rare and aggressive subtype of pancreatic adenocarcinoma. It constitutes less than 1% of all pancreatic malignant tumours [149].

Its histogenesis is not clear, as at the time of diagnosis, it presents with a large size and its relation to the pancreatic duct is difficult to establish. About 20% of cases seem to arise from mucinous or intraductal papillary mucinous neoplasms (IPMNs) [150] and it has been hypothesised that it has an epithelial origin with a mesenchymal transition [150,151]. The epithelial to mesenchymal transition is a transient and reversible transformation which is normally activated during embryonic development and tissue repair but also during carcinogenesis [152,153]. Through this step, tumoral cells acquire mesenchymal features that enable them to invade adjacent vessels and distant organs [154].

Two phenotypes have been described [155], a pure form containing only osteoclast-like giant cells, with a better prognosis than the mixed form, a combination of undifferentiated carcinoma of the pancreas and osteoclast-like giant cells forming a very aggressive tumour with a poor outcome. This mixed form constitutes a distinct variant from undifferentiated carcinoma of the pancreas [156]. UCOGC may occur in association with PDAC [157].

UCOGC occurs more commonly in women (women:men ratio of 13:8) with higher prevalence in middle-aged and elderly patients [158].

Presenting symptoms are non-specific and consist of upper abdominal pain, weight loss and/or anorexia. Jaundice and steatorrhoea have been described in 25% of cases [159].

CA 19-9 and CEA serum levels have been reported to be increased in some patients [160].

Favoured locations are the body and tail of the pancreas [157].

Biliary ducts and pancreatic duct dilatation may occur [151,158,159], as UCOGC seems prone to grow intraductally [151].

At presentation, UCOGCs are usually large lesions [161], locally aggressive, with a tendency to invade adjacent structures. Lymph node involvement and distant metastases are rarely encountered [151,161].

On cross-sectional imaging, appearance may vary and it displays non-specific features, either hypovascular [158] or hypervascular [162]. Hypervascular behaviour may be explained by a relationship to giant cell tumours of the bone, also hypervascular, so enhancement is proportionate to the volume of the osteoclastic cell component [151]. Haemorrhage [163], cystic changes [162], necrosis [158] calcification [164] and vascular invasion may occur [163].

UCOGC may be misdiagnosed as PDAC, mucinous carcinoma [165], SPT [158], pNEN [166] and pancreatic pseudocyst [167].

Diagnosis follows histological examination after EUS biopsy. Surgical resection is the treatment of choice. The efficacy of chemotherapy and radiotherapy has not been proved yet.

Its prognosis is variable, ranging from a few months to up to ten years as reported in the literature [168]. It was traditionally considered worse than that of PDAC [169,170] due to the advanced stage at diagnosis [165] and its tendency to recur even after complete resection [165,171].

Another analysis result of another series concluded that the prognosis (5-year survival >50%) is considerably better than that of PDAC [150]. It has been hypothesised that these discordant prognosis results are probably due to the use of wrong terminology [172] and it is clear that true UCOGCs have a more indolent behaviour [164], especially the pure form [173].

The underlying reasons for the better prognosis compared to PDAC may be its slower local spread, more indolent nature, better response to surgery and/or chemotherapy, less nodal involvement and fewer distant metastases [174].

The most important criterion for prognosis is the presence of an associated PDAC [173].

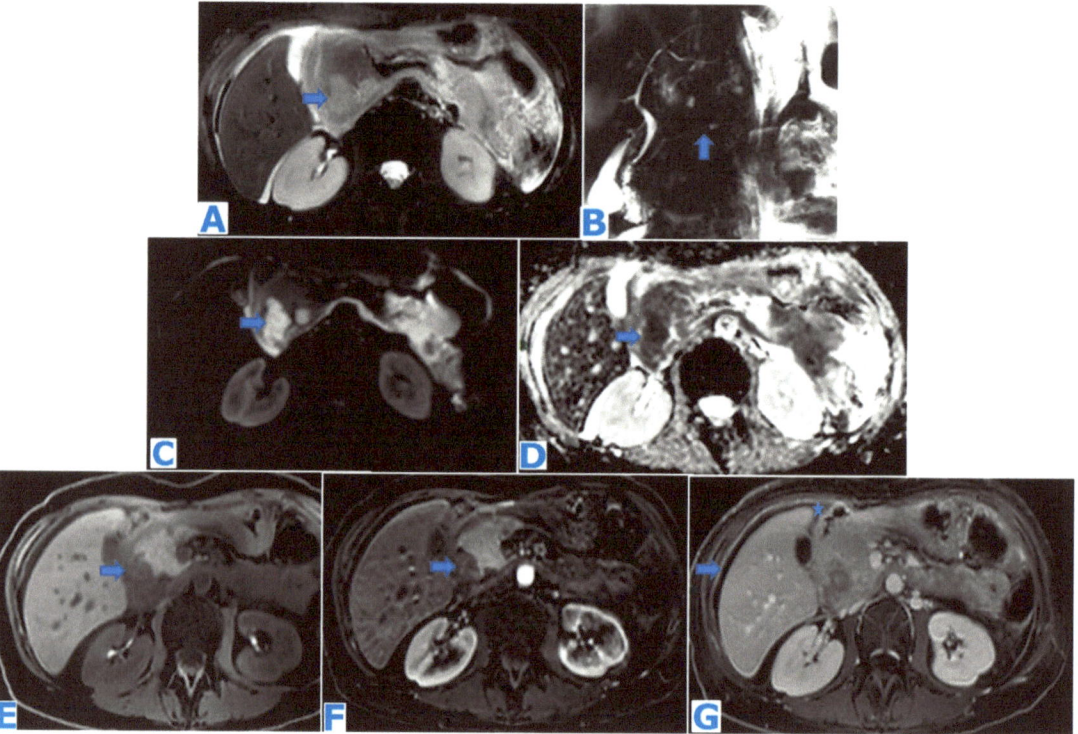

Figure 11. (**A**): axial FST2WI, (**B**): MRCP, (**C**): DWI, (**D**): ADC, (**E**): NEC axial FST1WI, (**F**): axial CE pancreatic parenchymal phase FST1WI, (**G**): axial CE portal venous phase FST1WI. UCOGC in a 45-year-old patient who presented with bloating. A cephalic pancreatic mass was identified, hyperintense in T2WIs (arrow in (**A**)), with MPD integrity (arrow in (**B**)) and no biliary duct dilatation, diffusion restriction (arrows in (**C**,**D**)) and scarce progressive enhancement in the dynamic sequences (arrows in (**E**–**G**)). These non-specific features did not fulfil PDAC diagnostic criteria. Ascites (* in (**G**)) and peritoneal deposits (arrow in (**G**)) were also found. Histology examination following EUS-guided FNB revealed a UCOGC.

4.3. Pancreatic Adenosquamous Carcinoma (Figure 12)

Pancreatic adenosquamous carcinoma (PASC) is a rare and aggressive variant of PDAC which is frequently misdiagnosed as such on imaging or even histopathologically. Its actual prevalence is thus inexact and has been reported to range from 0.38 to 10% [175–177]. A squamous cell component of at least 30% among glandular elements of PDAC has been a requisite for the diagnosis [178,179], although the required percentage recently has been questioned, as the proportion of squamous carcinoma does not have a clinical correlation and its evaluation remains subjective [180–183].

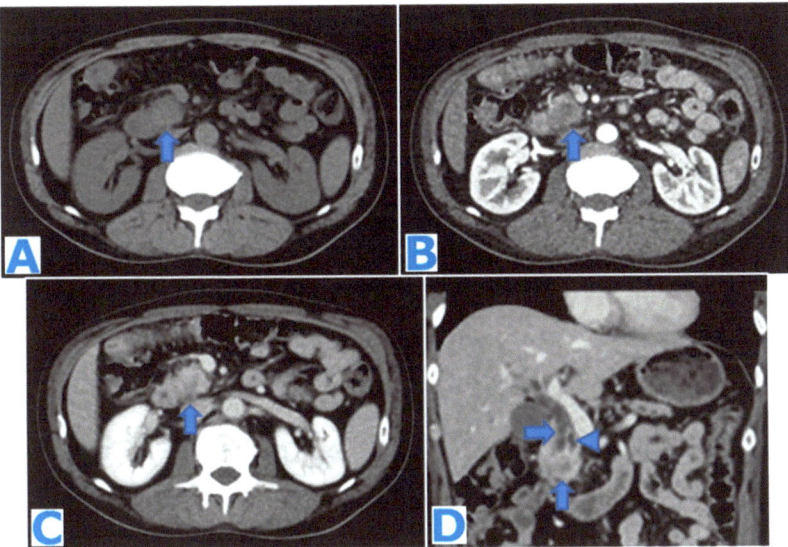

Figure 12. (**A**): axial NCE-CT, (**B**): axial CE pancreatic parenchymal phase CT, (**C**): axial CE portal venous phase CT, (**D**): CE portal phase CT coronal MPR. Adenosquamous carcinoma. A 60-year-old patient with elevated liver enzymes was discovered to have a pancreatic mass during an ultrasound. Note the subtle contour abnormalities of the pancreatic head on the unenhanced CT (arrow in (**A**)) and the progressively enhancing lesion (arrow in (**B**,**C**)). Observe the biliary duct (arrow in (**D**)) and the upstream MPD dilatation (arrowhead in (**D**)). EUS-guided FNA concluded moderately differentiated adenocarcinoma and, since the tumour was resectable, the patient underwent surgery. Histological examination proved it to be a PASC. Retrospectively, it shows a greater enhancement than a typical PDAC.

As squamous cells are not found in normal pancreatic tissue, the pathophysiology remains a mystery. Three hypotheses have been reported. The leading theory proposes that since squamous cells are found in the setting of chronic pancreatitis or in the event of tumour ductal obstruction and these conditions are associated with PDAC, squamous carcinoma could arise from a preexisting adenocarcinoma, through metaplastic changes [179,181,184,185]. PASC could also be the result of two different neoplastic pancreatic cell lines merging [184,186,187] or even having a common origin, as the third theory implies, where certain pluripotential primitive cells would differentiate into adenocarcinoma and others into squamous cell carcinoma, resulting in a tumour with both cell types [179,184].

Squamous carcinoma tends to show intercellular bridges and/or focal keratin pearl formation within its cells. However, PASC frequently presents as a poorly differentiated tumour and the use of immunochemistry is often needed to confirm the differentiation [188].

Elevated levels of CA 19-9 and CEA are found in most patients [189]. Hypercalcemia of malignancy is found in some cases, probably related to high serum levels of parathyroid hormone-related protein [190–192].

There is a higher prevalence in men and average age at presentation is 68 years [175].

Presenting symptoms are non-specific and indistinguishable from those of PDAC (abdominal pain, weight loss, anorexia and jaundice) [186,193].

Most frequently, at presentation, PASC is locally advanced or has distant metastases [194]: liver, lung [195,196] and even bone and skin [197–199].

Like PDAC, the head of the pancreas is the most common location but it arises within the body–tail more often than PDAC [175].

It is frequently associated with MPD dilatation and CBD dilatation when found within the head.

PASC tends to be larger than PDAC. It appears as a round lobulated mass with extensive central necrosis which causes an hyperintensity in T2WIs greater than that of PDAC [200] and a fibrous capsule that enhances progressively. Enhancement is overall considered to be greater than that of PDAC [201]. Another presenting imaging feature which may be helpful to distinguish it from PDAC is the frequently associated portal vein tumour thrombus [189,201–203].

Diagnosis may be achieved presurgically through an EUS-guided biopsy.

Complete resection is the only potentially curative treatment, although only 15–20% of patients are surgical candidates. A less favourable outcome has traditionally been associated with PASC, compared to PDAC, with a worse survival in patients who have undergone resection [204]. However, surgical resection has been shown to significantly improve median patient survival: median overall survival after surgery is 12 months, while in PDAC it is 16 months [175]. On the other end of the differentiation spectrum, squamous cell carcinoma appears to be an even more aggressive tumour, with worse survival data, which might suggest that the squamous element is a worsening prognosis factor [204].

4.4. Colloid Carcinoma (Figure 13)

Colloid carcinoma (CC) of the pancreas, alternatively referred to as mucinous non-cystic carcinoma, is a rare variant of ductal adenocarcinoma, which occurs with a rate of 1% of all pancreatic tumours [205,206].

Its hallmark is the abundant presence of extracellular mucin (adding up to at least 50% of the tumour), with malignant cells floating within it [207]. This mucinous component is the reason why it was previously categorised as mucinous cystadenoma or signet-ring cell carcinoma of the pancreas [206].

It appears that there is a slightly higher prevalence in men [205,208,209] and age at presentation ranges within the seventh decade [205].

Tumour markers (including CEA and CA 19-9) are usually elevated [205].

Presenting symptoms resemble those associated with PDAC: abdominal pain, jaundice and weight loss [179]. Almost half of patients with CC present a history of pancreatitis [209].

Most colloid carcinomas are associated with intestinal-type invasive IPMN although they may also arise de novo [210,211], and these types occur most frequently within the head of the pancreas [211,212]. Another less frequent association has been described with mucinous cystic tumours, involving preferably the tail of the pancreas [205].

CC is a slow-growing tumour that shows local invasion rather than disseminated disease [212]. Lymph node metastases and vascular invasion occur less frequently in CC than in PDAC [213,214].

The presence of dilatation of the main pancreatic duct will depend on whether the CC derives from an IPMN; if so, the tumour will be intraluminal, either the main or branch duct, and there will be downstream MPD dilatation [213]. If the tumour is unrelated to an IPMN, no dilatation will be found. Bile duct dilatation may occur in tumours arising from the head of the pancreas.

The reported tumour size at presentation ranges from 1 to 16cm [205,206]. Usually, they present on CT with a lobulated appearance and slightly ill-defined margins [215]. Calcifications are often found [215]. In T2WIs, CC shows very bright signal intensity with internal septa and a salt and pepper appearance, these features being consistent with the abundant mucin lakes with floating stroma and tumour cells [210]. Enhancement will happen typically progressively so at a delayed phase it will be more conspicuous. Enhancement will be observed internally in a sponge-like fashion, due to the enhancing stroma amidst the mucin lakes, which will enhance poorly and peripherally, associated with induced desmoplastic reaction [210,215].

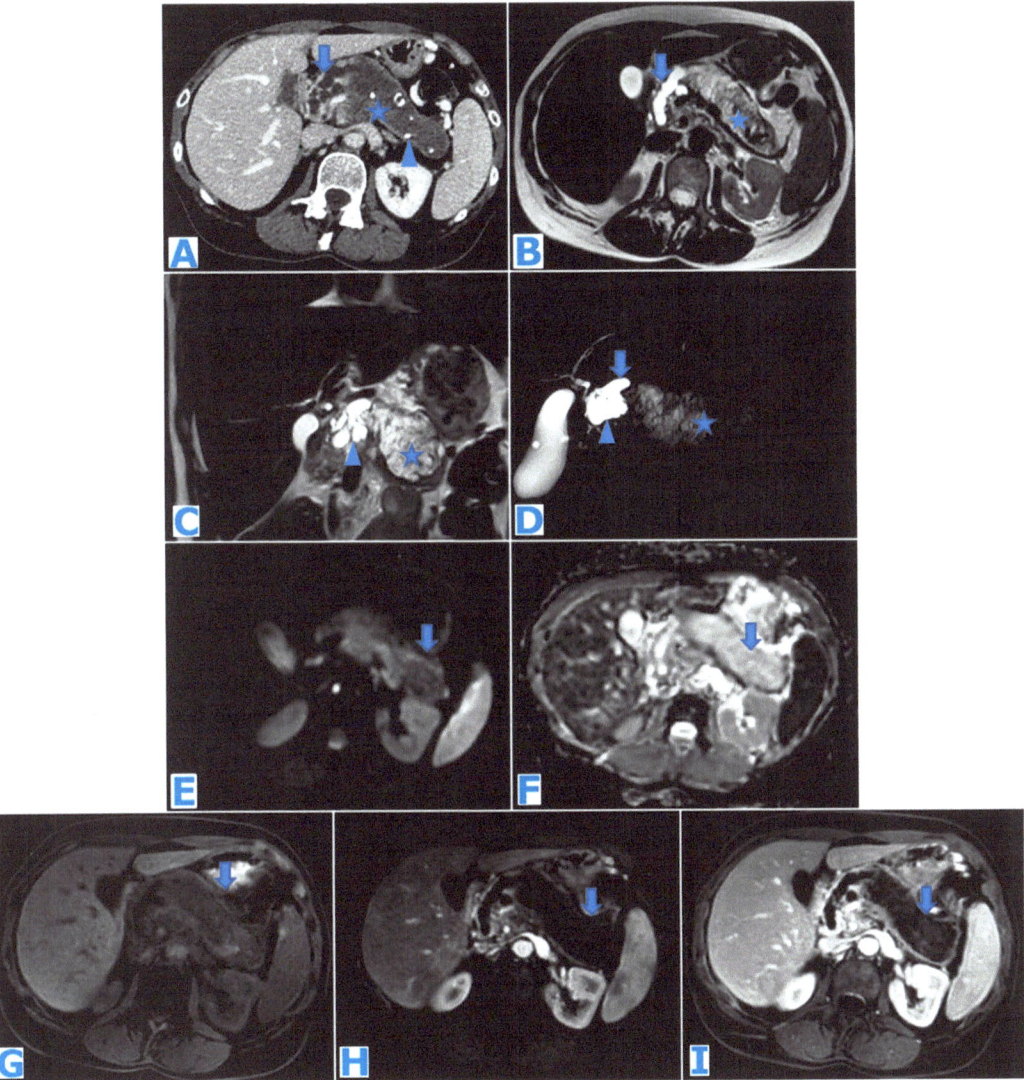

Figure 13. (**A**): axial CE portal venous phase CT, (**B**): axial T2WI, (**C**): coronal T2WI, (**D**): MRCP, (**E**): DWI, (**F**): ADC, (**G**): axial NCE FST1WI, (**H**): CE pancreatic parenchymal phase FST1WI, (**I**): axial CE portal venous phase FST1WI. Colloid carcinoma. Patient is a 52-year-old woman with left upper quadrant pain for the previous six months and weight loss (15 kg). Blood laboratory tests are anodyne. Observe the intraluminal mass within the body and distal pancreas (* in (**A–D**)), notice its salt and pepper pattern in T2WIs (* in (**B,C**)) and how it is partly calcified (arrowhead in (**A**)). The lesion is associated with downstream MPD dilatation (arrow in (**A,B,D**)) and side branch ecstasy (arrowhead in (**C,D**)). There is no diffusion restriction (arrow in (**E,F**)). In the dynamic sequences following intravenous contrast administration, the tumour shows gradual enhancement of the periphery and the subtle septa (arrows in (**G–I**)). Patient underwent a cephalic duodenopancreatectomy and diagnosis was pathologically proven.

CC has an indolent behaviour, and its prognosis is superior to PDAC: 5-year survival rates of 40–60% vs. 10–15%, respectively [216,217]. One of the reasons explaining this better prognosis is the mucin, which surrounds the cells and acts as a barrier preventing their spread [207,216]. The other reason lies within the surface glycoproteins present in colloid carcinoma: MUC1 is present in PDAC on the luminal aspect or throughout the cells, whereas CC expresses MUC1 on the basal surface [218]. Also, another surface glycoprotein found in CC, MUC2, not found in PDAC, has been described to have tumour suppressor activity [215].

A misleading cystic appearance due to the abundant mucin production may cause a misdiagnosis of cystic tumours, such as IPMN or a mucinous cystic adenocarcinoma [219]. Hallmarks to distinguish IPMN-unrelated colloid carcinomas from IPMN in cross-sectional images are an absence of communication with the MPD and of intraductal papillary components and a lack of downstream pancreatic ductal dilatation, features that can be successfully assessed with MRCP. Also, the typical papillary bulging into the duodenal lumen and spillage of mucin from the ampulla of Vater, typical findings on endoscopic retrograde cholangiopancreatography (ERCP), will not be present in CC [210,220]. Mucinous cystic adenocarcinomas, on the other hand, are large well-defined unilocular or macrocystic lesions with enhancing soft tissue components, different from the not-so-well-defined CC with progressive internal enhancement, besides the fact that the target populations are women.

In the event of an intraluminal CC communicating with the MPD, features will be difficult to distinguish from invasive IPMN on cross-sectional imaging and ERCP will be essential to rule IPMN out.

Even though FNA is useful to describe the large amounts of mucin, it may not provide enough data to complete the diagnosis [221]. The presence of malignant epithelial cells within a mucin magma should provide definitive diagnosis [179]. However, given the rarity of this entity, CCs are typically diagnosed during histological examination following surgery.

Surgery is recommended as the only curative treatment in eligible patients [221]. A recent study has suggested that adjuvant chemotherapy may not be effective for CC [222]. The survival rate has been reported to be better than for PDAC (5-year survival rate of 57%) [223]. Long-term surveillance is recommended to detect recurrence [221].

4.5. Primary Pancreatic Leiomyosarcoma (Figures 14 and 15)

Primary pancreatic leiomyosarcoma (PPLM) belongs to the group of malignant mesenchymal tumours that may originate in the pancreas, along with malignant peripheral nerve sheath tumours, undifferentiated pleomorphic sarcomas, liposarcomas, rhabdomyosarcomas, solitary fibrous tumour and primitive neuroectodermal tumours (PNETs), among which it ranks first in frequency [224]. It is a very rare and aggressive tumour, which accounts only for 0.1% of malignant pancreatic neoplasms [225].

Its cells show smooth muscle features [226], a fact that has given rise to theories regarding the walls of intrapancreatic vessels or the smooth muscle cells of the pancreatic ducts as possible origins [226]. These theories may be the rationale behind the close relationship between the tumour and the vessels/duct [226–229].

It occurs most frequently during the fifth decade; gender predominance is not clear [226,230–232]. An association with East Asian ethnicity has been recently proposed, with a higher prevalence of regional invasion [233].

Presenting symptoms are non-specific and variable, and the most frequently encountered complaints are abdominal pain/tenderness, weight loss and a palpable abdominal mass [229].

Since it is a mesenchymal tumour, there is no association with tumour markers.

No preferred site within the pancreas has been described [226], and there is similar incidence between the head and the body–tail [232].

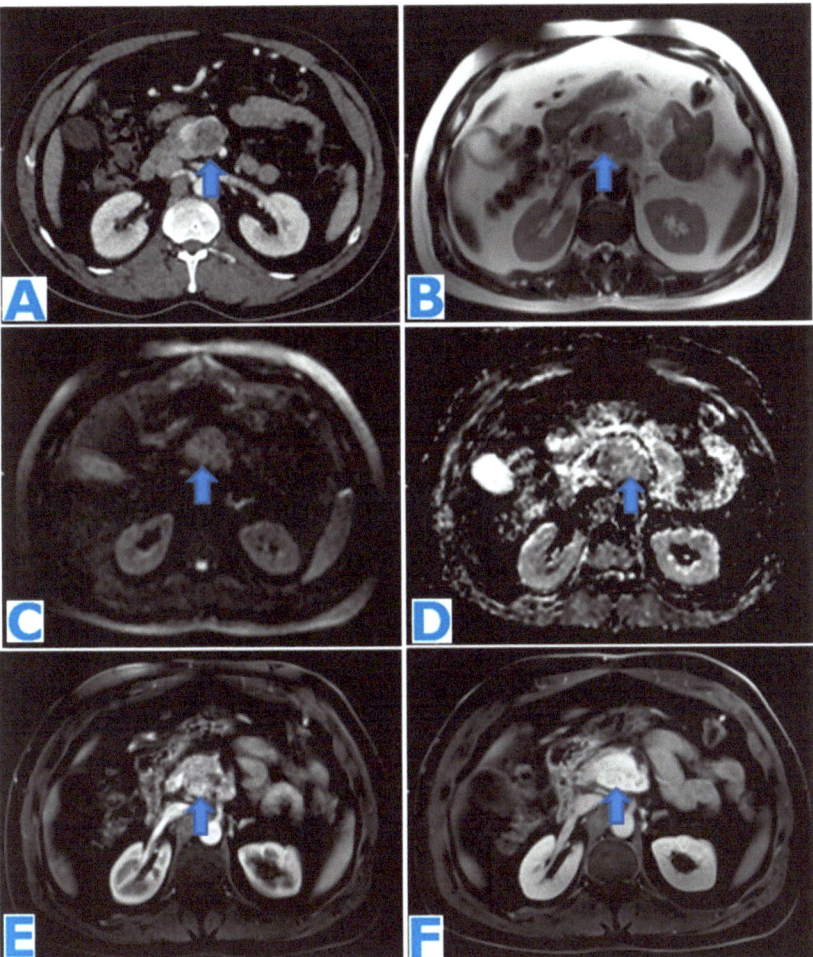

Figure 14. (**A**): axial CE portal venous phase CT, (**B**): axial T2WI, (**C**): DWI, (**D**): ADC, (**E**): axial CE pancreatic parenchymal phase FST1WI, (**F**): axial CE portal venous phase FST1WI. Primary pancreatic leiomyosarcoma incidentally discovered in a 53-year-old patient during a routine check-up. Note the heterogeneous mass within the pancreatic isthmus (arrow in (**B**)) with compression of the superior mesenteric and splenic vein (arrow in (**A**)). No biliary or pancreatic duct dilatation is observed. The lesion shows diffusion restriction (arrow in (**C,D**)) and hypervascularity, with progressive enhancement following intravenous contrast administration (arrow in (**E,F**)). EUS-guided FNB concluded PPLM. The patient underwent radiotherapy before surgery but then refused to be operated upon and developed hepatic and muscular metastases (not shown here). Stable disease was achieved with chemotherapy for five years, but it is currently progressing.

It is locally very aggressive and, since it is usually discovered at a late stage, invasion of neighbouring organs and vessels is a frequent feature. It is prone to metastasise to the liver, and lung metastases are also frequently present at diagnosis [232,234]. However, lymphatic spread is rare [226,229], a fact that could be helpful for differential diagnosis.

PPLMs have been described in the literature as non-specific masses on CT/MR, with size ranging from 3–25cm [230], that, as volume increases, become heterogeneous, with haemorrhagic, necrotic and cystic components, due to degenerative changes [232,235].

Peripheric enhancement is present with a large central non-enhancing component [235,236]. These features may lead to misdiagnosis of a large leiomyosarcoma as a pseudocyst [229] or a cystoadenocarcinoma [237].

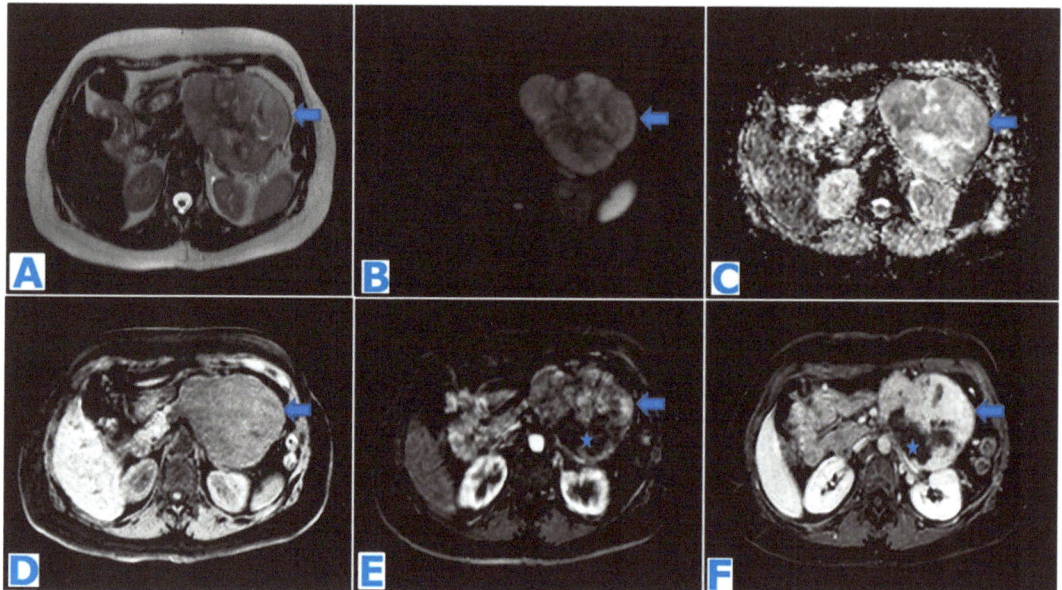

Figure 15. (**A**): axial T2WI, (**B**): DWI, (**C**): ADC, (**D**): axial NCE FST1WI, (**E**): axial CE pancreatic parenchymal phase FST1WI, (**F**): axial CE portal venous phase FST1WI. Primary pancreatic leiomyosarcoma incidentally discovered in a 50-year-old female patient during an ultrasound for a urinary infection. Observe the large heterogeneous mass in T2WI (arrow in (**A**)) within the distal pancreas, with diffusion restriction (arrow in (**B**,**C**)). The sequences following intravenous contrast administration show the central cystic/necrotic component (* in (**E**,**F**)) and the solid and progressively peripheral enhancement (arrow in (**D**–**F**)). Resectability criteria were fulfilled, and patient underwent distal pancreatectomy. Histological examination concluded PPLM.

Usually, there is no associated MPD dilatation. However, tumours arising from smooth cells of the pancreatic duct have been described [238].

It has been proposed that diagnosis should be entertained when confronted with a mass that fulfils the following criteria: large size, increased enhancement and absence of biliary duct dilatation [236] and other authors have added the presence of cystic/necrotic components to the list [239,240].

Differential diagnosis includes the far more frequent PDAC, and, less frequently, pNEN [240–242], a metastasis to the pancreas from another known primary tumour [240,243] and, more rarely, an invading leiomyosarcoma originating from adjacent organs and simulating a pancreatic primary tumour [244]. An isolated metastasis to the pancreas from a distant leiomyosarcoma is extremely rare [245], with female genital tract, gastrointestinal tract, soft tissues of the extremities and retroperitoneum as most common sites of origin [246].

Diagnosis is usually achieved after histological examinations and immunohistochemical staining [232], following surgery or intraoperative biopsy. EUS-guided FNA often comes up with false negative results due to the cystic and fibrous nature of the lesion [235,247].

In the absence of organ/vessel invasion or distant metastases, radical resection with negative margins stands as the only potentially curative treatment [248].

Radiation and chemotherapy have not achieved clinical success, as for other leiomyosarcomas [249–251].

It is usually associated with a poor outcome; the median survival time in a series of 49 cases [252] was 48 months.

4.6. Primary and Secondary Pancreatic Lymphoma (Figures 16–18)

Primary pancreatic lymphoma (PPL) is an extremely rare non-epithelial tumour that accounts for less than 0.5% of all pancreatic tumours and 1% of all extranodal lymphomas [253].

PPL occurs most commonly in middle-aged patients (mean age 53 years) [254], especially Caucasians [255], and with a male prevalence [254]. It is frequently associated with immunosuppression that seems to favour the disease [256].

Patients mainly complain of abdominal pain at diagnosis. Other presenting symptoms are jaundice, which is relatively common, pancreatitis and/or gastric or duodenal obstruction [110,257]. Fever, chills, night sweats and weight loss are associated with systemic non-Hodgkin lymphoma (constituting the classic B symptoms) but are rare in PPL [254].

The most frequent subtype is B-cell non-Hodgkin lymphoma [255].

CA 19-9 usually ranges within normal limits [254], even though PPL-associated biliary dilatation may cause a mild elevation of CA 19-9 [252]; LDH is often elevated [256]. Thus, the combination of increased LDH serum levels without concurrent increased CA 19-9 should favour the diagnosis of pancreatic lymphoma [255,258].

Different morphologic patterns have been described [259], the most common is a solitary focal mass. A diffuse infiltration with pancreatic enlargement, a peripheral involvement and a multinodular type comprehend the rest of the presentations.

The focal pattern occurs mainly within the head, as the part that contains the largest concentration of lymphoid tissue [255,260]. It is depicted as a bulky, well-circumscribed mass, ranging between 2 and 14 cm [255]. It is homogeneous, and it shows progressive and delayed but limited homogeneous enhancement, to a lesser degree compared to the preserved pancreatic parenchyma [259]. Characteristically, necrosis and calcification are hardly ever present [261], although necrosis may happen secondary to concomitant acute pancreatitis, or due to a duodenal fistula causing an intratumoral collection [262]. Compared to the preserved pancreatic parenchyma, PPL is usually hypointense in T1WIs and hyperintense in T2WIs [262]. The hallmark on MR imaging is the significant diffusion restriction, similar to that of the spleen.

The infiltrative pattern leads to a diffuse, ill-defined enlargement of the pancreas and may mimic acute pancreatitis [263]. However, even if both the focal and diffuse patterns may be associated with stranding of the peripancreatic fat [264], it is minimal, unlike the marked inflammation associated with acute pancreatitis. Moreover, the typical peripancreatic collections and a concordant clinical history are absent.

Peripheral involvement occurs rarely, as a focally enlarged hypointense pancreas in T1- and T2WIs, and with a capsule-like rim, which may mimic autoimmune pancreatitis [265].

The multinodular pattern is similar to the solitary focal mass, but the lesions are smaller [254]. Differential diagnosis includes multiple metastases from hypovascular tumours and multifocal autoimmune pancreatitis.

Despite the large size previously mentioned, the main pancreatic duct is usually not dilated [254] and pancreatic atrophy is not present [264]. Nevertheless, mild pancreatic duct dilatation may still be found so its presence should not rule out the possibility of pancreatic lymphoma [261]. The biliary duct has been described for a considerable number of patients [261]. However, even if present, biliary and/or pancreatic ductal obstruction will be disproportionately milder than expected, considering the size of the mass.

As with lymphomas elsewhere, PPL may infiltrate surrounding organs, not respecting anatomic boundaries, and may displace and encase adjacent vessels but will not invade or cause stenosis or occlusion [254]. No irregularities within the vessel wall are found [257,258].

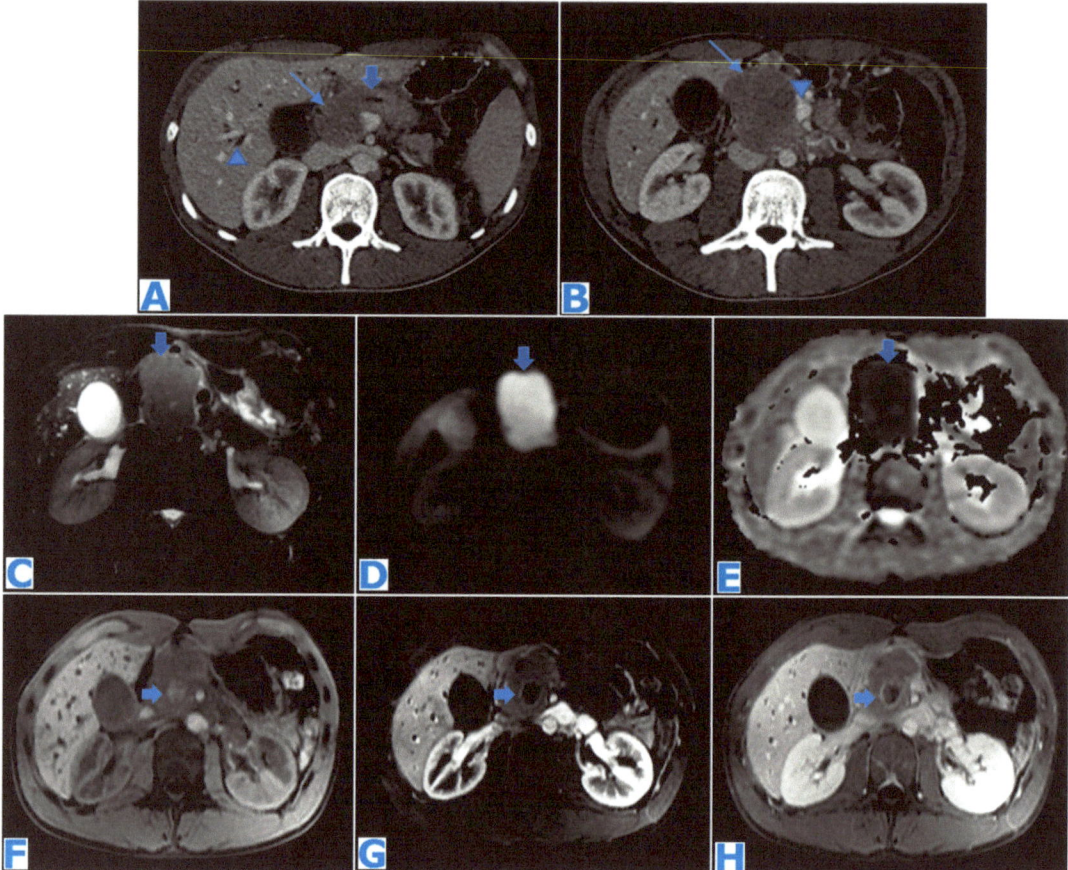

Figure 16. (**A,B**): axial CE portal venous phase CT. (**C**): axial FST2WI, (**D**): DWI, (**E**): ADC, (**F**): axial NCE FST1WI, (**G**): axial CE pancreatic parenchymal phase FST1WI, (**H**): axial CE portal venous phase FST1W1. Primary pancreatic lymphoma (focal form) in a 26-year-old patient with obstructive jaundice. CT revealed a hypovascular mass in the head of the pancreas (thin arrows in (**A,B**)), with minimal bile (arrowhead in (**A**)) and MPD dilatation (thick arrow in (**A**)), no distal parenchymal atrophy and abutment of the superior mesenteric vein (arrowhead in (**B**)). Note in the T2WI a homogeneous slightly hyperintense mass (arrow in (**C**)) with marked diffusion restriction (arrows in (**D,E**)) and its hypovascularity following intravenous contrast administration. Considering the tumour size, its homogeneity, marked diffusion restriction, growth pattern and hypovascularity with minimal MPD and biliary dilatation, lymphoma was one of the top possibilities on the differential diagnosis list. Note a small haematoma in the center of the mass (arrows on (**F–H**)) secondary to a EUS-guided biopsy, which concluded Burkitt lymphoma. The patient was successfully treated with chemotherapy, obtaining a complete remission.

A small volume of retroperitoneal lymphadenopathy is frequently found to be associated, both peripancreatic and around the aorta and cava vein. If present below the renal veins, pancreatic ductal adenocarcinoma can be confidently excluded [259,266,267].

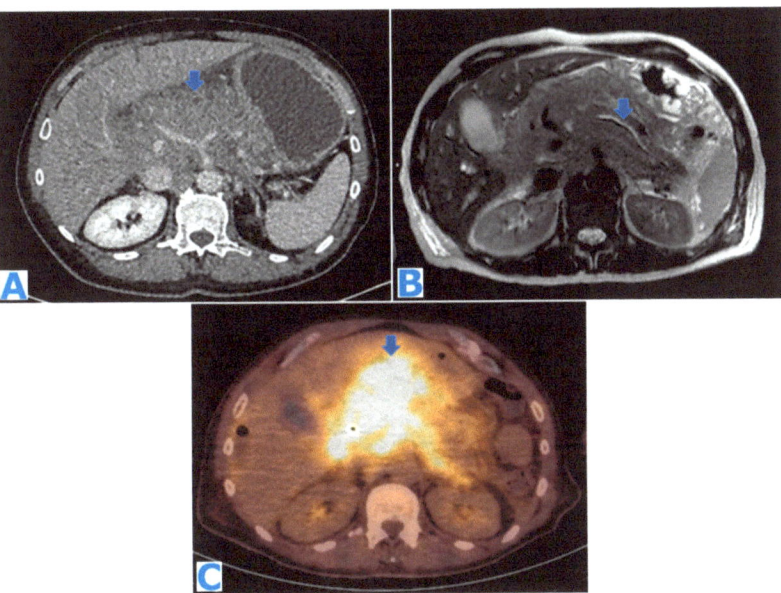

Figure 17. (**A**): axial CE portal venous phase CT, (**B**): axial T2WI, (**C**): FDG-PET-CT. Primary pancreatic lymphoma (diffuse form) in a 65-year-old alcoholic patient referred to our institution after being diagnosed with a pancreatic mass. An ill-defined infiltrating pancreatic mass is observed (arrow in (**A**)), with no biliary or pancreatic duct dilatation (observe the MPD's normal appearance, arrow in (**B**)). The mass shows an intense hypermetabolic uptake on the FDG-PET-CT (arrow in (**C**)). Biopsy revealed a high-grade PPL with diffuse big cell B lymphoma and Burkitt-like components.

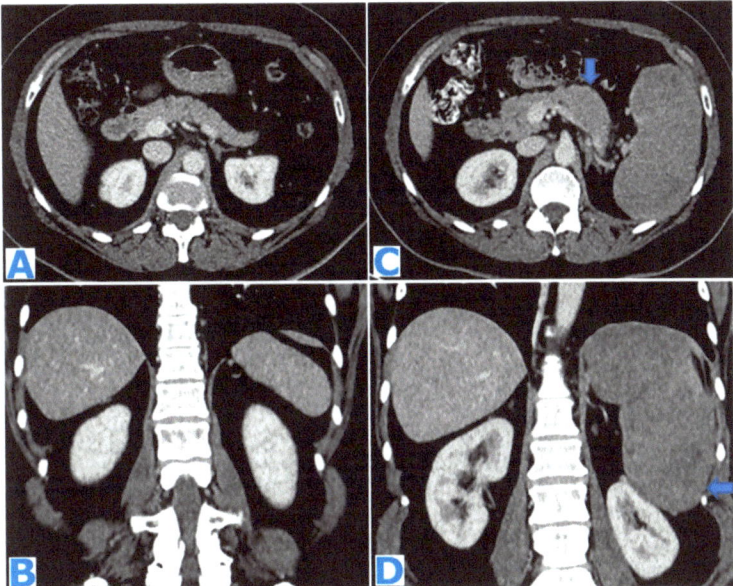

Figure 18. Images from 2017, (**A**,**B**): axial and coronal CE portal venous phase CT MPR. Images from 2022, (**C**,**D**): axial and coronal CE portal venous phase CT MPR. Secondary pancreatic lymphoma in

a 60-year-old patient with a known glomus jugulotympanicum paraganglioma on surveillance. Note the normal appearance of pancreas and the spleen (**A**,**B**) on the prior CT. Abdominal adenopathies were found (not shown). Observe the spleen enlargement (arrow in (**D**)), with focal lesions. Hepatoduodenal and retroperitoneal adenopathies were also found (not shown). Note the isoenhancing mass within the body of the pancreas (arrow in (**C**)). EUS-guided FNB revealed a diffuse large B-cell SPL.

Secondary pancreatic lymphoma (SPL) is a direct involvement of the pancreas from peripancreatic adenopathies and, as opposed to the primary tumour, occurs more frequently, in up to 30% of lymphoma patients [257], especially in widespread nodal or extranodal disease [268]. Even in this scenario, a predominant involvement of the pancreas is quite uncommon [269]. The most common type is diffuse large B-cell non-Hodgkin lymphoma [270]. SPL may also show the different presentation patterns previously described [259]. It may be difficult to distinguish on imaging from the diffuse form of PPL, but the clinical setting is different.

PPL may be misdiagnosed as PDAC, as they share imaging features. Differentiation becomes critical as PPL is highly sensitive to chemotherapy and does not require surgery. Diagnosis is achieved after EUS-guided biopsy. Long-term regression or remission is frequently achieved, with survival rates similar to those of nodal non-Hodgkin lymphoma [255]. However, relapses occur frequently [271], especially at distant sites, like the central nervous system [255,257,272], and prolonged follow-up is recommended.

4.7. Pancreatic Metastases (Figures 19–22)

Metastases to the pancreas are uncommon, only accounting for 2–5% of pancreatic malignancies [273]. They mostly occur secondary to intra-abdominal tumours [274], including RCC, colon and gastric cancer [275,276], although lung cancer also ranks high among the most frequent sites of origin [276].

PM may invade the epithelium of the pancreatic duct and mimic PDAC symptoms, namely, jaundice and abdominal pain as the most common presenting signs [276,277]. However, PM may also be asymptomatic and incidentally identified during the initial workup of the primary tumour or during surveillance. There may be a latency period from the diagnosis of the primary tumour to the detection of PM, which in the case of clear cell renal or breast carcinoma may be quite long, up to 21 years after surgery of RCC [276–278].

PMs are commonly associated with widespread disease, at a late stage, and more than 90% of patients have extrapancreatic disease [279]. However, it should be noted that in more than half of PM cases, the pancreas is the only organ metastatically involved [280], especially in RCC [281].

There is no location predilection within the pancreas [282]. In the particular case of PM from lung cancers, the head seems to be a favoured site as 76% of small cell lung carcinomas, the histological type mostly associated with PM [283], arise there [284].

Cancer antigens have little diagnostic reliability [285]. In an analysis of series with 192 cases in total, CA 19-9 was elevated in 8–28% of cases, but this may be related to the gastrointestinal origin of most of the primary tumours included and unrelated to PM [286].

Three patterns of metastatic involvement have been described. The most common appearance (50–75%) is the single pattern, depicting a solitary, localised and well-defined lesion. The second most common is the diffuse infiltration that causes a generalised enlargement of the pancreas (15–44%). The remaining pattern (5–10%) is represented by several nodules, which can coalesce into larger masses [280,287].

Dilatation of the main pancreatic or bile ducts is uncommon [288].

PMs typically appear hypointense in FST1WIs compared to normal parenchyma and may show moderate hyperintensity in T2WIs [289] although they may also appear hypointense, especially in the diffuse infiltration pattern. The behaviour after intravenous contrast injection relates to size: even though most of the lesions are hypovascular, lesions smaller than 1.5 cm may be hypervascular and larger lesions may show a rim of enhancement due to central necrosis [290,291]. This peripheral enhancement pattern has been described as a frequent finding (41%) [263,292], especially in PMs from RCC. The rationale behind this enhancement pattern is that the periphery of the lesion receives more blood than the center, since PMs nurture themselves by parasitising blood supply from the surrounding parenchyma.

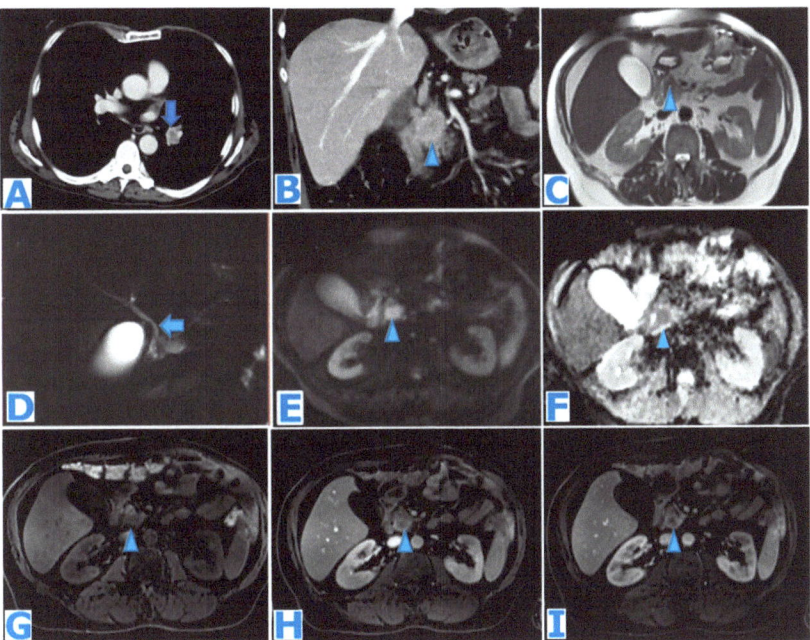

Figure 19. (**A**): axial CE-CT, (**B**): coronal MPR CE portal venous phase CT, (**C**): axial T2WI, (**D**): MRCP, (**E**): DWI, (**F**): ADC, (**G**): axial NCE FST1WI, (**H**): axial CE arterial phase FST1WI, (**I**): axial CE portal venous phase FST1WI. Solitary PM from lung adenocarcinoma in a 56-year-old patient with advanced stage disease and hyperbilirubinemia. Observe the primary tumour within the left hilum (arrow in (**A**)). The patient also presented peritoneal and bone metastases, not shown. A mass was found within the head of the pancreas (arrowhead in (**B**)), with no MPD dilatation (arrowhead in (**C**)). However, the lesion was associated with discreet common bile duct dilatation (arrow in (**D**)). Observe the diffusion restriction (arrowhead in (**E**,**F**)) and the progressive peripheral enhancement following intravenous contrast administration (arrowhead in (**G**–**I**)) with central necrosis. Note the resemblance to the primary tumour (arrow in (**A**)). EUS-guided FNB confirmed a PM from an adenocarcinoma of pulmonary origin.

As in any other organ, PM features resemble those of the primary tumour, e.g., PMs from RCC are often hypervascular [293]. PMs from melanoma, due to the paramagnetic effect of melanin, show a high signal intensity in T1WIs and low signal intensity in T2WIs [294]. PMs from dermatofibrosarcoma are usually hypointense in T1WIs, slightly hyperintense in T2WIs and show a spoke wheel-like enhancement [295].

At least one third of PMs are misdiagnosed as primary tumours [296]. Differential diagnosis of hypervascular PM should include primary pancreatic NET, intrapancreatic accessory spleen and vascular lesions [292]. Hypovascular PMs need to be differentiated from PDAC, lymphoma and focal pancreatitis [297,298]. Peripheral enhancement is a useful sign to differentiate PM from PDAC [263]; other distinguishing features are absence of dilatation of the upstream pancreatic duct and/or bile ducts, parenchymal atrophy and absence of vessel involvement [293,294].

The treatment of choice in eligible patients is pancreatic metastasectomy. However, its success depends on the biology of the primary tumour. According to most large studies, the best long-term survival predictor is the type of cancer [275,299]. PMs from RCC achieve the best outcome (61% 5-year survival) [274] and surgery is the treatment of choice if all metastatic lesions can be resected, although there is a high rate of recurrence (33–42% of patients who undergo pancreatic metastasectomy). On the other end of the spectrum, lung carcinoma is associated with the worst survival (0%) [300].

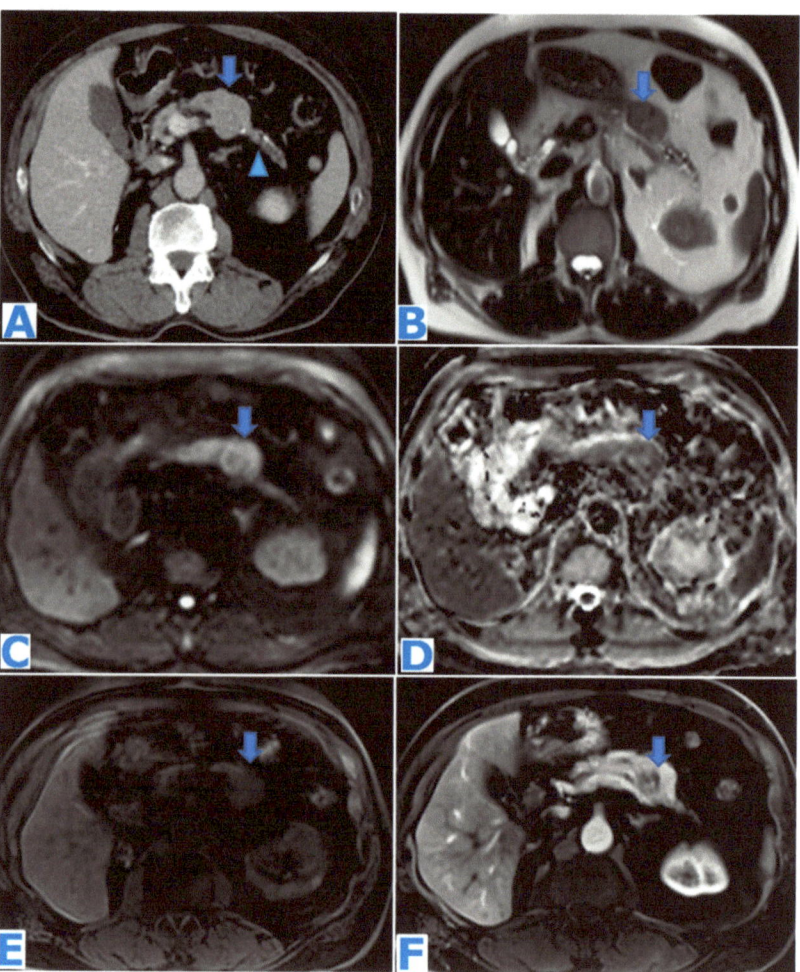

Figure 20. (**A**): axial CE-CT, (**B**): axial T2WI, (**C**): DWI, (**D**): ADC, (**E**): axial NCE FST1W1, (**F**): axial CE arterial phase FST1W1. Solitary PM from a known RCC discovered during follow-up in a 56-year-old patient who underwent a right nephrectomy 10 years prior. A homogeneous mass was found within the body of the pancreas (arrow in (**A**,**B**)), with discrete pancreatic duct dilatation and distal parenchymal atrophy (arrowhead in (**A**)). The mass showed diffusion restriction (arrow in (**C**,**D**)) and marked peripheral enhancement (arrow in (**E**,**F**)). An EUS-guided FNB showed rare epithelial cells and concluded haemorrhagic cyst. Given the discordance between the images and the histological report, the MDT decided to perform a left pancreatectomy and the histological examination concluded RCC metastasis.

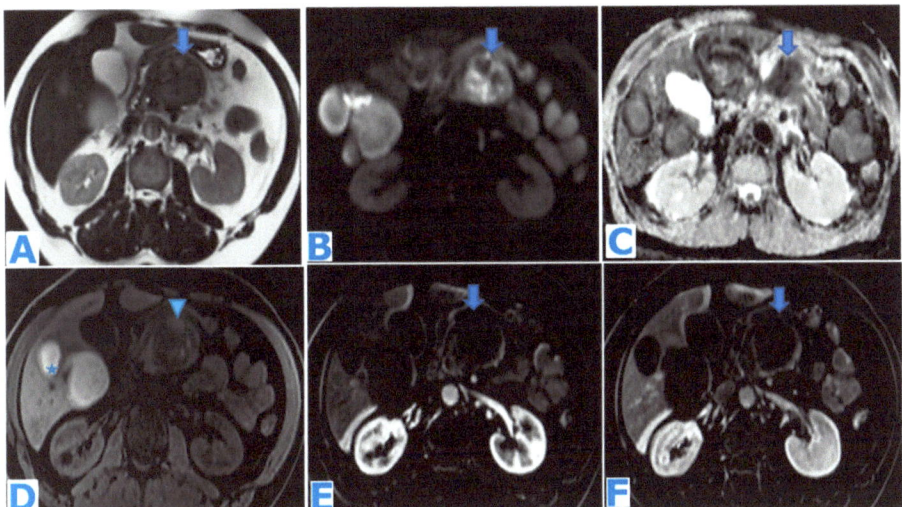

Figure 21. (**A**): axial T2WI, (**B**): DWI, (**C**): ADC, (**D**): NCE FST1W1, (**E**): CE arterial phase FST1W1 subtraction, (**F**): CE portal venous phase FST1W1 subtraction. PM from a known malignant skin melanoma in a 54-year-old patient who presented with acute abdominal pain. A heterogeneous mass was found within the body of the pancreas (arrow in (**A**)), showing diffusion restriction (arrow in (**B**,**C**)) and no pancreatic duct dilatation. The lesion showed hyperintense content in T1WIs (arrowhead in (**D**)) compatible with melanin, with scarce enhancement after intravenous contrast administration (arrow in (**E**,**F**)). There were also several melanin-containing hepatic lesions (* in (**D**)). Diagnosis of pancreatic and hepatic metastases was proven by biopsy.

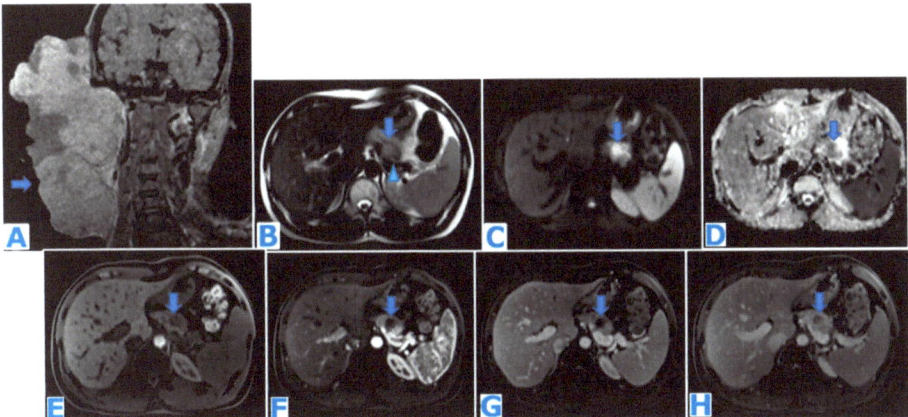

Figure 22. (**A**): image from 2016: coronal CE T1WI. Images from 2021: (**B**): axial T2WI, (**C**): DWI, (**D**): ADC, (**E**): NCE FST1WI, (**F–H**): axial CE dynamic FST1WI (pancreatic parenchymal, portal venous and delayed venous phase). PM from a facial DFSP in a 35-year-old patient who presented with elevated pancreatic enzymes on a check-up, five years after the primary tumour diagnosis (arrow in (**A**)). Five solid lesions were found within the pancreas, of which only one is shown, slightly hyperintense in T2WIs (arrow in (**B**)) with minimal MPD dilatation (arrowhead in (**B**)), diffusion restriction (arrow in (**C**,**D**)) and a hypovascular behaviour following intravenous contrast administration with progressive enhancement (corresponding to the fibrous content) (arrow in (**E–H**)). Histological examination following EUS-FNB concluded PM from DFSP.

5. Conclusions

Several rare focal and diffuse lesions may be found in the pancreas, either incidentally discovered, related to specific or, most frequently, non-specific clinical symptoms and biological abnormalities, or in the setting of a known oncologic condition. These lesions are associated with different behaviours, which range from benign to very aggressively malignant and, therefore, they are associated with different prognosis. Cross-sectional imaging findings combined with the clinico-biological setting contribute substantially to achieving the correct diagnosis. Typical imaging features related to the appearance of the lesion on cross-section imaging modalities in addition to indirect associated signs, such as the presence/absence of biliary and/or pancreatic duct dilatation, invasion of adjacent organs, peripancreatic vascular involvement or loco-regional lymph nodal invasion together with the presence of distant metastases, are crucial to correctly address the diagnosis.

Nevertheless, challenging cases occur, in which imaging features remain indeterminate and there is no typical clinical or biological presentation, and thus EUS-FNA/FNB is required to obtain histologically proven confirmation of the nature of the lesion, which is mandatory for optimal patient management.

Supplementary Materials: The following supporting information can be downloaded at: https://www.mdpi.com/article/10.3390/diagnostics13162719/s1, Table S1: Benign Lesions; Table S2: Potentially Malignant Lesions; Table S3: Malignant Lesions.

Funding: This review received no external funding.

Acknowledgments: The authors are grateful to Valérie Vilgrain for contributing with the colloid carcinoma case and Pedro Veron Guembe for his help with editing.

Conflicts of Interest: The authors declare no conflict of interest.

References

1. Fletcher, J.G.; Wiersema, M.J.; Farrell, M.A.; Fidler, J.L.; Burgart, L.J.; Koyama, T.; Johnson, C.D.; Stephens, D.H.; Ward, E.M.; Harmsen, W.S. Pancreatic malignancy: Value of arterial, pancreatic, and hepatic phase imaging with multi-detector row CT. *Radiology* **2003**, *229*, 81–90. [CrossRef] [PubMed]
2. Dodds, W.J.; Taylor, A.J.; Erickson, S.J.; Stewart, E.T.; Lawson, T.L. Radiologic imaging of splenic anomalies. *AJR Am. J. Roentgenol.* **1990**, *155*, 805–810. [CrossRef]
3. Lehtinen, S.J.; Schammel, C.M.; Devane, M.; Trocha, S.D. Intrapancreatic accessory spleen presenting as a pancreatic mass. *J. Gastrointest. Oncol.* **2013**, *4*, E23–E26.
4. Lake, S.T.; Johnson, P.T.; Devane, M.; Trocha, S.D. CT of splenosis: Patterns and pitfalls. *AJR Am. J. Roentgenol.* **2012**, *199*, W686–W693. [CrossRef] [PubMed]
5. White, J.D.; West, A.N.; Priebat, D.A. Splenosis mimicking an intra-abdominal malignancy. *Am. J. Med.* **1989**, *87*, 687–690. [CrossRef]
6. Abu Hilal, M.; Harb, A.; Zeidan, B.; Steadman, B.; Primrose, J.N.; Pearce, N.W. Hepatic splenosis mimicking HCC in a patient with hepatitis C liver cirrhosis and mildly raised alpha feto protein; the important role of explorative laparoscopy. *World J. Surg. Oncol.* **2009**, *7*, 1. [CrossRef] [PubMed]
7. Ding, Q.; Ren, Z.; Da Rold, A.; Guerriero, S.; Pariset, S.; Buffone, A.; Tedeschi, U. A rare diagnosis for a pancreatic mass: Splenosis. *J. Gastrointest. Surg.* **2004**, *8*, 915–916.
8. Halpert, B.; Gyorkey, F. Lesions observed in accessory spleens of 311 patients. *Am. J. Clin. Pathol.* **1959**, *32*, 165–168. [CrossRef]
9. Kim, S.H.; Lee, J.M.; Han, J.K.; Lee, J.Y.; Kim, K.W.; Cho, K.C.; Choi, B.I. Intrapancreatic accessory spleen: Findings on MR Imaging, CT, US and scintigraphy, and the pathologic analysis. *Korean J. Radiol.* **2008**, *9*, 162–174. [CrossRef] [PubMed]
10. Varga, I.; Galfiova, P.; Adamkov, M.; Danisovic, L.; Polak, S.; Kubikova, E.; Galbavy, S. Congenital anomalies of the spleen from an embryological point of view. *Med. Sci. Monit.* **2009**, *15*, RA269–RA276. [PubMed]
11. Kawamoto, S.; Johnson, P.T.; Hall, H.; Cameron, J.L.; Hruban, R.H.; Fishman, E.K. Intrapancreatic accessory spleen: CT appearance and differential diagnosis. *Abdom. Imaging* **2012**, *37*, 812–827. [CrossRef]
12. Glazer, G.M.; Axel, L.; Goldberg, H.I.; Moss, A.A. Dynamic CT of the normal spleen. *AJR Am. J. Roentgenol.* **1981**, *137*, 343–346. [CrossRef]
13. Ding, Q.; Ren, Z.; Wang, J.; Ma, X.; Zhang, J.; Sun, G.; Zuo, C.; Gu, H.; Jiang, H. Intrapancreatic accessory spleen: Evaluation with CT and MRI. *Exp. Ther. Med.* **2018**, *16*, 3623–3631. [CrossRef]
14. Lin, W.C.; Lee, R.C.; Chiang, J.H.; Wei, C.J.; Chu, L.S.; Liu, R.S.; Chang, C.Y. MR features of abdominal splenosis. *AJR Am. J. Roentgenol.* **2003**, *180*, 493–496. [CrossRef] [PubMed]

15. Davidson, E.D.; Campbell, W.G.; Hersh, T. Epidermoid splenic cyst occurring in an intrapancreatic accessory spleen. *Dig. Dis. Sci.* **1980**, *25*, 964–967. [CrossRef]
16. Hu, S.; Zhu, L.; Song, Q.; Chen, K. Epidermoid cyst in intrapancreatic accessory spleen: Computed tomography findings and clinical manifestation. *Abdom. Imaging* **2012**, *37*, 828–833. [CrossRef]
17. Okura, N.; Mori, K.; Morishita, Y.; Oda, T.; Tanoi, T.; Minami, M. Inflammatory pseudotumor of the intrapancreatic accessory spleen: Computed tomography and magnetic resonance imaging findings. *Jpn. J. Radiol.* **2012**, *30*, 171–175. [CrossRef]
18. Mariani, G.; Bruselli, L.; Kuwert, T.; Kim, E.E.; Flotats, A.; Israel, O.; Dondi, M.; Watanabe, N. A review on the clinical uses of SPECT/CT. *Eur. J. Nucl. Med. Mol. Imaging* **2010**, *37*, 1959–1985. [CrossRef]
19. Barquilla-Cordero, P.; Chiquero-Palomo, M.; Martín-Noguerol, E.; Pacheco-Gómez, N.; Vinagre-Rodríguez, G.; Moyano-Calvente, S.L.; Molina-Infante, J. Tuberculosis pancreática primaria en un paciente inmunocompetente: Primer caso comunicado en España. *Gastroenterol. Hepatol.* **2010**, *33*, 582–585. [CrossRef]
20. Panic, N.; Maetzel, H.; Bulajic, M.; Radovanovic, M.; Löhr, J.-M. Pancreatic tuberculosis: A systematic review of symptoms, diagnosis and treatment. *United Eur. Gastroenterol. J.* **2020**, *8*, 396–402. [CrossRef]
21. De Backer, A.I.; Mortelé, K.J.; Bomans, P.; De Keulenaer, B.L.; Vanschoubroeck, I.J.; Kockx, M.M. Tuberculosis of the pancreas: MRI features. *AJR Am. J. Roentgeno* **2005**, *184*, 50–54. [CrossRef]
22. Pandita, K.K.; Sarla, D.S. Isolated pancreatic tuberculosis. *Indian. J. Med. Microbiol.* **2009**, *27*, 259–260. [CrossRef] [PubMed]
23. Baraboutis, I.; Skoutelis, A. Isolated tuberculosis of pancreas. *J. Pancreas* **2004**, *5*, 155–158.
24. Xia, F.; Poon, R.T.; Wang, S.G.; Bie, P.; Huang, X.Q.; Dong, J.H. Tuberculosis of pancreas and peripancreatic lymph nodes in immunocompetent patients: Experience from China. *World J. Gastroenterol.* **2003**, *9*, 1361–1364. [CrossRef] [PubMed]
25. Nagar, A.M.; Raut, A.A.; Morani, A.C.; Sanghvi, D.A.; Desai, C.S.; Thapar, V.B. Pancreatic Tuberculosis: A Clinical and Imaging Review of 32 Cases. *J. Comput. Assist. Tomogr.* **2009**, *33*, 136–141. [CrossRef] [PubMed]
26. Knowles, K.F.; Saltman, D.; Robson, H.G.; Lalonde, R. Tuberculous pancreatitis. *Tubercle* **1990**, *71*, 65–68. [CrossRef]
27. Radin, D.R. Intraabdominal Mycobacterium tuberculosis vs Mycobacterium avium-intracellulare infections in patients with AIDS: Distinction based on CT findings. *AJR Am. J. Roentgenol.* **1991**, *156*, 487–491. [CrossRef]
28. Tetlezi, J.P.; Pisegna, J.R.; Barkin, J.S. Tuberculous pancreatic abscess as a manifestation of AIDS. *Am. J. Gastroenterol.* **1989**, *84*, 581–582.
29. Levine, R.; Tenner, S.; Steinberg, W.; Ginsberg, A.; Borum, M.; Huntington, D. Tuberculous abscess of the pancreas. Case report and review of literature. *Dig. Dis. Sci.* **1992**, *37*, 141–144. [CrossRef]
30. Puri, R.; Thandassery, R.B.; Eloubeidi, M.A.; Sud, R. Diagnosis of isolated pancreatic tuberculosis: The role of EUS-guided FNA cytology. *Gastrointest. Endosc.* **2012**, *75*, 900–904. [CrossRef]
31. Pombo, F.; Díaz Candamio, M.J.; Rodriguez, E.; Pombo, S. Pancreatic tuberculosis. CT findings. *Abdom. Imaging* **1998**, *23*, 394–397. [CrossRef]
32. Ladas, S.D.; Vaidakis, E.; Lariou, C.; Anastasiou, K.; Chalevelakis, G.; Kintzonidis, D.; Raptis, S.A. Pancreatic tuberculosis in non-immunocompromised patients: Reports of two cases and a literature review. *Eur. J. Gastroenterol. Hepatol.* **1998**, *10*, 973–976. [CrossRef]
33. Dou, Y.; Liang, Z. Pancreatic tuberculosis: A computed tomography imaging review of thirteen cases. *Radiol. Infect. Dis.* **2019**, *6*, 31–37. [CrossRef]
34. Fischer, G.; Spengler, U.; Nuebrand, M.; Sauerbruch, T. Isolated tuberculosis of the pancreas masquerading as a pancreatic mass. *Am. J. Gastroenterol.* **1995**, *90*, 2227–2230.
35. Rana, S.S.; Sharma, V.; Sampath, S.; Sharma, R.; Mittal, B.R.; Bhasin, D.K. Vascular invasion does not discriminate between pancreatic tuberculosis and pancreatic malignancy: A case series. *Ann. Gastroenterol.* **2014**, *27*, 395–398.
36. Sharma, V.; Rana, S.S.; Kumar, A.; Bhasin, D.K. Pancreatic tuberculosis. *J. Gastroenterol. Hepatol.* **2016**, *31*, 310–318. [CrossRef] [PubMed]
37. Ibrahim, G.F.; Al-Nakshabandi, N.A. Pancreatic tuberculosis: Role of multidetector computed tomography. *Can. Assoc. Radiol. J.* **2011**, *62*, 260–264. [CrossRef]
38. D'Cruz, S.; Sachdev, A.; Kaur, L.; Handa, U.; Bhalla, A.; Lehl, S.S. Fine needle aspiration diagnosis of isolated pancreatic tuberculosis. A case report and review of literature. *J. Pancreas* **2003**, *4*, 158–162.
39. Kimura, W.; Moriya, T.; Hirai, I.; Hanada, K.; Abe, H.; Yanagisawa, A.; Fukushima, N.; Ohike, N.; Shimizu, M.; Hatori, T.; et al. Multicenter study of serous cystic neoplasm of the Japan pancreas society. *Pancreas* **2012**, *41*, 380–387. [CrossRef]
40. Demesmaker, V.; Abou-Messaoud, F.; Parent, M.; Vanhoute, B.; Maassarani, F.; Kothonidis, K. Pancreatic solid serous cystadenoma: A rare entity that can lead to a futile surgery. *J. Surg. Case Rep.* **2019**, *12*, 360. [CrossRef]
41. Compagno, J.; Oertel, J.E. Microcystic adenoma of the pancreas (glycogen-rich cystadenoma): A clinicopathologic study of 34 cases. *Am. J. Clin. Pathol.* **1978**, *69*, 289–298. [CrossRef] [PubMed]
42. Chu, L.C.; Singhi, A.D.; Haroun, R.R.; Hruban, R.H.; Fishman, E.K. The many faces of pancreatic serous cystadenoma: Radiologic and pathologic correlation. *Diagn. Interv. Imaging* **2017**, *98*, 191–202. [CrossRef]
43. Jais, B.; Rebours, V.; Malleo, G.; Salvia, R.; Fontana, M.; Maggino, L.; Bassi, C.; Manfredi, R.; Moran, R.; Lennon, A.M.; et al. Serous cystic neoplasm of the pancreas: A multinational study of 2622 patients under the auspices of the International Association of Pancreatology and European Pancreatic Club (European Study Group on Cystic Tumors of the Pancreas). *Gut* **2016**, *65*, 305–312. [CrossRef]

44. Okumura, Y.; Noda, T.; Eguchi, H.; Iwagami, Y.; Yamada, D.; Asaoka, T.; Kawamoto, K.; Gotoh, K.; Kobayashi, S.; Umeshita, K.; et al. Middle segment pancreatectomy for a solid serous cystadenoma diagnosed by MRCP and review of the literature: A case report. *Mol. Clin. Oncol.* **2018**, *8*, 675–682. [CrossRef]
45. Kishida, Y.; Matsubayashi, H.; Okamura, Y.; Uesaka, K.; Sasaki, K.; Sawai, H.; Imai, K.; Ono, H. A case of solid-type serous cystadenoma mimicking neuroendocrine tumor of the pancreas. *J. Dig. Dis.* **2014**, *15*, 211–215. [CrossRef]
46. Sun, H.Y.; Kim, S.H.; Kim, M.A.; Lee, J.Y.; Han, J.K.; Choi, B.I. CT imaging spectrum of pancreatic serous tumors: Based on new pathologic classification. *Eur. J. Radiol.* **2010**, *75*, 45–55. [CrossRef]
47. Stern, J.R.; Frankel, W.L.; Ellison, E.C.; Bloomston, M. Solid serous microcystic adenoma of the pancreas. *World J. Surg. Oncol.* **2007**, *5*, 26. [CrossRef]
48. European Study Group on Cystic Tumours of the Pancreas: European evidence-based guidelines on pancreatic cystic neoplasms. *Gut* **2018**, *67*, 789–804. [CrossRef] [PubMed]
49. Ganeshan, D.M.; Paulson, E.; Tamm, E.P.; Taggart, M.W.; Balachandran, A.; Bhosale, P. Solid pseudo-papillary tumors of the pancreas: Current update. *Abdom. Imaging* **2013**, *38*, 1373–1382. [CrossRef] [PubMed]
50. De Robertis, R.; Marchegiani, G.; Catania, M.; Ambrosetti, M.C.; Capelli, P.; Salvia, R.; D'Onofrio, M. Solid Pseudopapillary Neoplasms of the Pancreas: Clinicopathologic and Radiologic Features According to Size. *AJR Am. J. Roentgenol.* **2019**, *213*, 1073–1080. [CrossRef]
51. Canzonieri, V.; Berretta, M.; Buonadonna, A.; Libra, M.; Vasquez, E.; Barbagallo, E.; Bearz, A.; Berretta, S. Solid pseudopapillary tumour of the pancreas. *Lancet Oncol.* **2003**, *4*, 255–256. [CrossRef] [PubMed]
52. Cienfuegos, J.A.; Lozano, M.D.; Rotellar, F.; Martí, P.; Pedano, N.; Arredondo, J.; Bellver, M.; Sola, J.J.; Pardo, F. Solid pseudopapillary tumor of the pancreas (SPPT). Still an unsolved enigma. *Rev. Esp. Enferm. Dig.* **2010**, *102*, 722–728. [CrossRef] [PubMed]
53. Kosmahl, M.; Seada, L.S.; Jänig, U.; Harms, D.; Klöppel, G. Solid-pseudopapillary tumor of the pancreas: Its origin revisited. *Virchows Arch.* **2000**, *436*, 473–480. [CrossRef] [PubMed]
54. Machado, M.C.; Machado, M.A.; Bacchella, T.; Jukemura, J.; Almeida, J.L.; Cunha, J.E. Solid pseudopapillary neoplasm of the pancreas: Distinct patterns of onset, diagnosis, and prognosis for male versus female patients. *Surgery* **2008**, *143*, 29–34. [CrossRef]
55. Papavramidis, T.; Papavramidis, S. Solid pseudopapillary tumors of the pancreas: Review of 718 patients reported in English literature. *J. Am. Coll. Surg.* **2005**, *200*, 965–972. [CrossRef]
56. Orlando, C.A.; Bowman, R.L.; Loose, J.H. Multicentric papillary-cystic neoplasm of the pancreas. *Arch. Pathol. Lab. Med.* **1991**, *115*, 958–960.
57. Salvia, R.; Bassi, C.; Festa, L.; Falconi, M.; Crippa, S.; Butturini, G.; Brighenti, A.; Capelli, P.; Pederzoli, P. Clinical and biological behavior of pancreatic solidpseudopapillary tumors: Report on 31 consecutive patients. *J. Surg. Oncol.* **2007**, *95*, 304–310. [CrossRef]
58. Adams, A.L.; Siegal, G.P.; Jhala, N.C. Solid pseudopapillary tumor of the pancreas: A review of salient clinical and pathologic features. *Adv. Anat. Pathol.* **2008**, *15*, 39–45. [CrossRef]
59. Huang, S.C.; Wu, T.H.; Chen, C.C.; Chen, T.C. Spontaneous rupture of solid pseudopapillary neoplasm of the pancreas during pregnancy. *Obs. Gynecol.* **2013**, *121*, 486–488. [CrossRef]
60. Mirapoğlu, S.L.; Aydogdu, I.; Gucin, Z.; Yilmaz, T.F.; Umutoglu, T.; Kilincaslan, H. Traumatic rupture of solid pseudopapillary tumors of the pancreas in children: A case report. *Mol. Clin. Oncol.* **2016**, *5*, 587–589. [CrossRef]
61. Hibi, T.; Ojima, H.; Sakamoto, Y.; Kosuge, T.; Shimada, K.; Sano, T.; Sakamoto, M.; Kitajima, M.; Yamasaki, S. A solid pseudopapillary tumor arising from the greater omentum followed by multiple metastases with increasing malignant potential. *J. Gastroenterol.* **2006**, *41*, 276–281. [CrossRef] [PubMed]
62. Chen, J.; Zong, L.; Wang, P.; Liu, Y.; Zhang, H.; Chang, X.; Lu, Z.; Li, W.; Ma, Y.; Yu, S.; et al. Solid Pseudopapillary Neoplasms of the Pancreas: Clinicopathologic Analysis and a Predictive Model. *Mod. Pathol.* **2023**, *36*, 100141. [CrossRef] [PubMed]
63. Wu, H.; Huang, Y.F.; Liu, X.H.; Xu, M.H. Extrapancreatic solid pseudopapillary neoplasm followed by multiple metastases: Case report. *World J. Gastrointest. Oncol.* **2017**, *9*, 497–501. [CrossRef]
64. Miyazaki, Y.; Miyajima, A.; Maeda, T.; Yuge, K.; Hasegawa, M.; Kosaka, T.; Kikuchi, E.; Kameyama, K.; Jinzaki, M.; Nakagawa, K.; et al. Extrapancreatic solid pseudopapillary tumor: Case report and review of the literature. *Int. J. Clin. Oncol.* **2012**, *17*, 165–168. [CrossRef]
65. Deshpande, V.; Oliva, E.; Young, R.H. Solid pseudopapillary neoplasm of the ovary: A report of 3 primary ovarian tumors resembling those of the pancreas. *Am. J. Surg. Pathol.* **2010**, *34*, 1514–1520. [CrossRef] [PubMed]
66. Walter, T.; Hommell-Fontaine, J.; Hervieu, V.; Adham, M.; Poncet, G.; Dumortier, J.; Lombard-Bohas, C.; Scoazec, J.Y. Primary malignant solid pseudopapillary tumors of the gastroduodenal area. *Clin. Res. Hepatol. Gastroenterol.* **2011**, *35*, 227–233. [CrossRef] [PubMed]
67. Buetow, P.C.; Buck, J.L.; Pantongrag-Brown, L.; Beck, K.G.; Ros, P.R.; Adair, C.F. Solid and papillary epithelial neoplasm of the pancreas: Imaging-pathologic correlation on 56 cases. *Radiology* **1996**, *199*, 707–711. [CrossRef]
68. Alexandrescu, D.T.; O'Boyle, K.; Feliz, A.; Fueg, A.; Wiernik, P.H. Metastatic solid-pseudopapillary tumour of the pancreas: Clinico-biological correlates and management. *Clin. Oncol.* **2005**, *17*, 358–363. [CrossRef]

69. Lee, J.H.; Yu, J.S.; Kim, H.; Kim, J.K.; Kim, T.H.; Kim, K.W.; Park, M.S.; Kim, J.H.; Kim, Y.B.; Park, C. Solid pseudopapillary carcinoma of the pancreas: Differentiation from benign solid pseudopapillary tumour using CT and MRI. *Clin. Radiol.* **2008**, *63*, 1006–1014. [CrossRef]
70. Hassan, I.; Celik, I.; Nies, C.; Zielke, A.; Gerdes, B.; Moll, R.; Ramaswamy, A.; Wagner, H.J.; Bartsch, D.K. Successful treatment of solid-pseudopapillary tumor of the pancreas with multiple liver metastases. *Pancreatology* **2005**, *5*, 289–294. [CrossRef]
71. Zhan, H.; Cheng, Y.; Wang, L.; Su, P.; Zhong, N.; Zhang, Z. Clinicopathological Features and Treatment Outcomes of Solid Pseudopapillary Neoplasms of the Pancreas: A 10-Year Case Series from a Single Center. *J. Laparoendosc. Adv. Surg. Tech.* **2019**, *29*, 600–607. [CrossRef] [PubMed]
72. Beltrame, V.; Pozza, G.; Dalla Bona, E.; Fantin, A.; Valmasoni, M.; Sperti, C. Solid-Pseudopapillary Tumor of the Pancreas: A Single Center Experience. *Gastroenterol. Res. Pract.* **2016**, *2016*, 4289736. [CrossRef] [PubMed]
73. Wright, M.J.; Javed, A.A.; Saunders, T.; Zhu, Y.; Burkhart, R.A.; Yu, J. Surgical Resection of 78 Pancreatic Solid Pseudopapillary Tumors: A 30-Year Single Institutional Experience. *J. Gastrointest. Surg.* **2020**, *24*, 874–881. [CrossRef]
74. Ventriglia, A.; Manfredi, R.; Mehrabi, S.; Boninsegna, E.; Negrelli, R.; Pedrinolla, B.; Pozzi Mucelli, R. MRI features of solid pseudopapillary neoplasm of the pancreas. *Abdom. Imaging* **2014**, *39*, 1213–1220. [CrossRef]
75. Chae, S.H.; Lee, J.M.; Baek, J.H.; Shin, C.I.; Yoo, M.H.; Yoon, J.H.; Kim, J.H.; Han, J.K.; Choi, B.I. Magnetic resonance imaging spectrum of solid pseudopapillary neoplasm of the pancreas. *J. Comput. Assist. Tomogr.* **2014**, *38*, 249–257. [CrossRef]
76. Guerrache, Y.; Soyer, P.; Dohan, A.; Faraoun, S.A.; Laurent, V.; Tasu, J.P.; Aubé, C.; Cazejust, J.; Boudiaf, M.; Hoeffel, C. Solid-pseudopapillary tumor of the pancreas: MR imaging findings in 21 patients. *Clin. Imaging* **2014**, *38*, 475–482. [CrossRef] [PubMed]
77. Coleman, K.M.; Doherty, M.C.; Bigler, S.A. Solid-pseudopapillary tumor of the pancreas. *Radiographics* **2003**, *23*, 1644–1648. [CrossRef]
78. Baek, J.H.; Lee, J.M.; Kim, S.H.; Kim, S.J.; Kim, S.H.; Lee, J.Y.; Han, J.K.; Choi, B.I. Small ($\leq$3 cm) Solid Pseudopapillary Tumors of the Pancreas at Multiphasic Multidetector CT 1. *Radiology* **2010**, *257*, 97–106. [CrossRef]
79. Liu, M.; Liu, J.; Hu, Q.; Xu, W.; Liu, W.; Zhang, Z.; Sun, Q.; Qin, Y.; Yu, X.; Ji, S.; et al. Management of solid pseudopapillary neoplasms of pancreas: A single center experience of 243 consecutive patients. *Pancreatology* **2019**, *19*, 681–685. [CrossRef]
80. Morito, A.; Eto, K.; Matsuishi, K.; Hamasaki, H.; Morita, K.; Ikeshima, S.; Horino, K.; Shimada, S.; Baba, H. A case of repeat hepatectomy for liver mastasis from solid pseudopapillary neoplasm of the pancreas: A case report. *Surg. Case Rep.* **2021**, *7*, 60. [CrossRef]
81. Law, J.K.; Ahmed, A.; Singh, V.K.; Akshintala, V.S.; Olson, M.T.; Raman, S.P.; Ali, S.Z.; Fishman, E.K.; Kamel, I.; Canto, M.I.; et al. A systematic review of solid-pseudopapillary neoplasms: Are these rare lesions? *Pancreas* **2014**, *43*, 331–337. [CrossRef] [PubMed]
82. Yang, F.; Jin, C.; Long, J.; Yu, X.J.; Xu, J.; Di, Y.; Li, J.; de Fu, L.; Ni, Q.X. Solid pseudopapillary tumor of the pancreas: A case series of 26 consecutive patients. *Am. J. Surg.* **2009**, *198*, 210–215. [CrossRef] [PubMed]
83. Devi, J.; Sathyalakshmi, R.; Chandramouleeswari, K.; Devi, N.R. Pancreatic schwannoma—A rare case report. *J. Clin. Diagn. Res.* **2014**, *8*, FD15–FD16.
84. Antinheimo, J.; Sankila, R.; Carpén, O.; Pukkala, E.; Sainio, M.; Jääskeläinen, J. Population-based analysis of sporadic and type 2 neurofibromatosis-associated meningiomas and schwannomas. *Neurology* **2000**, *54*, 71–76. [CrossRef] [PubMed]
85. Zhang, X.; Siegelman, E.S.; Lee, M.K., 4th; Tondon, R. Pancreatic schwannoma, an extremely rare and challenging entity: Report of two cases and review of literature. *Pancreatology* **2019**, *19*, 729–737. [CrossRef]
86. Varshney, V.K.; Yadav, T.; Elhence, P.; Sureka, B. Preoperative diagnosis of pancreatic schwannoma—Myth or reality. *J. Cancer Res. Ther.* **2020**, *16*, S222–S226. [CrossRef]
87. Kinhal, V.A.; Ravishankar, T.H.; Melapure, A.I.; Jayaprakasha, G.; Range Gowda, B.C.; Manjunath. Pancreatic schwannoma: Report of a case and review of literature. *Indian J. Surg.* **2010**, *72*, 296–298. [CrossRef]
88. Ma, Y.; Shen, B.; Jia, Y.; Luo, Y.; Tian, Y.; Dong, Z.; Chen, W.; Li, Z.P.; Feng, S.T. Pancreatic schwannoma: A case report and an updated 40-year review of the literature yielding 68 cases. *BMC Cancer* **2017**, *14*, 853.
89. Wang, H.; Zhang, B.B.; Wang, S.F.; Zhong, J.J.; Zheng, J.M.; Han, H. Pancreatic schwannoma: Imaging features and pathological findings. *Hepatobiliary Pancreat. Dis. Int. HBPD INT* **2020**, *19*, 200–202. [CrossRef]
90. Tofigh, A.M.; Hashemi, M.; Honar, B.N.; Solhjoo, F. Rare presentation of pancreatic schwannoma: A case report. *J. Med. Case Rep.* **2008**, *12*, 268. [CrossRef]
91. Abu-Zaid, A.; Azzam, A.; Abou Al-Shaar, H.; Alshammari, A.M.; Amin, T.; Mohammed, S. Pancreatic tail schwannoma in a 44-year-old male: A case report and literature review. *Case Rep. Oncol. Med.* **2013**, *2013*, 416713. [CrossRef] [PubMed]
92. Moriya, T.; Kimura, W.; Hirai, I.; Takeshita, A.; Tezuka, K.; Watanabe, T.; Mizutani, M.; Fuse, A. Pancreatic schwannoma: Case report and an updated 30-year review of the literature yielding 47 cases. *World J. Gastroenterol.* **2012**, *18*, 1538–1544. [CrossRef] [PubMed]
93. Novellas, S.; Chevallier, P.; Saint Paul, M.C.; Gugenheim, J.; Bruneton, J.N. MRI features of a pancreatic schwannoma. *Clin. Imaging* **2005**, *29*, 434–436. [CrossRef]
94. Yu, R.S.; Sun, J.Z. Pancreatic schwannoma: CT findings. *Abdom. Imaging* **2006**, *31*, 103–105. [CrossRef] [PubMed]
95. Hamada, K.; Ueda, T.; Higuchi, I.; Inoue, A.; Tamai, N.; Myoi, A.; Tomita, Y.; Aozasa, K.; Yoshikawa, H.; Hatazawa, J. Peripheral nerve schwannoma: Two cases exhibiting increased FDG uptake in early and delayed PET imaging. *Skelet. Radiol.* **2005**, *34*, 52–57. [CrossRef] [PubMed]

96. Birk, H.; Zygourakis, C.C.; Kliot, M. Developing an algorithm for cost-effective, clinically judicious management of peripheral nerve tumors. *Surg. Neurol. Int.* **2016**, *7*, 80.
97. Wang, S.; Xing, C.; Wu, H.; Dai, M.; Zhao, Y. Pancreatic schwannoma mimicking pancreatic cystadenoma: A case report and literature review of the imaging features. *Medicine* **2019**, *98*, e16095. [CrossRef]
98. Shimizu, K.; Shiratori, K.; Toki, F.; Suzuki, M.; Imaizumi, T.; Takasaki, K.; Kobayashi, M.; Hayashi, N. Nonfunctioning islet cell tumor with a unique pattern of tumor growth. *Dig. Dis. Sci.* **1999**, *44*, 547–551. [CrossRef]
99. Akatsu, T.; Wakabayashi, G.; Aiura, K.; Suganuma, K.; Takigawa, Y.; Wada, M.; Kawachi, S.; Tanabe, M.; Ueda, M.; Shimazu, M.; et al. Intraductal growth of a nonfunctioning endocrine tumor of the pancreas. *J. Gastroenterol.* **2004**, *39*, 584–588. [CrossRef]
100. Fassan, M.; Pizzi, S.; Pasquali, C.; Parenti, A.R. Pancreatic endocrine tumor in multiple endocrine neoplasia type 1syndrome with intraductal growth into the main pancreatic duct. *Pancreas* **2009**, *38*, 341–342. [CrossRef]
101. Inagaki, M.; Watanabe, K.; Yoshikawa, D.; Suzuki, S.; Ishizaki, A.; Matsumoto, K.; Haneda, M.; Tokusashi, Y.; Miyokawa, N.; Sato, S.; et al. A malignant nonfunctioning pancreatic endocrine tumor with unique pattern of intraductal growth. *J. Hepatobiliary Pancreat. Surg.* **2007**, *14*, 318–323. [CrossRef] [PubMed]
102. Kawakami, H.; Kuwatani, M.; Hirano, S.; Kondo, S.; Nakanishi, Y.; Itoh, T.; Asaka, M. Pancreatic endocrine tumors with intraductal growth into the main pancreatic duct and tumor thrombus within the portal vein: A case report and review of the literature. *Int. Med.* **2007**, *46*, 273–277. [CrossRef] [PubMed]
103. Kitami, C.E.; Shimizu, T.; Sato, O.; Kurosaki, I.; Mori, S.; Yanagisawa, Y.; Ajioka, Y.; Hatakeyama, K. Malignant islet cell tumor projecting into the main pancreatic duct. *J. Hepatobiliary Pancreat. Surg.* **2000**, *7*, 529–533. [CrossRef]
104. Terada, T.; Kawaguchi, M.; Furukawa, K.; Sekido, Y.; Osamura, Y. Minute mixed ductal-endocrine carcinoma of the pancreas with predominant intraductal growth. *Pathol. Int.* **2002**, *52*, 740–746. [CrossRef]
105. D'Onofrio, M.; Capelli, P.; Pederzoli, P. *Imaging and Pathology of Pancreatic Neoplasms. A Pictorial Atlas*, 1st ed.; Springer Science + Business Media: Milan, Italy, 2015.
106. Yazawa, N.; Imaizumi, T.; Okada, K.; Matsuyama, M.; Dowaki, S.; Tobita, K.; Ohtani, Y.; Ogoshi, K.; Hirabayashi, K.; Makuuchi, H. Nonfunctioning pancreatic endocrine tumor with extension into the main pancreatic duct: Report of a case. *Surg. Today* **2011**, *41*, 737–740. [CrossRef] [PubMed]
107. Chetty, R.; El-Shinnawy, I. Intraductal pancreatic neuroendocrine tumor. *Endocr. Pathol.* **2009**, *20*, 262–266. [CrossRef]
108. Ciaravino, V.; De Robertis, R.; Tinazzi Martini, P.; Cardobi, N.; Cingarlini, S.; Amodio, A.; Landoni, L.; Capelli, P.; D'Onofrio, M. Imaging presentation of pancreatic neuroendocrine neoplasms. *Insights Imaging* **2018**, *9*, 943–953. [CrossRef]
109. Klemperer, P.; Coleman, B.R. Primary neoplasms of the pleura. A report of five cases. *Am. J. Ind. Med.* **1992**, *22*, 4–31. [CrossRef]
110. Manning, M.A.; Paal, E.E.; Srivastava, A.; Mortele, K.J. Nonepithelial Neoplasms of the Pancreas, Part 2: Malignant Tumors and Tumors of Uncertain Malignant Potential From the Radiologic Pathology Archives. *Radiographics* **2018**, *38*, 1047–1072. [CrossRef]
111. Taguchi, Y.; Hara, T.; Tamura, H.; Ogiku, M.; Watahiki, M.; Takagi, T.; Harada, T.; Miyazaki, S.; Hayashi, T.; Kanai, T.; et al. Malignant solitary fibrous tumor of the pancreas: A case report. *Surg. Case Rep.* **2020**, *136*, 287. [CrossRef]
112. Li, J.; Li, J.; Xiong, Y.; Xu, T.; Xu, J.; Li, Q.; Yang, G. Atypical/malignant solitary fibrous tumor of the pancreas with spleen vein invasion: Case report and literature review. *Medicine* **2020**, *99*, e19783. [CrossRef] [PubMed]
113. Fung, E.C.; Crook, M.A. Doege-Potter syndrome and 'big-IGF2': A rare cause of hypoglycaemia. *Ann. Clin. Biochem.* **2011**, *48 Pt 2*, 95–96. [CrossRef] [PubMed]
114. Shanbhogue, A.K.; Prasad, S.R.; Takahashi, N.; Vikram, R.; Zaheer, A.; Sandrasegaran, K. Somatic and visceral solitary fibrous tumors in the abdomen and pelvis: Cross-sectional imaging spectrum. *Radiographics* **2011**, *31*, 393–408. [CrossRef] [PubMed]
115. Huang, S.C.; Huang, H.Y. Solitary fibrous tumor: An evolving and unifying entity with unsettled issues. *Histol. Histopathol.* **2019**, *34*, 313–334.
116. Ginat, D.T.; Bokhari, A.; Bhatt, S.; Dogra, V. Imaging features of solitary fibrous tumors. *AJR Am. J. Roentgenol.* **2011**, *196*, 487–495. [CrossRef] [PubMed]
117. Martin-Broto, J.; Mondaza-Hernandez, J.L.; Moura, D.S.; Hindi, N. A Comprehensive Review on Solitary Fibrous Tumor: New Insights for New Horizons. *Cancers* **2021**, *13*, 2913. [CrossRef]
118. Srinivasan, V.D.; Wayne, J.D.; Rao, M.S.; Zynger, D.L. Solitary fibrous tumor of the pancreas: Case report with cytologic and surgical pathology correlation and review of the literature. *J. Pancreas* **2008**, *9*, 526–530.
119. Davanzo, B.; Emerson, R.E.; Lisy, M.; Koniaris, L.G.; Kays, J.K. Solitary fibrous tumor. *Transl. Gastroenterol. Hepatol.* **2018**, *3*, 94. [CrossRef]
120. Kayani, B.; Sharma, A.; Sewell, M.D.; Platinum, J.; Olivier, A.; Briggs, T.W.R.; Eastwood, D.M. A Review of the Surgical Management of Extrathoracic Solitary Fibrous Tumors. *Am. J. Clin. Oncol.* **2018**, *41*, 687–694. [CrossRef]
121. Robinson, L.A. Solitary fibrous tumor of the pleura. *Cancer Control* **2006**, *13*, 264–269. [CrossRef]
122. Ordóñez, N.G. Pancreatic acinar cell carcinoma. *Adv. Anat. Pathol.* **2001**, *8*, 144–159. [PubMed]
123. Toll, A.D.; Hruban, R.H.; Ali, S.Z. Acinar cell carcinoma of the pancreas: Clinical and cytomorphologic characteristics. *Korean J. Pathol.* **2013**, *47*, 93–99. [CrossRef] [PubMed]
124. Chaudhary, P. Acinar Cell Carcinoma of the Pancreas: A Literature Review and Update. *Indian J. Surg.* **2015**, *77*, 226–231. [CrossRef] [PubMed]

125. Lack, E.E.; Cassady, J.R.; Levey, R.; Vawter, G.F. Tumors of the exocrine pancreas in children and adolescents. A clinical and pathologic study of eight cases. *Am. J. Surg. Pathol.* **1983**, *7*, 319–327. [CrossRef]
126. Bhosale, P.; Balachandran, A.; Wang, H.; Wei, W.; Hwang, R.F.; Fleming, J.B.; Varadhachary, G.; Charnsangavej, C.; Tamm, E. CT imaging features of acinar cell carcinoma and its hepatic metastases. *Abdom. Imaging* **2013**, *38*, 1383–1390. [CrossRef]
127. Klimstra, D.S.; Heffess, C.S.; Oertel, J.E.; Rosai, J. Acinar cell carcinoma of the pancreas. A clinicopathologic study of 28 cases. *Am. J. Surg. Pathol.* **1992**, *16*, 815–837. [CrossRef]
128. Hsu, M.Y.; Pan, K.T.; Chu, S.Y.; Hung, C.F.; Wu, R.C.; Tseng, J.H. CT and MRI features of acinar cell carcinoma of the pancreas with pathological correlations. *Clin. Radiol.* **2010**, *65*, 223–229. [CrossRef]
129. Fabre, A.; Sauvanet, A.; Flejou, J.F.; Belghiti, J.; Palazzo, L.; Ruszniewski, P.; Degott, C.; Terris, B. Intraductal acinar cell carcinoma of the pancreas. *Virchows Arch.* **2001**, *438*, 312–315. [CrossRef]
130. Calimano-Ramirez, L.F.; Daoud, T.; Gopireddy, D.R.; Morani, A.C.; Waters, R.; Gumus, K.; Klekers, A.R.; Bhosale, P.R.; Virarkar, M.K. Pancreatic acinar cell carcinoma: A comprehensive review. *World J. Gastroenterol.* **2022**, *28*, 5827–5844. [CrossRef]
131. Borowicz, J.; Morrison, M.; Hogan, D.; Miller, R. Subcutaneous fat necrosis/panniculitis and polyarthritis associated with acinar cell carcinoma of the pancreas: A rare presentation of pancreatitis, panniculitis and polyarthritis syndrome. *J. Drugs Dermatol.* **2010**, *9*, 1145–1150.
132. Radin, D.R.; Colletti, P.M.; Forrester, D.M.; Tang, W.W. Pancreatic acinar cell carcinoma with subcutaneous and intraosseous fat necrosis. *Radiology* **1986**, *158*, 67–68. [CrossRef] [PubMed]
133. Burns, W.A.; Matthews, M.J.; Hamosh, M.; Weide, G.V.; Blum, R.; Johnson, F.B. Lipase-secreting acinar cell carcinoma of the pancreas with polyarthropathy. A light and electron microscopic, histochemical, and biochemical study. *Cancer* **1974**, *33*, 1002–1009. [CrossRef] [PubMed]
134. Cingolani, N.; Shaco-Levy, R.; Farruggio, A.; Klimstra, D.S.; Rosai, J. Alpha-fetoprotein production by pancreatic tumors exhibiting acinar cell differentiation: Study of five cases, one arising in a mediastinal teratoma. *Hum. Pathol.* **2000**, *31*, 938–944. [CrossRef] [PubMed]
135. Raman, S.P.; Hruban, R.H.; Cameron, J.L.; Wolfgang, C.L.; Fishman, E.K. Pancreatic imaging mimics: Part 2, pancreatic neuroendocrine tumors and their mimics. *AJR Am. J. Roentgenol.* **2012**, *199*, 309–318. [CrossRef]
136. Raman, S.P.; Hruban, R.H.; Cameron, J.L.; Wolfgang, C.L.; Kawamoto, S.; Fishman, E.K. Acinar cell carcinoma of the pancreas: Computed tomography features—A study of 15 patients. *Abdom. Imaging* **2013**, *38*, 137–143. [CrossRef]
137. Chiou, Y.Y.; Chiang, J.H.; Hwang, J.I.; Yen, C.H.; Tsay, S.H.; Chang, C.Y. Acinar cell carcinoma of the pancreas: Clinical and computed tomography manifestations. *J. Comput. Assist. Tomogr.* **2004**, *28*, 180–186. [CrossRef]
138. Thompson, E.D.; Wood, L.D. Pancreatic Neoplasms With Acinar Differentiation: A Review of Pathologic and Molecular Features. *Arch. Pathol. Lab. Med.* **2020**, *144*, 808–815. [CrossRef]
139. Tatli, S.; Mortele, K.J.; Levy, A.D.; Glickman, J.N.; Ros, P.R.; Banks, P.A.; Silverman, S.G. CT and MRI features of pure acinar cell carcinoma of the pancreas in adults. *AJR Am. J. Roentgenol.* **2005**, *184*, 511–519. [CrossRef]
140. Javadi, S.; Menias, C.O.; Korivi, B.R.; Shaaban, A.M.; Patnana, M.; Alhalabi, K.; Elsayes, K.M. Pancreatic Calcifications and Calcified Pancreatic Masses: Pattern Recognition Approach on CT. *Am. J. Roentgenol.* **2017**, *209*, 77–87. [CrossRef]
141. Klöppel, G.; Kosmahl, M. Cystic lesions and neoplasms of the pancreas. The features are becoming clearer. *Pancreatology* **2001**, *1*, 648–655. [CrossRef]
142. Mergo, P.J.; Helmberger, T.K.; Buetow, P.C.; Helmberger, R.C.; Ros, P.R. Pancreatic neoplasms: MR imaging and pathologic correlation. *Radiographics* **1997**, *17*, 281–301. [CrossRef] [PubMed]
143. Cantisani, V.; Mortele, K.J.; Levy, A.; Glickman, J.N.; Ricci, P.; Passariello, R.; Ros, P.R.; Silverman, S.G. MR imaging features of solid pseudopapillary tumor of the pancreas in adult and pediatric patients. *Am. J. Roentgenol.* **2003**, *181*, 395–401. [CrossRef] [PubMed]
144. Solcia, E.; Capella, C.; Kloppel, G. Tumors of the exocrine pancreas. In *Atlas of Tumor Pathology: Tumors of the Pancreas*; Rosai, J., Sorbin, L., Eds.; Armed Forces Institute of Pathology: Washington, DC, USA, 1997; pp. 31–144.
145. Distler, M.; Rückert, F.; Dittert, D.D.; Stroszczynski, C.; Dobrowolski, F.; Kersting, S.; Grützmann, R. Curative resection of a primarily unresectable acinar cell carcinoma of the pancreas after chemotherapy. *World J. Surg. Oncol.* **2009**, *7*, 22. [CrossRef] [PubMed]
146. Mortenson, M.M.; Katz, M.H.; Tamm, E.P.; Bhutani, M.S.; Wang, H.; Evans, D.B.; Fleming, J.B. Current diagnosis and management of unusual pancreatic tumors. *Am. J. Surg.* **2008**, *196*, 100–113. [CrossRef]
147. Matos, J.M.; Schmidt, C.M.; Turrini, O.; Agaram, N.P.; Niedergethmann, M.; Saeger, H.D.; Merchant, N.; Johnson, C.S.; Lillemoe, K.D.; Grützmann, R. Pancreatic acinar cell carcinoma: A multi-institutional study. *J. Gastrointest. Surg.* **2009**, *13*, 1495–1502. [CrossRef]
148. Wang, Y.; Wang, S.; Zhou, X.; Zhou, H.; Cui, Y.; Li, Q.; Zhang, L. Acinar cell carcinoma: A report of 19 cases with a brief review of the literature. *World J. Surg. Oncol.* **2016**, *14*, 172. [CrossRef]
149. Kamisawa, T.; Wood, L.D.; Itoi, T.; Takaori, K. Pancreatic cancer. *Lancet* **2016**, *388*, 73–85. [CrossRef]
150. Muraki, T.; Reid, M.D.; Basturk, O.; Jang, K.T.; Bedolla, G.; Bagci, P.; Mittal, P.; Memis, B.; Katabi, N.; Bandyopadhyay, S.; et al. Undifferentiated Carcinoma With Osteoclastic Giant Cells of the Pancreas: Clinicopathologic Analysis of 38 Cases Highlights a More Protracted Clinical Course Than Currently Appreciated. *Am. J. Surg. Pathol.* **2016**, *40*, 1203–1216. [CrossRef]

151. Jo, S. Huge undifferentiated carcinoma of the pancreas with osteoclast-like giant cells. *World J. Gastroenterol.* **2014**, *20*, 2725–2730. [CrossRef]
152. Kalluri, R.; Weinberg, R.A. The basics of epithelial-mesenchymal transition. *J. Clin. Investig.* **2010**, *119*, 1420–1428. [CrossRef]
153. Nieto, M.A.; Huang, R.Y.; Jackson, R.A.; Thiery, J.P. EMT: 2016. *Cell* **2016**, *166*, 21–45. [CrossRef] [PubMed]
154. Lambert, A.W.; Pattabiraman, D.R.; Weinberg, R.A. Emerging Biological Principles of Metastasis. *Cell* **2017**, *168*, 670–691. [CrossRef] [PubMed]
155. Joo, Y.E.; Heo, T.; Park, C.H.; Lee, W.S.; Kim, H.S.; Kim, J.C.; Koh, Y.S.; Choi, S.K.; Cho, C.K.; Rew, J.S.; et al. A case of osteoclast-like giant cell tumor of the pancreas with ductal adenocarcinoma: Histopathological, immunohistochemical, ultrastructural and molecular biological studies. *J. Korean Med. Sci.* **2005**, *20*, 516–520. [CrossRef] [PubMed]
156. Nagtegaal, I.D.; Odze, R.D.; Klimstra, D.; Paradis, V.; Rugge, M.; Schirmacher, P.; Washington, K.M.; Carneiro, F.; Cree, I.A. WHO Classification of Tumours Editorial Board. The 2019 WHO classification of tumours of the digestive system. *Histopathology* **2020**, *76*, 182–188. [CrossRef] [PubMed]
157. Cavalcanti, E.; Schena, N.; Serino, G.; Lantone, G.; Armentano, R. Assessment and management of undifferentiated carcinoma with osteoclastic like giant cells of the pancreas: A case report and revision of literature. *BMC Gastroenterol.* **2021**, *21*, 247. [CrossRef]
158. Yang, K.Y.; Choi, J.I.; Choi, M.H.; Park, M.Y.; Rha, S.E.; Byun, J.Y.; Jung, E.S.; Lall, C. Magnetic resonance imaging findings of undifferentiated carcinoma with osteoclast-like giant cells of pancreas. *Clin. Imaging* **2016**, *40*, 148–151. [CrossRef]
159. Maksymov, V.; Khalifa, M.A.; Bussey, A.; Carter, B.; Hogan, M. Undifferentiated (anaplastic) carcinoma of the pancreas with osteoclast-like giant cells showing various degree of pancreas duct involvement. A case report and literature review. *JOP* **2011**, *12*, 170–176.
160. Yazawa, T.; Watanabe, A.; Araki, K.; Segawa, A.; Hirai, K.; Kubo, N.; Igarashi, T.; Tsukagoshi, M.; Ishii, N.; Hoshino, K.; et al. Complete resection of a huge pancreatic undifferentiated carcinoma with osteoclast-like giant cells. *Int. Cancer Conf. J.* **2017**, *6*, 193–196. [CrossRef]
161. Gao, H.Q.; Yang, Y.M.; Zhuang, Y.; Liu, P. Locally advanced undifferentiated carcinoma with osteoclast-like giant cells of the pancreas. *World J. Gastroenterol.* **2015**, *21*, 694–698. [CrossRef]
162. Sakhi, R.; Hamza, A.; Khurram, M.S.; Ibrar, W.; Mazzara, P. Undifferentiated carcinoma of the pancreas with osteoclast-like giant cells reported in an asymptomatic patient: A rare case and literature review. *Autops. Case Rep.* **2017**, *7*, 51–57. [CrossRef]
163. Togawa, Y.; Tonouchi, A.; Chiku, T.; Sano, W.; Doki, T.; Yano, K.; Uno, H.; Muronoi, T.; Kaneoya, K.; Shinagawa, T.; et al. A case report of undifferentiated carcinoma with osteoclast-like giant cells of the pancreas and literature review. *Clin. J. Gastroenterol.* **2010**, *3*, 195–203. [CrossRef] [PubMed]
164. Ichikawa, T.; Federle, M.P.; Ohba, S.; Ohtomo, K.; Sugiyama, A.; Fujimoto, H.; Haradome, H.; Araki, T. Atypical exocrine and endocrine pancreatic tumors (anaplastic, small cell, and giant cell types): CT and pathologic features in 14 patients. *Abdom. Imaging* **2000**, *25*, 409–419. [CrossRef] [PubMed]
165. Wada, T.; Itano, O.; Oshima, G.; Chiba, N.; Ishikawa, H.; Koyama, Y.; Du, W.; Kitagawa, Y. A male case of an undifferentiated carcinoma with osteoclast-like giant cells originating in an indeterminate mucin-producing cystic neoplasm of the pancreas. A case report and review of the literature. *World J. Surg. Oncol.* **2011**, *9*, 100. [CrossRef] [PubMed]
166. Sato, K.; Urakawa, H.; Sakamoto, K.; Ito, E.; Hamada, Y.; Yoshimitsu, K. Undifferentiated carcinoma of the pancreas with osteoclast-like giant cells showing intraductal growth and intratumoral hemorrhage: MRI features. *Radiol. Case Rep.* **2019**, *14*, 1283–1287. [CrossRef] [PubMed]
167. Oehler, U.; Jurs, M.; Kloppel, G.; Helpap, B. Osteoclast-like giant cell tumour of the pancreas presenting as a pseudocyst-like lesion. *Virchows Arch.* **1997**, *431*, 215–218. [CrossRef]
168. Molberg, K.H.; Heffess, C.; Delgado, R.; Albores-Saavedra, J. Undifferentiated carcinoma with osteoclast-like giant cells of the pancreas and periampullary region. *Cancer* **1998**, *82*, 1279–1287. [CrossRef]
169. Zou, X.P.; Yu, Z.L.; Li, Z.S.; Zhou, G.Z. Clinicopathological features of giant cell carcinoma of the pancreas. *Hepatobiliary Pancreat. Dis. Int.* **2004**, *3*, 300–302.
170. Paal, E.; Thompson, L.D.; Frommelt, R.A.; Przygodzki, R.M.; Heffess, C.S. A clinicopathologic and immunohistochemical study of 35 anaplastic carcinomas of the pancreas with a review of the literature. *Ann. Diagn. Pathol.* **2001**, *5*, 129–140. [CrossRef]
171. Hirano, H.; Morita, K.; Tachibana, S.; Okimura, A.; Fujisawa, T.; Ouchi, S.; Nakasho, K.; Ueyama, S.; Nishigami, T.; Terada, N. Undifferentiated carcinoma with osteoclast-like giant cells arising in a mucinous cystic neoplasm of the pancreas. *Pathol. Int.* **2008**, *58*, 383–389. [CrossRef]
172. Demetter, P.; Maréchal, R.; Puleo, F.; Delhaye, M.; Debroux, S.; Charara, F.; Gomez Galdon, M.; Van Laethem, J.L.; Verset, L. Undifferentiated Pancreatic Carcinoma with Osteoclast-like Giant Cells: What Do We Know So Far? *Front. Oncol.* **2021**, *11*, 630086. [CrossRef]
173. Luchini, C.; Pea, A.; Lionheart, G.; Mafficini, A.; Nottegar, A.; Veronese, N.; Chianchiano, P.; Brosens, L.A.; Noë, M.; Offerhaus, G.J.A.; et al. Pancreatic undifferentiated carcinoma with osteoclast-like giant cells is genetically similar to, but clinically distinct from, conventional ductal adenocarcinoma. *J. Pathol.* **2017**, *243*, 148–154. [CrossRef]
174. Moore, J.C.; Bentz, J.S.; Hilden, K.; Adler, D.G. Osteoclastic and pleomorphic giant cell tumors of the pancreas: A review of clinical, endoscopic, and pathologic features. *World J. Gastrointest. Endosc.* **2010**, *2*, 15–19. [CrossRef] [PubMed]

175. Boyd, C.A.; Benarroch-Gampel, J.; Sheffield, K.M.; Cooksley, C.D.; Riall, T.S. 415 patients with adenosquamous carcinoma of the pancreas: A population-based analysis of prognosis and survival. *J. Surg. Res.* **2012**, *174*, 12–19. [CrossRef] [PubMed]
176. Borazanci, E.; Millis, S.Z.; Korn, R.; Han, H.; Whatcott, C.J.; Gatalica, Z.; Barrett, M.T.; Cridebring, D.; Von Hoff, D.D. Adenosquamous carcinoma of the pancreas: Molecular characterization of 23 patients along with a literature review. *World J. Gastrointest. Oncol.* **2015**, *7*, 132–140. [CrossRef] [PubMed]
177. Simone, C.G.; Zuluaga Toro, T.; Chan, E.; Feely, M.M.; Trevino, J.G.; George, T.J., Jr. Characteristics and outcomes of adenosquamous carcinoma of the pancreas. *Gastrointest. Cancer Res.* **2013**, *6*, 75–79. [CrossRef]
178. Herxheimer, G. Über heterologe Cancroide. *Beitr. Pathol. Anat.* **1907**, *41*, 348–412.
179. Hruban, R.H.; Pitman, M.B.; Klimstra, D.S. *Tumors of the Pancreas, Afip Atlas of Tumor Pathology, 4th Series Fascicle 6*, 6th ed.; American Registry of Pathology: Washington, DC, USA, 2007.
180. Voong, K.R.; Davison, J.; Pawlik, T.M.; Uy, M.O.; Hsu, C.C.; Winter, J.; Hruban, R.H.; Laheru, D.; Rudra, S.; Swartz, M.J.; et al. Resected pancreatic adenosquamous carcinoma: Clinicopathologic review and evaluation of adjuvant chemotherapy and radiation in 38 patients. *Hum. Pathol.* **2010**, *41*, 113–122. [CrossRef]
181. Kardon, D.E.; Thompson, L.D.; Przygodzki, R.M.; Heffess, C.S. Adenosquamous carcinoma of the pancreas: A clinicopathologic series of 25 cases. *Mod. Pathol.* **2001**, *14*, 443–451. [CrossRef]
182. Yamaguchi, K.; Enjoji, M. Adenosquamous carcinoma of the pancreas: A clinicopathologic study. *J. Surg. Oncol.* **1991**, *47*, 109–116. [CrossRef]
183. Murakami, Y.; Yokoyama, T.; Yokoyama, Y.; Kanehiro, T.; Uemura, K.; Sasaki, M.; Morifuji, M.; Sueda, T. Adenosquamous carcinoma of the pancreas: Preoperative diagnosis and molecular alterations. *J. Gastroenterol.* **2003**, *38*, 1171–1175. [CrossRef]
184. Trikudanathan, G.; Dasanu, C.A. Adenosquamous carcinoma of the pancreas: A distinct clinicopathologic entity. *South. Med. J.* **2010**, *103*, 903–910. [CrossRef] [PubMed]
185. Momosaki, S.; Yano, H.; Kojiro, M. Establishment of a human hepatic adenosquamous carcinoma cell line (KMC-2) and its response to cytokines. *Pathol. Int.* **1995**, *45*, 137–146. [CrossRef] [PubMed]
186. Madura, J.A.; Jarman, B.T.; Doherty, M.G.; Yum, M.N.; Howard, T.J. Adenosquamous carcinoma of the pancreas. *Arch. Surg.* **1999**, *134*, 599–603. [CrossRef] [PubMed]
187. Kovi, J. Adenosquamous carcinoma of the pancreas: A light and electron microscopic study. *Ultrastruct. Pathol.* **1982**, *3*, 17–23. [CrossRef]
188. Xiong, Q.; Zhang, Z.; Xu, Y.; Zhu, Q. Pancreatic Adenosquamous Carcinoma: A Rare Pathological Subtype of Pancreatic Cancer. *J. Clin. Med.* **2022**, *11*, 7401. [CrossRef]
189. Yin, Q.; Wang, C.; Wu, Z.; Wang, M.; Cheng, K.; Zhao, X.; Yuan, F.; Tang, Y.; Miao, F. Adenosquamous carcinoma of the pancreas: Multidetector-row computed tomographic manifestations and tumor characteristics. *J. Comput. Assist. Tomogr.* **2013**, *37*, 125–133. [CrossRef] [PubMed]
190. Inoue, T.; Nagao, S.; Tajima, H.; Okudaira, K.; Hashiguchi, K.; Miyazaki, J.; Matsuzaki, K.; Tsuzuki, Y.; Kawaguchi, A.; Itoh, K.; et al. Adenosquamous pancreatic cancer producing parathyroid hormone-related protein. *J. Gastroenterol.* **2004**, *39*, 176–180. [CrossRef] [PubMed]
191. Kobayashi, N.; Higurashi, T.; Iida, H.; Mawatari, H.; Endo, H.; Nozaki, Y.; Tomimoto, A.; Yoneda, K.; Akiyama, T.; Fujita, K.; et al. Adenosquamous carcinoma of the pancreas associated with humoral hypercalcemia of malignancy (HHM). *J. Hepatobiliary Pancreat. Surg.* **2008**, *15*, 531–535. [CrossRef]
192. López-Tomassetti-Fernández, E.M.; Favre-Rizzo, J.; Delgado-Plasencia, L.; Hernández-Hernández, J.R. Hypercalcemia associated with adenosquamous pancreatic carcinoma: A reason to initiate palliative treatment. *Rev. Esp. Enferm. Dig.* **2013**, *105*, 425–428. [CrossRef]
193. Hsu, J.T.; Chen, H.M.; Wu, R.C.; Yeh, C.N.; Yeh, T.S.; Hwang, T.L.; Jan, Y.Y.; Chen, M.F. Clinicopathologic features and outcomes following surgery for pancreatic adenosquamous carcinoma. *World J. Surg. Oncol.* **2008**, *6*, 95. [CrossRef]
194. Ducreux, M.; Cuhna, A.S.; Caramella, C.; Hollebecque, A.; Burtin, P.; Goéré, D.; Seufferlein, T.; Haustermans, K.; Van Laethem, J.L.; Conroy, T.; et al. ESMO Guidelines Committee. Cancer of the pancreas: ESMO Clinical Practice Guidelines for diagnosis, treatment and follow-up. *Ann. Oncol.* **2015**, *26* (Suppl. 5), v56–v68. [CrossRef] [PubMed]
195. Wahab, A.; Gonzalez, J.J.; Devarkonda, V.; Saint-Phard, T.; Singh, T.; Adekolujo, O.S. Squamous cell carcinoma-A rare pancreatic exocrine malignancy. *Cancer Biol. Ther.* **2019**, *20*, 593–596. [CrossRef] [PubMed]
196. Itani, K.M.; Karni, A.; Green, L. Squamous cell carcinoma of the pancreas. *J. Gastrointest. Surg.* **1999**, *3*, 512–515. [CrossRef] [PubMed]
197. Horino, K.; Takamori, H.; Ikuta, Y.; Nakahara, O.; Chikamoto, A.; Ishiko, T.; Beppu, T.; Baba, H. Cutaneous metastases secondary to pancreatic cancer. *World J. Gastrointest. Oncol.* **2012**, *4*, 176–180. [CrossRef] [PubMed]
198. Zhou, H.Y.; Wang, X.B.; Gao, F.; Bu, B.; Zhang, S.; Wang, Z. Cutaneous metastasis from pancreatic cancer: A case report and systematic review of the literature. *Oncol. Lett.* **2014**, *8*, 2654–2660. [CrossRef]
199. Miyahara, M.; Hamanaka, Y.; Kawabata, A.; Sato, Y.; Tanaka, A.; Yamamoto, A.; Ueno, N.; Nishihara, K.; Suzuki, T. Cutaneous metastases from pancreatic cancer. *Int. J. Pancreatol.* **1996**, *20*, 127–130. [CrossRef]
200. Ding, Y.; Zhou, J.; Sun, H.; He, D.; Zeng, M.; Rao, S. Contrast-enhanced multiphasic CT and MRI findings of adenosquamous carcinoma of the pancreas. *Clin. Imaging* **2013**, *37*, 1054–1060. [CrossRef]

201. Toshima, F.; Inoue, D.; Yoshida, K.; Yoneda, N.; Minami, T.; Kobayashi, S.; Ikdeda, H.; Matsui, O.; Gabata, T. Adenosquamous carcinoma of pancreas: CT and MR imaging features in eight patients, with pathologic correlations and comparison with adenocarcinoma of pancreas. *Abdom. Radiol.* **2016**, *41*, 508–520. [CrossRef]
202. De Moura, D.T.H.; Coronel, M.; Chacon, D.A.; Tanigawa, R.; Chaves, D.M.; Matuguma, S.E.; Dos Santos, M.E.L.; Jukemura, J.; De Moura, E.G.H. Primary adenosquamous cell carcinoma of the pancreas: The use of endoscopic ultrasound guided—Fine needle aspiration to establish a definitive cytologic diagnosis. *Rev. Gastroenterol. Peru* **2017**, *37*, 370–373.
203. Martínez de Juan, F.; Reolid Escribano, M.; Martínez Lapiedra, C.; Maia de Alcantara, F.; Caballero Soto, M.; Calatrava Fons, A.; Machado, I. Pancreatic adenosquamous carcinoma and intraductal papillary mucinous neoplasm in a *CDKN2A* germline mutation carrier. *World J. Gastrointest. Oncol.* **2017**, *9*, 390–396. [CrossRef]
204. Paramythiotis, D.; Kyriakidis, F.; Karlafti, E.; Didangelos, T.; Oikonomou, I.M.; Karakatsanis, A.; Poulios, C.; Chamalidou, E.; Vagionas, A.; Michalopoulos, A. Adenosquamous carcinoma of the pancreas: Two case reports and review of the literature. *J. Med. Case Rep.* **2022**, *16*, 395. [CrossRef] [PubMed]
205. Liszka, L.; Zielinska-Pajak, E.; Pajak, J.; Gołka, D. Colloid carcinoma of the pancreas: Review of selected pathological and clinical aspects. *Pathology* **2008**, *40*, 655–663. [CrossRef] [PubMed]
206. Adsay, N.V.; Pierson, C.; Sarkar, F. Colloid (mucinous noncystic) carcinoma of the pancreas. *Am. J. Surg. Pathol.* **2001**, *25*, 26–42. [CrossRef]
207. Aaltonen, L.A.; Hamilton, S.R. *Pathology and Genetics of Tumours of the Digestive System*; World Health Organization, International Agency for Research on Cancer: Lyon, France, 2000; p. 314.
208. Waters, J.A.; Schnelldorfer, T.; Aguilar-Saavedra, J.R. Survival after resection for invasive intraductal papillary mucinous neoplasm and for pancreatic adenocarcinoma: A multi-institutional comparison according to American Joint Committee on Cancer Stage. *J. Am. Coll. Surg.* **2011**, *213*, 275–283. [CrossRef]
209. Whang, E.E.; Danial, T.; Dunn, J.C.; Ashley, S.W.; Reber, H.A.; Lewin, T.J.; Tompkins, R.K. The spectrum of mucin-producing adenocarcinoma of the pancreas. *Pancreas* **2000**, *21*, 147–151. [CrossRef]
210. Yoon, M.A.; Lee, J.M.; Kim, S.H.; Lee, J.Y.; Han, J.K.; Choi, B.I.; Choi, J.Y.; Park, S.H.; Lee, M.W. MRI features of pancreatic colloid carcinoma. *AJR Am. J. Roentgenol.* **2009**, *193*, W308–W313. [CrossRef]
211. Nakahashi, G.; Yamaguchi, R.; Watanabe, S. A case of rapid growing mucinous carcinoma of the pancreas without intraductal papillary mucinous neoplasm. *J. Biliary Tract. Pancreas* **2017**, *38*, 885–890.
212. Raut, C.P.; Cleary, K.R.; Staerkel, G.A.; Abbruzzese, J.L.; Wolff, R.A.; Lee, J.H.; Vauthey, J.N.; Lee, J.E.; Pisters, P.W.; Evans, D.B. Intraductal papillary mucinous neoplasms of the pancreas: Effect of invasion and pancreatic margin status on recurrence and survival. *Ann. Surg. Oncol.* **2006**, *13*, 582–594. [CrossRef]
213. Poultsides, G.A.; Reddy, S.; Cameron, J.L.; Hruban, R.H.; Pawlik, T.M.; Ahuja, N.; Jain, A.; Edil, B.H.; Iacobuzio-Donahue, C.A.; Schulick, R.D.; et al. Histopathologic basis for the favorable survival after resection of intraductal papillary mucinous neoplasm-associated invasive adenocarcinoma of the pancreas. *Ann. Surg.* **2010**, *251*, 470–476. [CrossRef]
214. Ren, F.Y.; Shao, C.W.; Zuo, C.J.; Lu, J.P. CT features of colloid carcinomas of the pancreas. *Chin. Med. J.* **2010**, *123*, 1329–1332.
215. Adsay, N.V.; Merati, K.; Nassar, H.; Shia, J.; Sarkar, F.; Pierson, C.R.; Cheng, J.D.; Visscher, D.W.; Hruban, R.H.; Klimstra, D.S. Pathogenesis of colloid (pure mucinous) carcinoma of exocrine organs: Coupling of gel-forming mucin (MUC2) production with altered cell polarity and abnormal cell-stroma interaction may be the key factor in the morphogenesis and indolent behavior of colloid carcinoma in the breast and pancreas. *Am. J. Surg. Pathol.* **2003**, *27*, 571–578. [PubMed]
216. Song, S.J.; Lee, J.M.; Kim, Y.J.; Kim, S.H.; Lee, J.Y.; Han, J.K.; Choi, B.I. Differentiation of intraductal papillary mucinous neoplasms from other pancreatic cystic masses: Comparison of multirow-detector CT and MR imaging using ROC analysis. *J. Magn. Reson. Imaging* **2007**, *26*, 86–93. [CrossRef]
217. Plerhoples, T.A.; Ahdoot, M.; DiMaio, M.A.; Pai, R.K.; Park, W.G.; Poultsides, G.A. Colloid carcinoma of the pancreas. *Dig. Dis. Sci.* **2011**, *56*, 1295–1298. [CrossRef] [PubMed]
218. Flor-de-Lima, B.S.; Freitas, P.; Couto, N.; Castillo-Martin, M.; Santiago, I. Pancreatic intraductal papillary mucinous neoplasm associated colloid carcinoma. *Radiol. Case Rep.* **2021**, *16*, 2989–2992. [CrossRef]
219. Schawkat, K.; Manning, M.A.; Glickman, J.N.; Mortele, K.J. Pancreatic Ductal Adenocarcinoma and Its Variants: Pearls and Perils. *Radiographics* **2020**, *40*, 1219–1239. [CrossRef] [PubMed]
220. Parwani, A.V.; Ali, S.Z. Pathologic quiz case: A 52-year-old woman with jaundice and history of necrotizing pancreatitis. Primary colloid carcinoma of the pancreas. *Arch. Pathol. Lab. Med.* **2005**, *129*, 255–256. [CrossRef]
221. Hirono, S.; Yamaue, H. Surgical strategy for intraductal papillary mucinous neoplasms of the pancreas. *Surg. Today* **2020**, *50*, 50–55. [CrossRef]
222. Marchegiani, G.; Andrianello, S.; Dal Borgo, C.; Secchettin, E.; Melisi, D.; Malleo, G.; Bassi, C.; Salvia, R. Adjuvant chemotherapy is associated with improved postoperative survival in specific subtypes of invasive intraductal papillary mucinous neoplasms (IPMN) of the pancreas: It is time for randomized controlled data. *HPB Oxf.* **2019**, *21*, 596–603. [CrossRef]
223. Sohn, T.A.; Yeo, C.J.; Cameron, J.L.; Koniaris, L.; Kaushal, S.; Abrams, R.A.; Sauter, P.K.; Coleman, J.; Hruban, R.H.; Lillemoe, K.D. Resected adenocarcinoma of the pancreas—616 patients: Results, outcomes, and prognostic indicators. *J. Gastrointest. Surg.* **2000**, *4*, 567–579. [CrossRef]
224. Youngwirth, L.M.; Freischlag, K.; Nussbaum, D.P.; Benrashid, E.; Blazer, D.G. Primary sarcomas of the pancreas: A review of 253 patients from the National Cancer Data Base. *Surg. Oncol.* **2018**, *27*, 676–680. [CrossRef]

225. Baylor, S.M.; Berg, J.W. Cross-classification and survival characteristics of 5,000 cases of cancer of the pancreas. *J. Surg. Oncol.* **1973**, *5*, 335–358. [CrossRef] [PubMed]
226. Kim, J.Y.; Song, J.S.; Park, H.; Byun, J.H.; Song, K.B.; Kim, K.P.; Kim, S.C.; Hong, S.M. Primary mesenchymal tumors of the pancreas: Single-center experience over 16 years. *Pancreas* **2014**, *43*, 959–968. [CrossRef] [PubMed]
227. Papalampros, A.; Vailas, M.G.; Deladetsima, I.; Moris, D.; Sotiropoulou, M.; Syllaios, A.; Petrou, A.; Felekouras, E. Irreversible electroporation in a case of pancreatic leiomyosarcoma: A novel weapon versus a rare malignancy? *World J. Surg. Oncol.* **2019**, *17*, 6. [CrossRef] [PubMed]
228. Søreide, J.A.; Undersrud, E.S.; Al-Saiddi, M.S.; Tholfsen, T.; Søreide, K. Primary Leiomyosarcoma of the Pancreas-a Case Report and a Comprehensive Review. *J. Gastrointest. Cancer* **2016**, *47*, 358–365. [CrossRef]
229. Zalatnai, A.; Kovács, M.; Flautner, L.; Sipos, B.; Sarkady, E.; Bocsi, J. Pancreatic leiomyosarcoma. Case report with immunohistochemical and flow cytometric studies. *Virchows Arch.* **1998**, *432*, 469–472. [CrossRef] [PubMed]
230. Sato, T.; Asanuma, Y.; Nanjo, H.; Arakawa, A.; Kusano, T.; Koyama, K.; Shindo, M. A resected case of giant leiomyosarcoma of the pancreas. *J. Gastroenterol.* **1994**, *29*, 223–227. [CrossRef]
231. Muhammad, S.U.; Azam, F.; Zuzana, S. Primary pancreatic leiomyosarcoma: A case report. *Cases J.* **2008**, *1*, 280. [CrossRef]
232. Singla, V.; Arora, A.; Tyagi, P.; Bansal, R.K.; Sharma, P.; Bansal, N.; Kumar, A. Rare cause of recurrent acute pancreatitis due to leiomyosarcoma. *Trop. Gastroenterol.* **2016**, *37*, 70–72. [CrossRef]
233. Xu, J.; Zhang, T.; Wang, T.; You, L.; Zhao, Y. Clinical characteristics and prognosis of primary leiomyosarcoma of the pancreas: A systematic review. *World J. Surg. Oncol.* **2013**, *11*, 290. [CrossRef]
234. Aleshawi, A.J.; Allouh, M.Z.; Heis, F.H.; Tashtush, N.; Heis, H.A. Primary Leiomyosarcoma of the Pancreas: A Comprehensive Analytical Review. *J. Gastrointest. Cancer* **2020**, *51*, 433–438. [CrossRef]
235. Zhang, H.; Jensen, M.H.; Farnell, M.B.; Smyrk, T.C.; Zhang, L. Primary leiomyosarcoma of the pancreas: Study of 9 cases and review of literature. *Am. J. Surg. Pathol.* **2010**, *34*, 1849–1856. [CrossRef] [PubMed]
236. Barral, M.; Faraoun, S.A.; Fishman, E.K.; Dohan, A.; Pozzessere, C.; Berthelin, M.A.; Bazeries, P.; Barat, M.; Hoeffel, C.; Soyer, P. Imaging features of rare pancreatic tumors. *Diagn. Interv. Imaging* **2016**, *97*, 1259–1273. [CrossRef] [PubMed]
237. Srivastava, D.N.; Batra, A.; Thulkar, S.; Julka, P.K. Leiomyosarcoma of pancreas: Imaging features. *Indian. J. Gastroenterol.* **2000**, *19*, 187–188.
238. Ishikawa, O.; Matsui, Y.; Aoki, Y.; Iwanaga, T.; Terasawa, T.; Wada, A. Leiomyosarcoma of the pancreas. Report of a case and review of the literature. *Am. J. Surg. Pathol.* **1981**, *5*, 597–602. [CrossRef] [PubMed]
239. Riddle, N.D.; Quigley, B.C.; Browarsky, I.; Bui, M.M. Leiomyosarcoma arising in the pancreatic duct: A case report and review of the current literature. *Case Rep. Med.* **2010**, *2010*, 252364. [CrossRef]
240. Kocakoc, E.; Havan, N.; Bilgin, M.; Atay, M. Primary pancreatic leiomyosarcoma. *Iran. J. Radiol.* **2014**, *11*, e4880. [CrossRef]
241. Machado, M.C.; Cunha, J.E.; Penteado, S.; Bacchella, T.; Jukemura, J.; Costa, A.C.; Halpern-Salomon, I. Preoperative diagnosis of pancreatic leiomyosarcoma. *Int. J. Pancreatol.* **2000**, *28*, 97–100. [CrossRef]
242. de la Santa, L.G.; Retortillo, J.A.; Miguel, A.C.; Klein, L.M. Radiology of pancreatic neoplasms: An update. *World J. Gastrointest. Oncol.* **2014**, *6*, 330–343. [CrossRef]
243. Viúdez, A.; De Jesus-Acosta, A.; Carvalho, F.L.; Vera, R.; Martín-Algarra, S.; Ramírez, N. Pancreatic neuroendocrine tumors: Challenges in an underestimated disease. *Crit. Rev. Oncol. Hematol.* **2016**, *101*, 193–206. [CrossRef]
244. Okun, S.D.; Lewin, D.N. Non-neoplastic pancreatic lesions that may mimic malignancy. *Semin. Diagn. Pathol.* **2016**, *33*, 31–42. [CrossRef]
245. Konstantinidis, I.T.; Dursun, A.; Zheng, H.; Wargo, J.A.; Thayer, S.P.; Fernandez-del Castillo, C.; Warshaw, A.L.; Ferrone, C.R. Metastatic tumors in the pancreas in the modern era. *J. Am. Coll. Surg.* **2010**, *211*, 749–753. [CrossRef] [PubMed]
246. Ogura, T.; Masuda, D.; Kurisu, Y.; Miyamoto, Y.; Hayashi, M.; Imoto, A.; Takii, M.; Takeuchi, T.; Inoue, T.; Tokioka, S.; et al. Multiple metastatic leiomyosarcoma of the pancreas: A first case report and review of the literature. *Intern. Med.* **2013**, *52*, 561–566. [CrossRef] [PubMed]
247. Lin, C.; Wang, L.; Sheng, J.; Zhang, D.; Guan, L.; Zhao, K.; Zhang, X. Transdifferentiation of pancreatic stromal tumor into leiomyosarcoma with metastases to liver and peritoneum: A case report. *BMC Cancer* **2016**, *16*, 947. [CrossRef] [PubMed]
248. Hébert-Magee, S.; Varadarajulu, S.; Frost, A.R.; Ramesh, J. Primary pancreatic leiomyosarcoma: A rare diagnosis obtained by EUS-FNA cytology. *Gastrointest. Endosc.* **2014**, *80*, 361–362. [CrossRef]
249. Aihara, H.; Kawamura, Y.J.; Toyama, N.; Mori, Y.; Konishi, F.; Yamada, S. A small leiomyosarcoma of the pancreas treated by local excision. *HPB* **2002**, *4*, 145–148. [CrossRef]
250. Milanetto, A.C.; Liço, V.; Blandamura, S.; Pasquali, C. Primary leiomyosarcoma of the pancreas: Report of a case treated by local excision and review of the literature. *Surg. Case Rep.* **2015**, *1*, 98. [CrossRef]
251. Hur, Y.H.; Kim, H.H.; Park, E.K.; Seoung, J.S.; Kim, J.W.; Jeong, Y.Y.; Lee, J.H.; Koh, Y.S.; Kim, J.C.; Kim, H.J.; et al. Primary leiomyosarcoma of the pancreas. *J. Korean Surg. Soc.* **2011**, *81* (Suppl. 1), S69–S73. [CrossRef]
252. Izumi, H.; Okada, K.; Imaizumi, T.; Hirabayashi, K.; Matsuyama, M.; Dowaki, S.; Tobita, K.; Makuuchi, H. Leiomyosarcoma of the pancreas: Report of a case. *Surg. Today* **2011**, *41*, 1556–1561. [CrossRef]
253. Battula, N.; Srinivasan, P.; Prachalias, A.; Rela, M.; Heaton, N. Primary pancreatic lymphoma: Diagnostic and therapeutic dilemma. *Pancreas* **2006**, *33*, 192–194. [CrossRef]

254. Kloppel, G.; Solcia, E.; Longnecker, D.S.; Capella, C.; Sobin, L.H. *Histological Typing of Tumours of the Exocrine Pancreas*; World Health Organization International Classification of Tumours; Springer: Berlin, Germany, 1996; pp. 11–20.
255. Sadot, E.; Yahalom, J.; Do, R.K.; Teruya-Feldstein, J.; Allen, P.J.; Gönen, M.; D'Angelica, M.I.; Kingham, T.P.; Jarnagin, W.R.; DeMatteo, R.P. Clinical features and outcome of primary pancreatic lymphoma. *Ann. Surg. Oncol.* **2015**, *22*, 1176–1184. [CrossRef]
256. Jones, W.F.; Sheikh, M.Y.; McClave, S.A. AIDS-related non-Hodgkin's lymphoma of the pancreas. *Am. J. Gastroenterol.* **1997**, *92*, 335–338.
257. Facchinelli, D.; Sina, S.; Boninsegna, E.; Borin, A.; Tisi, M.C.; Piazza, F.; Scapinello, G.; Maiolo, E.; Hohaus, S.; Zamò, A.; et al. Primary pancreatic lymphoma: Clinical presentation, diagnosis, treatment, and outcome. *Eur. J. Haematol.* **2020**, *105*, 468–475. [CrossRef]
258. Rad, N.; Khafaf, A.; Mohammad Alizadeh, A.H. Primary pancreatic lymphoma: What we need to know. *J. Gastrointest. Oncol.* **2017**, *8*, 749–757. [CrossRef]
259. Mishra, M.V.; Keith, S.W.; Shen, X.; Ad, V.B.; Champ, C.E.; Biswas, T. Primary pancreatic lymphoma. *Am. J. Clin. Oncol.* **2013**, *36*, 38–43. [CrossRef]
260. Fujinaga, Y.; Lall, C.; Patel, A.; Matsushita, T.; Sanyal, R.; Kadoya, M. MR features of primary and secondary malignant lymphoma of the pancreas: A pictorial review. *Insights Imaging* **2013**, *4*, 321–329. [CrossRef]
261. Merkle, E.M.; Bender, G.N.; Brambs, H.J. Imaging findings in pancreatic lymphoma: Differential aspects. *Am. J. Roentgenol.* **2000**, *174*, 671–675. [CrossRef]
262. Segaran, N.; Sandrasegaran, K.; Devine, C.; Wang, M.X.; Shah, C.; Ganeshan, D. Features of primary pancreatic lymphoma: A bi-institutional review with an emphasis on typical and atypical imaging features. *World J. Clin. Oncol.* **2021**, *12*, 823–832. [CrossRef]
263. Low, G.; Panu, A.; Millo, N.; Leen, E. Multimodality imaging of neoplastic and nonneoplastic solid lesions of the pancreas. *RadioGraphics* **2011**, *31*, 993–1015. [CrossRef]
264. Amodio, J.; Brodsky, J.E. Pediatric Burkitt lymphoma presenting as acute pancreatitis: MRI characteristics. *Pediatr. Radiol.* **2010**, *40*, 770–772. [CrossRef]
265. Boninsegna, E.; Zamboni, G.A.; Facchinelli, D.; Triantopoulou, C.; Gourtsoyianni, S.; Ambrosetti, M.C.; Veneri, D.; Ambrosetti, A.; Pozzi Mucelli, R. CT imaging of primary pancreatic lymphoma: Experience from three referral centres for pancreatic diseases. *Insights Imaging* **2018**, *9*, 17–24. [CrossRef]
266. Anand, D.; Lall, C.; Bhosale, P.; Ganeshan, D.; Qayyum, A. Current update on primary pancreatic lymphoma. *Abdom. Radiol.* **2016**, *41*, 347–355. [CrossRef] [PubMed]
267. Wallace, D.; Dang, N.; Dhawan, M.; Kulkarni, A. Diagnosis of a patient with primary pancreatic lymphoma. *Gastroenterol. Hepatol.* **2012**, *8*, 850–852.
268. Saif, M.W. Primary pancreatic lymphomas. *J. Pancreas* **2006**, *7*, 262–273.
269. Behrns, K.E.; Sarr, M.G.; Strickler, J.G. Pancreatic lymphoma: Is it a surgical disease? *Pancreas* **1994**, *9*, 662–667. [CrossRef]
270. Sadaf, S.; Loya, A.; Akhtar, N.; Yusuf, M.A. Role of endoscopic ultrasound guided-fine needle aspiration biopsy in the diagnosis of lymphoma of the pancreas: A clinicopathological study of nine cases. *Cytopathology* **2017**, *28*, 536–541. [CrossRef]
271. Freeman, C.; Berg, J.W.; Cutler, S.J. Occurrence and prognosis of extranodal lymphomas. *Cancer* **1972**, *29*, 252–260. [CrossRef]
272. Vitolo, U.; Seymour, J.F.; Martelli, M.; Illerhaus, G.; Illidge, T.; Zucca, E.; Campo, E.; Ladetto, M.; ESMO Guidelines Committee. Extranodal diffuse large B-cell lymphoma (DLBCL) and primary mediastinal B-cell lymphoma: ESMO Clinical Practice Guidelines for diagnosis, treatment and follow-up. *Ann. Oncol.* **2016**, *27* (Suppl. 5), 91–102. [CrossRef] [PubMed]
273. Ballarin, R.; Spaggiari, M.; Cautero, N.; De Ruvo, N.; Montalti, R.; Longo, C.; Pecchi, A.; Giacobazzi, P.; De Marco, G.; D'Amico, G.; et al. Pancreatic metastases from renal cell carcinoma: The state of the art. *World J. Gastroenterol.* **2011**, *17*, 4747–4756. [CrossRef] [PubMed]
274. Reddy, S.; Wolfgang, C.L. The role of surgery in the management of isolated metastases to the pancreas. *Lancet Oncol.* **2009**, *10*, 287–293. [CrossRef]
275. Reddy, S.; Edil, B.H.; Cameron, J.L.; Pawlik, T.M.; Herman, J.M.; Gilson, M.M.; Campbell, K.A.; Schulik, R.D.; Ahuja, N.; Wolfgang, C.L. Pancreatic resection of isolated metastases from nonpancreatic primary cancers. *Ann. Surg. Oncol.* **2008**, *15*, 3199–3206. [CrossRef]
276. Sweeny, A.D.; Fisher, W.E.; Wu, M.F.; Hilsenbeck, S.G.; Brunicardi, F.C. Value of pancreatic resection for cancer metastatic to the pancreas. *J. Surg. Res.* **2010**, *160*, 268–276. [CrossRef] [PubMed]
277. Showalter, S.L.; Hager, E.; Yeo, C.J. Metastatic disease to the pancreas and spleen. *Semin. Oncol.* **2008**, *35*, 160–171. [CrossRef] [PubMed]
278. Rypens, F.; Van Gansbeke, D.; Lambilliotte, J.P.; Van Regemorter, G.; Verhest, A.; Struyven, J. Pancreatic metastasis from renal cell carcinoma. *Br. J. Radiol.* **1992**, *65*, 547–548. [CrossRef] [PubMed]
279. Ferrozzi, F.; Bova, D.; Campodonico, F.; Chiara, F.D.; Passari, A.; Bassi, P. Pancreatic metastases: CT assessment. *Eur. Radiol.* **1997**, *7*, 241–245. [CrossRef] [PubMed]
280. Muranaka, T.; Teshima, K.; Honda, H.; Nanjo, T.; Hanada, K.; Oshiumi, Y. Computed tomography and histologic appearance of pancreatic metastases from distant sources. *Acta Radiol.* **1989**, *30*, 615–619. [CrossRef] [PubMed]
281. Cheng, S.K.; Chuah, K.L. Metastatic renal cell carcinoma to the pancreas: A review. *Arch. Pathol. Lab. Med.* **2016**, *140*, 598–602. [CrossRef]

282. Sikka, A.; Adam, S.Z.; Wood, C.; Hoff, F.; Harmath, C.B.; Miller, F.H. Magnetic resonance imaging of pancreatic metastases from renal cell carcinoma. *Clin. Imaging* **2015**, *39*, 945–953. [CrossRef]
283. Maeno, T.; Satoh, H.; Ishikawa, H.; Yamashita, Y.T.; Naito, T.; Fujiwara, M.; Kamma, H.; Ohtsuka, M.; Hasegawa, S. Patterns of pancreatic metastasis from lung cancer. *Anticancer Res.* **1998**, *18*, 2881–2884.
284. Woo, J.S.; Joo, K.R.; Woo, Y.S.; Jang, J.Y.; Chang, Y.W.; Lee, J.I.; Chang, R. Pancreatitis from metastatic small cell lung cancer: Successful treatment with endoscopic intrapancreatic stenting. *Korean J. Intern. Med.* **2006**, *21*, 256. [CrossRef]
285. Cwik, G.; Wallner, G.; Skoczylas, T.; Ciechanski, A.; Zinkiewicz, K. Cancer antigens 19-9 and 125 in the differential diagnosis of pancreatic mass lesions. *Arch. Surg.* **2006**, *141*, 968–973. [CrossRef]
286. Okamoto, T. Malignant biliary obstruction due to metastatic non-hepato-pancreato-biliary cancer. *World J. Gastroenterol.* **2022**, *28*, 985–1008. [CrossRef] [PubMed]
287. Ascenti, G.; Visalli, C.; Genitori, A.; Certo, A.; Pitrone, A.; Mazziotti, S. Multiple hypervascular pancreatic metastases from renal cell carcinoma: Dynamic MR and spiral CT in three cases. *Clin. Imaging* **2004**, *28*, 349–352. [CrossRef] [PubMed]
288. Galia, M.; Albano, D.; Picone, D.; Terranova, M.C.; Agrusa, A.; Di Buono, G.; Licata, A.; Lo Re, G.; La Grutta, L.; Midiri, M. Imaging features of pancreatic metastases: A comparison with pancreatic ductal adenocarcinoma. *Clin. Imaging* **2018**, *51*, 76–82. [CrossRef] [PubMed]
289. Kelekis, N.L.; Semelka, R.C.; Siegelman, E.S. MRI of pancreatic metastases from renal cancer. *J. Comput. Assist. Tomogr.* **1996**, *20*, 249–253. [CrossRef] [PubMed]
290. Crippa, S.; Angelini, C.; Mussi, C.; Bonardi, C.; Romano, F.; Sartori, P.; Uggeri, F.; Bovo, G. Surgical treatment of metastatic tumors to the pancreas: A single center experience and re-view of the literature. *World J. Surg.* **2006**, *30*, 1536–1542. [CrossRef]
291. Sperti, C.; Pasquali, C.; Liessi, G.; Pinciroli, L.; Decet, G.; Pedrazzoli, S. Pancreatic resection for metastatic tumors to the pancreas. *J. Surg. Oncol.* **2003**, *83*, 161–166. [CrossRef]
292. Law, C.H.; Wei, A.C.; Hanna, S.S.; Al-Zahrani, M.; Taylor, B.R.; Greig, P.D.; Langer, B.; Gallinger, S. Pancreatic resection for metastatic renal cell carcinoma: Presentation, treatment, and outcome. *Ann. Surg. Oncol.* **2003**, *10*, 922–926. [CrossRef]
293. Scatarige, J.C.; Horton, K.M.; Sheth, S.; Fishman, E.K. Pancreatic parenchymal metastases: Observations on helical CT. *Am. J. Roentgenol.* **2001**, *176*, 695–699. [CrossRef]
294. Atlas, S.W.; Braffmann, B.H.; LoBrutto, R.; Elder, D.E.; Herlyn, D. Human malignant melanomas with varying degrees of melanin content in nude mice: MR imaging, histopathology, and electron paramagnetic resonance. *J. Comput. Assist. Tomogr.* **1990**, *14*, 547–554. [CrossRef]
295. Wang, H.; Nie, P.; Dong, C.; Li, J.; Huang, Y.; Hao, D.; Xu, W. CT and MRI Findings of Soft Tissue Adult Fibrosarcoma in Extremities. *Biomed. Res. Int.* **2018**, *2018*, 6075705. [CrossRef]
296. Adsay, N.V.; Andea, A.; Basturk, O.; Kilinc, N.; Nassar, H.; Cheng, J.D. Secondary tumors of the pancreas: An analysis of a surgical and autopsy database and review of the literature. *Virchows Arch.* **2004**, *444*, 527–535. [CrossRef] [PubMed]
297. Tan, C.H.; Tamm, E.P.; Marcal, L.; Balachandran, A.; Charnsangavej, C.; Vikram, R.; Bhosale, P. Imaging features of hematogenous metastases to the pancreas: Pictorial essay. *Cancer Imaging* **2011**, *11*, 9–15. [CrossRef] [PubMed]
298. Palmowski, M.; Hacke, N.; Satzl, S.; Klauss, M.; Wente, M.N.; Neukamm, M.; Kleeff, J.; Hallscheidt, P. Metastasis to the pancreas: Characterization by morphology and contrast enhancement features on CT and MRI. *Pancreatology* **2008**, *8*, 199–203. [CrossRef]
299. Bahra, M.; Jacob, D.; Langrehr, J.M.; Glanemann, M.; Schumacher, G.; Lopez-Hänninen, E.; Neuhaus, P. Metastasen im Pankreas. Wann ist eine Resektion sinnvoll? *Chirurg* **2008**, *79*, 241–248. [CrossRef] [PubMed]
300. Bassi, C.; Butturini, G.; Falconi, M.; Sargenti, M.; Mantovani, W.; Pederzoli, P. High recurrence rate after atypical resection for pancreatic metastases from renal cell carcinoma. *Br. J. Surg.* **2003**, *90*, 555–559. [CrossRef] [PubMed]

Disclaimer/Publisher's Note: The statements, opinions and data contained in all publications are solely those of the individual author(s) and contributor(s) and not of MDPI and/or the editor(s). MDPI and/or the editor(s) disclaim responsibility for any injury to people or property resulting from any ideas, methods, instructions or products referred to in the content.

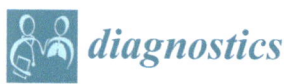

Review

The Spectrum of Solitary Benign Splenic Lesions—Imaging Clues for a Noninvasive Diagnosis

Sofia Gourtsoyianni [1], Michael Laniado [2], Luis Ros-Mendoza [3], Giancarlo Mansueto [4] and Giulia A. Zamboni [4,*]

[1] 1st Department of Radiology, School of Medicine, National and Kapodistrian University of Athens, Areteion Hospital, 76, Vas. Sophias Ave., 11528 Athens, Greece; sgty76@gmail.com
[2] Institute and Policlinic for Diagnostic and Interventional Radiology, University Hospital Carl Gustav Carus, TU Dresden, Fetscherstraße 74, 01307 Dresden, Germany; michael@laniado.de
[3] Department of Radiology, Miguel Servet University Hospital, Paseo Isabel la Católica 1-3, 50009 Zaragoza, Spain; lhrosmendoza@gmail.com
[4] Istituto di Radiologia, DAI Patologia e Diagnostica, Policlinico GB Rossi, AOUI Verona, 37134 Verona, Italy; giancarlo.mansueto@univr.it
* Correspondence: giulia.zamboni@univr.it

Abstract: Cross-sectional imaging of the upper abdomen, especially if intravenous contrast has been administered, will most likely reveal any acute or chronic disease harbored in the spleen. Unless imaging is performed with the specific purpose of evaluating the spleen or characterizing a known splenic lesion, incidentally discovered splenic lesions pose a small challenge. Solitary benign splenic lesions include cysts, hemangiomas, sclerosing angiomatous nodular transformation (SANT), hamartomas, and abscesses, among others. Sarcoidosis and tuberculosis, although predominantly diffuse micronodular disease processes, may also present as a solitary splenic mass lesion. In addition, infarction and rupture, both traumatic and spontaneous, may take place in the spleen. This review aims to describe the imaging features of the most common benign focal splenic lesions, with emphasis on the imaging findings as these are encountered on routine cross-sectional imaging from a multicenter pool of cases that, coupled with clinical information, can allow a definite diagnosis.

Keywords: spleen; benign; solitary; MRI; CT

1. Introduction

The spleen, often referred to as the forgotten organ, serves in adulthood as a filter for blood cells with additional important immune functions. As it is not essential for the preservation of vital life functions, it often receives limited attention from clinicians. Nevertheless, a wide range of diseases can affect the spleen, which might present as focal lesions on routine cross-sectional imaging, classified into six categories (Table 1).

Incidental splenic lesions, defined as lesions detected by imaging performed for a reason unrelated to the spleen, have not been evaluated in great detail and may equally excite and puzzle the reporting Radiologist. In a population-based whole-body magnetic resonance imaging (MRI) study of 2500 healthy individuals, 31.5% had incidental findings of potential clinical relevance, but only 12 involved the spleen with a reported likelihood of malignancy of only 1% [1]. Another study performed on trauma victims reported an incidence of less than 2% for splenic granulomas, hemangiomas, cysts, and abscesses, proving that most incidentally detected isolated splenic lesions are benign [2].

Unfortunately, due to overlapping imaging features, differentiation of benign from malignant splenic lesions may be challenging. Clinical history plays a pivotal role in incidental splenic lesion characterization, including pain related to the spleen, body temperature, immune status, and history of recent trauma. Significant predictors of malignant splenic lesions are the solid nature of the mass, lymph node enlargement, and/or the presence of underlying malignancy [3].

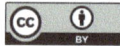

Table 1. Categories of focal splenic lesions.

Category	Lesion Type
Intermediate between benign and malignant	Inflammatory myofibroblastic tumor
Inflammatory	Sarcoidosis
Congenital/developmental	Lymphangioma Primary cyst
Acquired	False cyst Infarction
Vascular	Haemangioma Hamartoma Littoral cell angioma Sclerosing angiomatous nodular transformation (SANT)
Infectious	Pyogenic abscess Fungal abscess Tuberculosis Hydatid cyst
Malignant	Lymphoma Angiosarcoma Haemangiopericytoma Splenic metastasis

In this paper, cross-sectional imaging findings of the most common benign focal splenic lesions are reviewed, highlighting their key differences, as all typically present as hypodense on CT, with low signal intensity (SI) on T1 weighted images (WI) and most of the time hyperintense on T2-WI, exceptions listed in Table 2.

Table 2. Cross-sectional imaging characteristics of benign focal splenic lesions.

Lesion	CT	T1-WI	T2-WI	Enhancement
Inflammatory myofibroblastic tumor	LA	↓ SI	↓ SI	slow delayed
Sarcoidosis	LA	↓ SI	↓ SI	minimal delayed
Cyst	LA	↓ SI *	↑ SI	no
Lymphangioma	LA	↓ SI *	↑ SI with hypointense septa	no only septa
Infarct	nv	recent: ↑ SI old: iso/↓ SI	↑ SI	peripheral, wedge-shaped defect
Haemangioma	LA	↓ SI to isointense	↑ SI	variable marked
Hamartoma	LA/isoattenuating	↓ SI to isointense	mildly to moderate ↑ SI	heterogeneous non-enhancing central scar
Littoral cell angioma	LA	isointense	↓ SI	progressive enhancement
SANT	LA/isoattenuating	isointense	↓ SI with hyperintense septa	variable spoke-wheel
Pyogenic abscess	LA	↓ SI	↑ SI	peripheral rim
Fungal abscess	LA	intermediate SI	↑ SI	subtle rim
Tuberculosis	LA	↓ SI	↑ SI	peripheral

LA: Low attenuation. ↑ SI: increased signal intensity (hyperintense). ↓ SI: decreased signal intensity (hypointense). * unless hemorrhagic content/debris/high proteinaceous content. nv: not visible.

2. Normal Splenic Appearances with Different Imaging Modalities

2.1. US

Ultrasonography (US) is frequently the first imaging modality to assess the spleen because of its high diffusion and lack of ionizing radiation. In the hands of an experienced examiner, it has high reliability. On US, the splenic parenchyma is typically homogeneous, with finely textured internal echoes, and is slightly more echoic than the normal renal cortex, isoechoic to slightly hyperechoic compared to the liver parenchyma and hypoechoic compared to the pancreatic parenchyma. Color Doppler can be useful in the evaluation of vascular pathology in the splenic hilum. US can easily detect focal splenic lesions, but in most cases, these have a nonspecific appearance, and the diagnostic accuracy in the characterization is limited (30–75%). However, this has been reported to improve with the use of contrast-enhanced US [4]. The contrast medium currently available in Europe is Sonovue® (Bracco, Milan, Italy), an intravascular agent consisting of microbubbles (1–7 μm) containing Sulfur hexafluoride encapsulated by a phospholipid shell. The microbubbles remain inside the vessels for up to 7 min, after which they dissolve, with the gas exhaled through the lungs, while the shell gets metabolized, primarily by the liver. In order to avoid microbubble rupture under injection pressure, a needle with a diameter of 23 Gauge or larger must be used in adults to administer a bolus of 2 mL of ultrasonographic contrast medium, followed by approximately 10 mL of saline solution through an antecubital vein. A nonenhanced US examination is performed to identify the best scan view followed by arterial phase imaging at 12–20 s post-injection, during which the normal spleen demonstrates a zebra pattern, such as the one in CECT. During this phase, arterial vascular injuries may be detected. The venous phase starts after 40–60 s post-injection, being the optimal phase for organ injury detection. The healthy splenic parenchyma demonstrates a homogeneous enhancement for an extended period, approximately 5–7 min [5].

2.2. CT

On unenhanced CT, the spleen is homogeneous, has attenuation values ranging between 40 HU and 60 HU, and is hypodense or isodense to the liver parenchyma. On unenhanced images, calcifications can be easily detected. After intravenous contrast administration, the normal splenic parenchyma has a variable pattern of enhancement in the early and late arterial phases. The enhancement patterns include serpentine or mottled appearance and focal and diffuse heterogeneity because of variable flow rates through circulation in the white and red pulp, giving the typical "zebra-like" enhancement. In the portal-venous phase, the enhancement of the normal parenchyma becomes homogeneous.

2.3. MRI

Magnetic Resonance (MR), using a combination of T2-weighted, gradient-echo, and multiphasic contrast-enhanced imaging, provides superior lesion characterization compared with CT or US. On T1-weighted images (WI), the MR signal intensity of the splenic tissue is homogeneously low and equal to slightly less than that of the liver and muscle. On T2-WI, signal intensity is usually higher than that of the liver parenchyma. The spleen remains the brightest abdominal organ in T2-weighted images, even though signal intensity varies with patient age. Because the white pulp is not yet matured in the newborn, signal intensity is usually more hypointense than the normal liver parenchyma on T2-WI and more isointense on T1-WI. Splenic imaging characteristics evolve to the normal adult pattern within the first months of life. Normal splenic parenchyma tends to demonstrate a homogenously restricted diffusion on Diffusion-weighted imaging (DWI), i.e., high signal intensity on the highest b value obtained and low signal intensity on the corresponding ADC map [6]. Splenic lesions with a hyper- or isointense signal on high b-value DWI images (e.g., b 800) and iso- or hypointense signal on the corresponding ADC map compared to the normal splenic parenchyma are more likely malignant. Therefore, the addition of DWI to conventional MRI improves the prediction of malignant splenic lesions [7]. After dynamic administration of gadolinium contrast agents, the enhancement pattern of the spleen is similar to the contrast enhancement pattern on CT, appearing inhomogeneous in the arterial phase and homogeneous in the portal venous and equilibrium phases. A splenic lesion with low signal intensity on 3-min delayed images combined with arterial hypervascularity on dynamic MRI may predict the malignant nature of the splenic lesion, while the 3-min delayed phase low signal intensity and the presence of restricted diffusion raise the diagnostic performance for the discrimination of focal splenic lesions [8].

2.4. Nuclear Medicine

Nuclear medicine offers different radiopharmaceutical tracers to be used with conventional scintigraphy or Positron Emission Tomography (PET). Since Technetium Tc99m sulfur colloid accumulates in the liver and spleen through the uptake by the reticuloendothelial system, scintigraphy can be used to localize ectopic splenic tissue in cases of intrapancreatic accessory spleen, splenosis, or wandering spleen. PET with [18F]-Fluoro Deoxy Glucose (18F-FDG-PET) shows lower metabolism and tracer uptake of the normal spleen compared to the liver [9]. Diffusely increased splenic uptake is observed after administration of granulocyte colony-stimulating factor [10], but also in some cases of neoplastic (e.g., lymphomatous involvement) and inflammatory diseases (e.g., HIV, sarcoidosis) [11]. Focal tracer accumulation in the spleen occurs secondary to the presence of neoplastic or inflammatory lesions [12].

3. Lesion-Specific Imaging Characteristics

Inflammatory myofibroblastic tumor (IMT), formerly known as inflammatory pseudotumor, is an uncommon benign splenic lesion. It has been described in virtually all major organs with a few exceptions. In the liver and spleen, inflammatory pseudotumor is possibly linked to Epstein–Barr infection [13]. The prevalence is similar in both sexes, with a peak incidence in middle age. The lesions reported are usually large, measuring > 10 cm. It is composed of a combination of inflammatory and myofibroblastic spindle cells. Usually an incidental finding, it is included in the differential diagnosis of malignant splenic lesions, although currently, the World Health Organization classification of soft tissue tumors places IMTs in an intermediate category between benign and malignant, with metastases in less than 5% of extrasplenic cases [14,15]. In the US, inflammatory myofibroblastic tumors appear as solid hypoechoic masses. CT shows hypoattenuating hypoenhancing lesions, and stellate central calcifications seen on CT scans make the diagnosis very likely [16]. They present as hypointense masses both on T1-WI and T2-WI, with slow delayed enhancement (Figure 1) [17]. The diagnosis can be confirmed reliably only by histopathological and immunohistochemical evaluations. Although recurrence and metastatization have not been described for splenic inflammatory myofibroblastic tumors, patients must be followed up as these are considered tumors with intermediate malignant potential [14,17].

Sarcoidosis is a multisystem disease characterized by the presence of non-caseating granulomas. One-third of patients presenting with splenic sarcoidosis findings have normal chest radiography [18]. Splenic involvement has been reported in about 40% of cases of multisystem sarcoidosis, but isolated sarcoidosis of the spleen is extremely rare [19]. It may present either as splenomegaly or with multiple nodules, whereas a solitary splenic lesion is very rare. Patients with diffuse splenic granulomas have a worse prognosis in terms of persistent chronic sarcoidosis than patients without splenic involvement or patients with limited splenic disease [20]. Nodules appear hypodense on CT and have low SI both on T1-WI and T2-WI, with minimal delayed enhancement [21] (Figure 2). Nodules are best seen on T2-WI with fat saturation and on early gadolinium-enhanced T1–WI. MRI is said to be able to monitor disease activity, as during active inflammation, nodules demonstrate T2-WI hyperintensity due to edema and high vascular permeability, as well as restricted diffusion [22]. The main differential diagnosis includes infections, especially tuberculosis, and malignancies, especially lymphoma. The final diagnosis is based on three main criteria: a compatible presentation, the evidence of non-caseating granulomas on histological examination, and the exclusion of any alternative diagnosis [23].

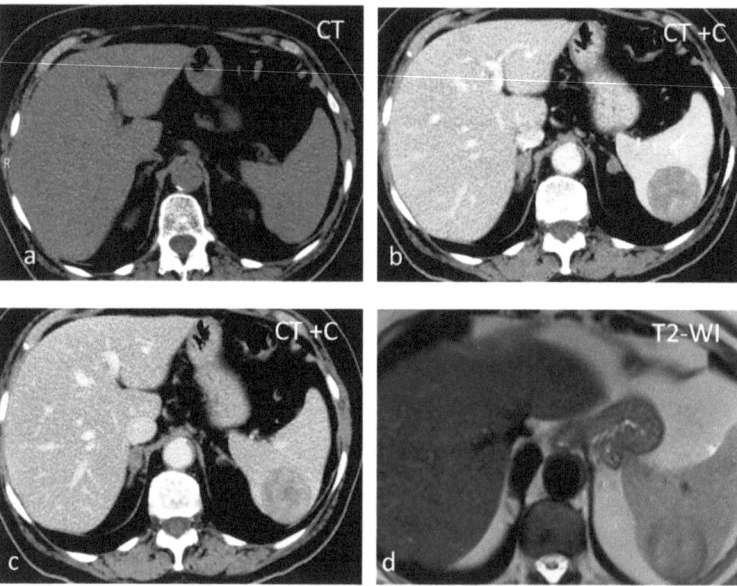

Figure 1. Large solid lesion, in keeping with an inflammatory myofibroblastic tumor, slightly hypodense in the non-contrast CT scan (**a**), depicting slightly heterogenous/patchy gradual enhancement pattern post-contrast enhancement (**b**,**c**). The lesion appears iso– to hypointense on T2-weighted MRI, more conspicuous than in the non-contrast CT scan (**d**).

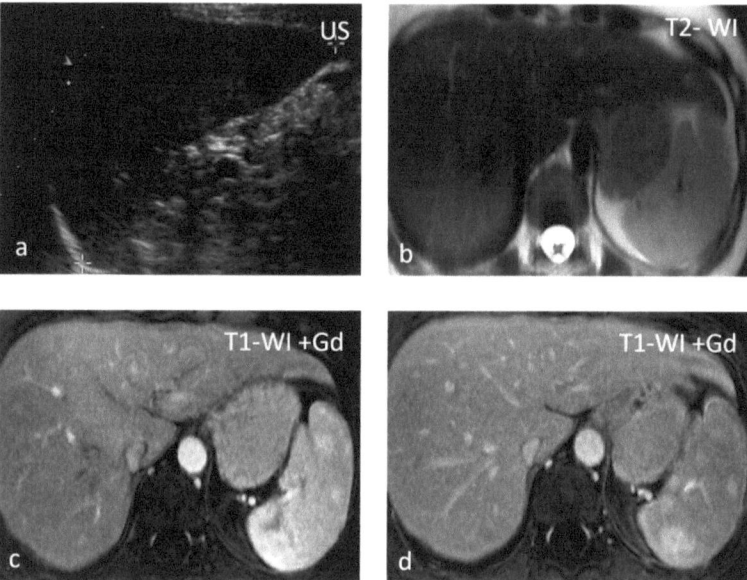

Figure 2. Sarcoidosis. US shows multiple hypoechoic nodules (**a**). The nodules appear slightly hypointense on T2 WI (**b**) and show mild delayed enhancement (**c**,**d**).

Lymphangioma, a vascular lesion like hemangioma, is a rare benign lesion that is commonly seen in children and exceptional in adults. In 60% of cases, the diagnosis is made before the age of 1 year. Lymphangioma is commonly subcapsular and may have satellite lesions [24]. Similarly to hemangiomas, lymphangiomas can involve the spleen exclusively, or they may be part of generalized angiomatosis, with lymphangiomas or hemangiomas involving several organs in the body [25]. US shows a rounded, well-defined hypoechoic lesion, possibly with internal septations and intralocular echogenic debris [26]. On CT, lymphangiomas appear as single or multiple thin-walled hypodense lesions with no enhancement in a typical subcapsular location [26]. Peripheral wall calcifications can be present. The lesion has typical benign cystic MRI features and may be multiloculated with hypointense thin septa (Figure 3), which may show enhancement. The management of choice for symptomatic, i.e., presenting with left upper quadrant pain and/or splenomegaly, lymphangiomas is splenectomy, as delay in therapeutic intervention can lead to life-threatening complications [24].

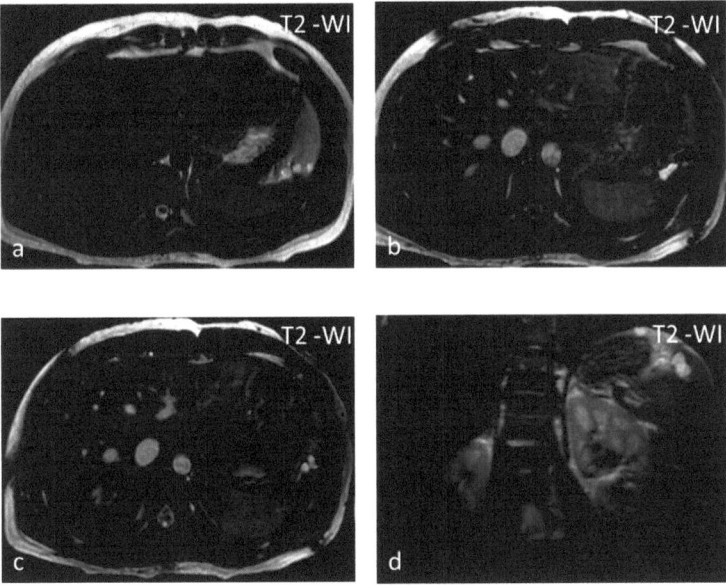

Figure 3. Lymphangiomas. Multiple, subcapsular, hyperintense lesions, one of which appears multiloculated with thin septa, are seen on axial T2-WI images (a–c) and coronal plane T2-WI image (d).

Cysts, most often solitary, are usually incidental findings, being asymptomatic [25]. Two categories exist: primary (true) and secondary (false). Primary cysts, also called epidermoid cysts, are congenital lesions with an epithelial lining, with a 20% prevalence in females. Possible explanations for the pathogenesis of true cyst include (1) infolding of peritoneal mesothelium after rupture of the splenic capsule, (2) collections of peritoneal mesothelial cells trapped in splenic sulci, or (3) origin from normal lymph spaces [27]. Primary splenic cysts constitute 10% of all nonparasitic cysts of the spleen. It is a rare condition with an incidence rate of 0.07%, as reported in a review of 42,327 autopsies [28]. Secondary cysts are lined by a fibrous wall and most often are post-traumatic. Rarely they may occur in splenic abscess or splenic infarction [29]. At ultrasound (US), cysts appear as well-defined rounded lesions with a thin wall and anechoic fluid content. They appear homogeneously hypoattenuating on CT and lack enhancement. Calcifications may be seen in the wall in post-traumatic cysts. Unless hemorrhage or debris is present, at MRI, splenic cysts appear hypointense on T1-WI and homogeneously hyperintense on T2-WI (Figure 4). Simple cysts, either primary or secondary, do not warrant further follow-up with imaging. However, due to the increased risk of complications (rupture, infection, hemorrhage), splenic cysts larger than 5 cm or symptomatic ones should be treated surgically, trying to preserve as much of the splenic parenchyma as possible [30].

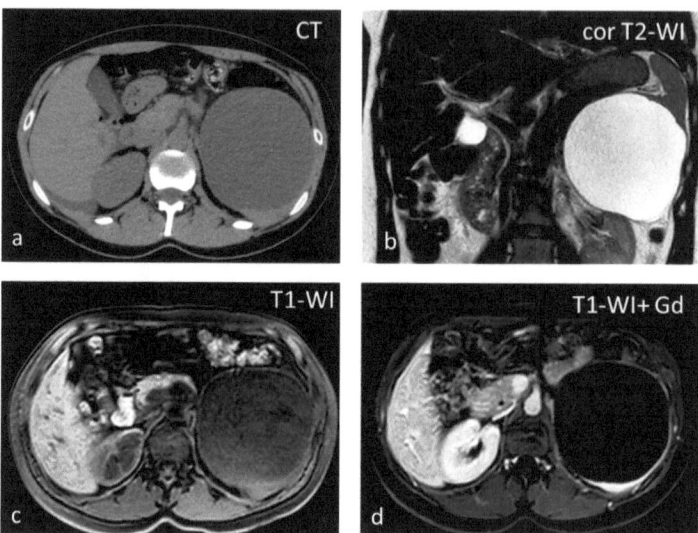

Figure 4. Large splenic cyst appearing homogeneously hypodense on non-contrast CT (**a**). The cyst content is homogeneously hyperintense on T2-WI (**b**) and hypointense on T1-WI (**c**). The cyst wall does not show significant enhancement (**d**).

Splenic infarct can be of either arterial or venous origin. Global infarction may be caused by occlusion of the splenic artery. Occlusion of a segmental artery leads to infarction if non-communicating branches are affected. Obstruction can be caused by cardiac emboli or local thrombosis, facilitated by systemic disorders such as vasculitides, hematologic disorders (e.g., sickle cell anemia), leukemia, or lymphoma. There is a great diversity of mechanisms and etiologies for splenic infarction, but it is a rare event with a reported incidence of only 0.016% of admissions to an academic general hospital over 10 years [31]. Acute splenic infarcts usually appear on US as wedge-shaped, peripheral hypoechoic lesions pointing toward the splenic hilum. Over time they become hyperechoic, simulating a pseudolesion; the lack of vascularity at color-Doppler aids in the differential diagnosis. On non-contrast CT, the detection of infarcts is difficult, while after intravenous contrast administration, they typically appear as peripheral, wedge-shaped defects (Figure 5). In the case of global infarction, peripheral contrast enhancement due to collateral flow from capsular vessels can be seen ("rim sign") [31]. The SI on T1-WI depends on the age of the lesion.

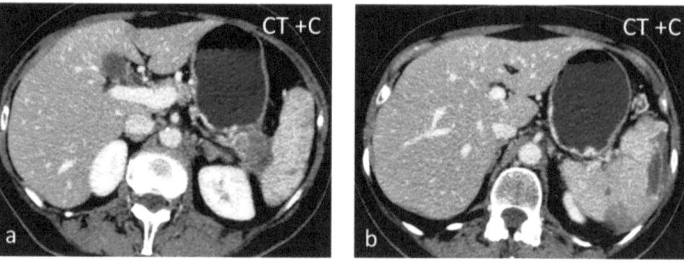

Figure 5. Splenic infarct. Axial CECT images (**a,b**) demonstrating peripheral hypoperfused area.

Hemangioma, although rare, is the most common splenic neoplasm and is found in up to 14% of patients at autopsy. It is formed by a proliferation of vascular channels, lined by a single layer of epithelium, and filled with blood. Hemangiomas are usually asymptomatic, solitary, or multiple. The natural course of hemangiomas is slow growth, and symptoms or complications, when present, occur late. Splenic hemangiomas may occur as part of generalized angiomatosis, as seen in Klippel–Trenaunay syndrome. Complications include rupture, hypersplenism, and malignant degeneration. Kasabach–Merritt syndrome, which involves the triad of anemia, thrombocytopenia, and coagulopathy, has been reported in patients with large hemangiomas [32]. Hemangiomas are round-shaped lesions with well-defined margins and a diameter <2 cm. Calcifications and cystic changes may be seen in up to 30% of cases. On US, hemangiomas have a variable appearance, being most commonly hyperechoic [32]. They appear hypoattenuating on non-contrast CT, hypo- to isointense on T1-WI, and hyperintense on T2-WI (Figure 6). Contrast enhancement can be immediate, homogeneous, and persistent or present as early peripheral enhancement with either uniform delayed enhancement or with fill-in and delayed enhancement of a central fibrous scar. Spontaneous rupture has been reported to occur in 25% of splenic hemangiomas, and treatment in such cases most often consists of splenectomy. In a study including 32 patients with splenic hemangiomas, 11 of the patients had splenic lesions characterized as such based on their typical imaging findings on CT and US alone, while all were managed successfully with observation [33].

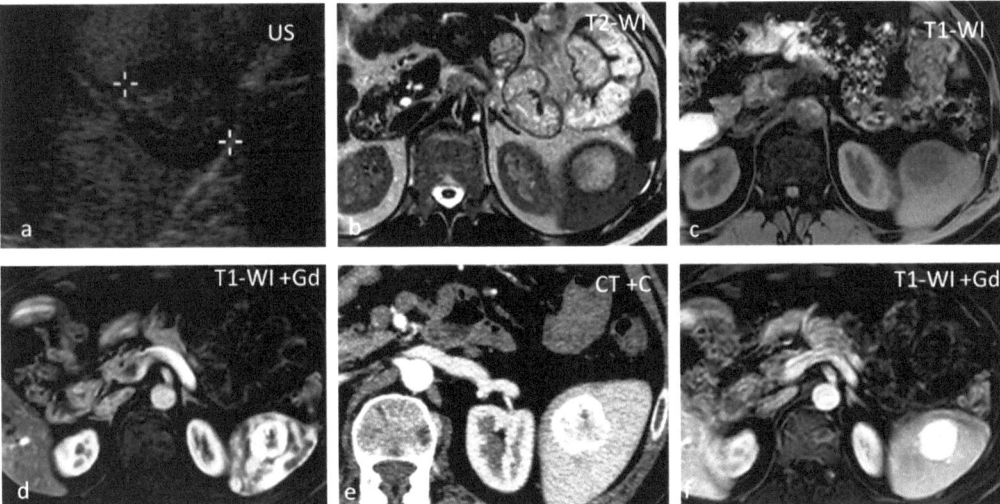

Figure 6. Hemangioma. A well-defined isoechoic splenic lesion with a hypoechoic rim on US (**a**). The lesion appears hyperintense on T2-WI with a thin hypointense rim (**b**) and hypointense on T1-WI (**c**), demonstrating strong peripheral enhancement in the early phases post intravenous contrast administration both at MRI (**d**) and CT (**e**), and homogeneous delayed enhancement (**f**).

Splenic hamartomas are very rare splenic lesions, with only around 200 cases reported since 1861 [34]. A review of the autopsy series has shown that the incidence of splenic hamartoma ranges from 0.024% to 0.13%. Hamartomas may occur at any age with equal gender predilection. Most patients have no symptoms, and the discovery of a splenic hamartoma usually is an incidental finding [32]. They present as solid, well-defined, round lesions, which may be associated with tuberous sclerosis. Females usually have larger hamartomas, which may reflect a hormonal influence. Some splenic hamartomas have rapid growth, and larger lesions may rupture [34]. On US, they appear as solid hypoechoic masses; when hemorrhage or cystic changes are present, they can be heterogeneous [35].

Color-Doppler shows rich vascularization. On CT, hamartomas are isodense or hypodense with heterogeneous enhancement. When isodense, they may be identified as focal contour deformities. Fat can be detected as areas with negative attenuation [35]. On MRI, hamartomas appear mildly hypointense to isointense on T1-WI and heterogeneously, mildly to moderately hyperintense on T2-WI, less than haemangiomas. They show diffuse, intense, heterogeneous enhancement in the early arterial phase. They become homogeneously isointense to slightly hyperintense in the delayed phase and reveal a non-enhancing central scar [36]. Although splenic hamartoma should be considered a differential diagnosis for all splenic masses, it is important to distinguish splenic hamartomas from splenic hemangiomas, the most common benign splenic lesions. In addition, despite specific imaging features of splenic hamartomas, it is difficult to rule out the possibility of a malignant neoplasm. Thus, the diagnosis must be confirmed by pathological examination [37].

Littoral cell angioma is another rare vascular tumor that often results in splenomegaly, with less than 150 cases reported in the literature. Due to increasing numbers of littoral cell angiomas described in association with autoimmune disorders (comorbidity rate, 12.2%) and tumors (comorbidity rate, 13.8%), an immune system dysfunction has been postulated as a possible crucial pathogenic mechanism [38,39]. Multiple hypoattenuating nodules of different sizes are seen on CT. When solitary, it is large with prolonged contrast enhancement. It is usually of low signal intensity on both T1 and T2-WI due to its hemosiderin content [38]. The lesion is listed in the differential diagnosis of both benign and malignant lesions; therefore, an imaging diagnosis is rarely obtained [40]. The gold standard treatment is splenectomy, followed by long-term follow-up.

Sclerosing Angiomatoid Nodular Transformation (SANT) is a rare benign vascular disorder of unknown cause, with the same prevalence as inflammatory pseudotumors and approximately 170 cases described in the scientific literature. SANT is almost exclusively described in the spleen, except for one reported in the adrenal gland [41]. Half of SANTs are asymptomatic, and half are diagnosed because of abdominal pain, pancytopenia, and splenomegaly. SANT is considered a disease of slight female preponderance. The patients usually present in the 30- to 60-year age group. Splenectomy is a useful and effective technique for the management of SANT. SANT patients have a good prognosis, with no recurrence after splenectomy [42]. SANT is formed by multiple coalescing angiomatoid nodules from the red pulp embedded within a dense fibrous stroma [42]. The nodules are constituted by irregular vascular spaces lined by thick endothelial cells; the fibrous bands coalesce to form a central stellate fibrous scar. SANT appears as a well-circumscribed, solitary round mass, typically 3–17 cm in size. It is often mistaken for a sclerosed hemangioma or an inflammatory pseudotumor and can mimic a malignancy [41]. On CT, they present as iso- to hypoattenuating masses, while they appear isointense on T1-WI but can show areas of hyperintensity or susceptibility if a hemorrhage is present. T2-WI shows a heterogeneous, predominantly hypointense mass with hyperintense septa radiating toward the center (Figure 7). Contrast enhancement may be peripheral with radiating lines (spoke-wheel pattern), rim-like, and progressive. In the delayed phase, SANTs appear homogeneous. Moderate and heterogeneous 18F-FDG avidity has also been reported [43].

Pyogenic abscesses are rare (incidence between 0.2 and 0.7% in autopsy series) and frequently unrecognized lesions that can be infective (from hematogenous spread or by direct extension), traumatic, post-infarction, or related to immunodeficiency. They can be solitary or multiple. In the majority of abscesses, streptococcus or staphylococcus is isolated. In the presence of a pyogenic splenic abscess without obvious etiology, it may be helpful to investigate bacterial endocarditis as a possible source of septic emboli [44]. On US, pyogenic abscesses appear as ill-defined hypoechoic or anechoic lesions with debris, fluid levels, and internal septations of varying thickness. Intralesional gas causing echogenic foci with 'dirty' shadowing is highly suggestive [45]. CT shows ill-defined lesions with inhomogeneous low attenuation (Figure 8). At MRI, they present with fluid lesion characteristics and show peripheral irregular rim enhancement [46].

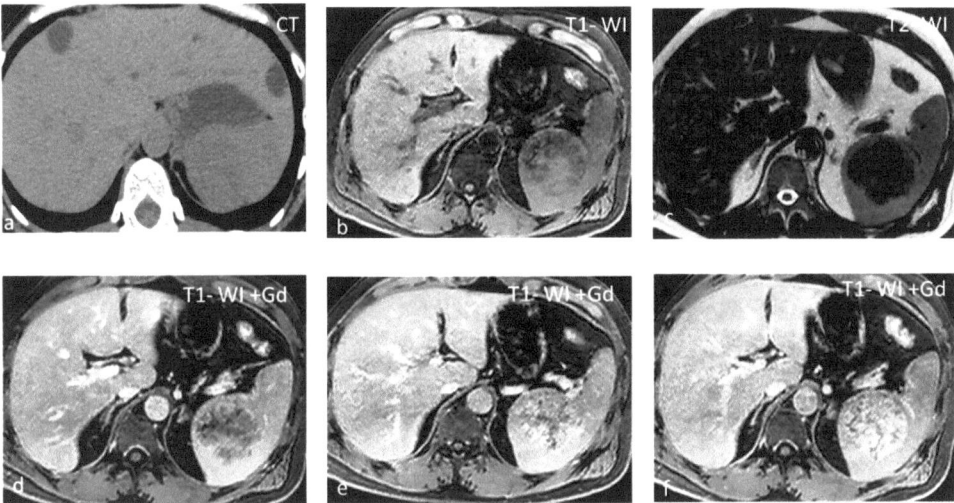

Figure 7. SANT appearing slightly hypodense on non-contrast CT (**a**) and isointense on T1-WI (**b**), with small areas of hyperintensity due to hemorrhage. On T2-WI (**c**), the lesion is heterogeneous, predominantly hypointense, with hyperintense radiating septa. After gadolinium administration, enhancement is progressive (**c**–**f**) along the radiating septa converging toward the center of the lesion.

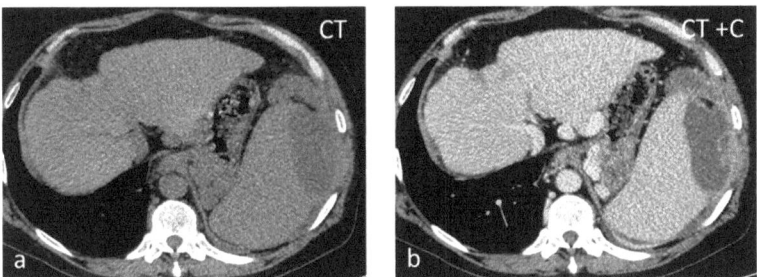

Figure 8. Thirty-seven-year-old male with HIV-HCV infection and splenic abscess from *E. coli*. The abscess appears as an ill-defined, subcapsular lesion with hypodense content on non-contrast CT (**a**) and thick irregular enhancing wall post intravenous contrast administration (**b**).

Fungal abscesses affect most commonly immunocompromised individuals. The most common infecting organisms are Candida albicans, Aspergillus fumigatus, and Cryptococcus neoformans [45]. Concurrent infection in the liver is very common in patients with splenic candidiasis [44]. The lesions are usually subcentimeter in size and multifocal. On US, fungal abscesses can demonstrate a "bulls-eye" appearance with a central hyperechoic inflammatory core surrounded by hypoechoic fibrotic tissue. CT usually shows multiple small low-attenuation lesions, occasionally with a central hyperdense focus. They have intermediate SI on T1-WI and high SI on T2-WI, with absent or subtle ring-like enhancement [45]. Associated parenchymal infarcts may also be observed in the course of the disease [44].

Splenic tuberculosis (TB) is rare, with few cases reported usually encountered in immunosuppressed individuals, although some case reports have been published on splenic TB in immunocompetent hosts [47]. Splenic TB more frequently occurs as part of a disseminated disease than in an isolated form. The most common symptoms that patients present with are fever (82.3%), fatigue and weight loss (44.12%), and splenomegaly (13.2–100%).

Different pathological forms of splenic involvement are described, including miliary tuberculosis, nodular tuberculosis, tuberculous spleen abscess, calcific tuberculosis, and mixed-type tuberculosis [47,48]. Solitary/macronodular TB enters into the differential diagnosis with primary and secondary splenic tumors and with abscesses. Its diameter ranges between 1 and 3 cm. The lesions are hyperechoic in the earlier stage and hypoechoic in the stage of caseating necrosis [26]. On CT, they appear hypodense with a rather heterogeneous enhancement pattern and central irregular necrosis. At a more advanced stage, the lesions can calcify, while associated findings include abdominal lymphadenopathy, high-attenuation ascites with nodular peritoneal thickening, and focal hepatic lesions. Splenectomy is the gold standard not only for diagnosis but also for treatment. In selected cases, a four-drug regimen of anti-tubercular treatment may be an alternative to surgery [49].

Hydatid cysts may occasionally involve the spleen, especially in endemic areas. Isolated hydatid of the spleen is rare, even in endemic regions, constituting 0.8–4% of all cases of human hydatid, while it constitutes 5.8% of all cases of abdominal hydatid. The diagnosis of cystic echinococcosis rests mainly on imaging, with immunodiagnostics playing only an ancillary role due to limitations in sensitivity and specificity [50]. The spleen represents the third most commonly involved organ in the body after the liver and lung [51]. According to a classification initially developed for liver hydatid cysts based on US and later expanded to include CT and other organs such as the spleen, five different types of hydatid cysts are differentiated: type I—univesicular cyst; type II—univesicular cyst with membrane detachment; type III—multivesicular cyst; type IV—pseudotumoral cyst; and type V—fully calcified cyst [52]. In a small series of 10 splenic hydatid cases, four were type I, and three cases each were type II and III, respectively [51]. On US, a mixed pattern of echogenicity may be produced by infolding membranes and dense debris [25]. On CT, this translates into high attenuation, while ring-like calcifications may also be seen in the periphery.

4. Conclusions

Benign focal splenic lesions, mostly detected incidentally, are not uncommon. Imaging can often only provide a differential diagnosis rather than a single definite diagnosis. Radiologists should be familiar with the characteristic imaging findings of different benign solitary splenic lesions, which, together with the clinical context, will aid them in giving the correct diagnosis and avoid overtreatment and unnecessary follow-up scans.

Funding: This research received no external funding.

Conflicts of Interest: The authors declare no conflict of interest.

References

1. Hegenscheid, K.; Seipel, R.; Schmidt, C.O.; Völzke, H.; Kühn, J.-P.; Biffar, R.; Kroemer, H.K.; Hosten, N.; Puls, R. Potentially relevant incidental findings on research whole-body MRI in the general adult population: Frequencies and management. *Eur. Radiol.* **2013**, *23*, 816–826. [CrossRef]
2. Ekeh, A.P.; Walusimbi, M.; Brigham, E.; Woods, R.J.; McCarthy, M.C. The Prevalence of Incidental Findings on Abdominal Computed Tomography Scans of Trauma Patients. *J. Emerg. Med.* **2010**, *38*, 484–489. [CrossRef] [PubMed]
3. Jang, S.; Kim, J.H.; Hur, B.Y.; Ahn, S.J.; Joo, I.; Kim, M.J.; Han, J.K. Role of CT in Differentiating Malignant Focal Splenic Lesions. *Korean J. Radiol.* **2018**, *19*, 930–937. [CrossRef]
4. Stang, A.; Keles, H.; Hentschke, S.; von Seydewitz, C.U.; Dahlke, J.; Malzfeldt, E.; Braumann, D. Differentiation of Benign from Malignant Focal Splenic Lesions Using Sulfur Hexafluoride–Filled Microbubble Contrast-Enhanced Pulse-Inversion Sonography. *Am. J. Roentgenol.* **2009**, *193*, 709–721. [CrossRef]
5. Iacobellis, F.; Schillirò, M.L.; Di Serafino, M.; Borzelli, A.; Grimaldi, D.; Verde, F.; Caruso, M.; Orabona, G.D.; Rinaldo, C.; Sabatino, V.; et al. Multimodality ultrasound assessment of the spleen: Normal appearances and emergency abnormalities. *J. Clin. Ultrasound* **2023**, *51*, 543–559. [CrossRef] [PubMed]
6. Yoshikawa, T.; Kawamitsu, H.; Mitchell, D.G.; Ohno, Y.; Ku, Y.; Seo, Y.; Fujii, M.; Sugimura, K. ADC Measurement of Abdominal Organs and Lesions Using Parallel Imaging Technique. *Am. J. Roentgenol.* **2006**, *187*, 1521–1530. [CrossRef]
7. Jang, K.M.; Kim, S.H.; Hwang, J.; Lee, S.J.; Kang, T.W.; Lee, M.W.; Choi, D. Differentiation of Malignant from Benign Focal Splenic Lesions: Added Value of Diffusion-Weighted MRI. *Am. J. Roentgenol.* **2014**, *203*, 803–812. [CrossRef]

8. Choi, S.Y.; Kim, S.H.; Jang, K.M.; Kang, T.; Song, K.D.; Moon, J.Y.; Choi, Y.H.; Lee, B.R. The value of con-trast-enhanced dynamic and diffusion-weighted MR imaging for distinguishing benign and malignant splenic masses. *Br. J. Radiol.* **2016**, *89*, 20160054. [CrossRef] [PubMed]
9. Cheng, G.; Alavi, A.; Lim, E.; Werner, T.J.; Del Bello, C.V.; Akers, S.R. Dynamic Changes of FDG Uptake and Clearance in Normal Tissues. *Mol. Imaging Biol.* **2013**, *15*, 345–352. [CrossRef]
10. Sugawara, Y.; Zasadny, K.R.; Kison, P.V.; Baker, L.H.; Wahl, R.L. Splenic fluorodeoxyglucose uptake increased by granulocyte colony-stimulating factor therapy: PET imaging results. *J. Nucl. Med.* **1999**, *40*, 1456–1462. [PubMed]
11. Liu, Y. Clinical significance of diffusely increased splenic uptake on FDG-PET. *Nucl. Med. Commun.* **2009**, *30*, 763–769. [CrossRef] [PubMed]
12. Metser, U.; Even-Sapir, E. The Role of 18F-FDG PET/CT in the Evaluation of Solid Splenic Masses. *Semin. Ultrasound CT MRI* **2006**, *27*, 420–425. [CrossRef]
13. Bui, P.L.; Vicens, R.A.; Westin, J.R.; Jensen, C.T. Multimodality imaging of Epstein–Barr virus-associated inflammatory pseudotumor-like follicular dendritic cell tumor of the spleen: Case report and literature review. *Clin. Imaging* **2015**, *39*, 525–528. [CrossRef]
14. IARC. WHO Classification of Soft tissue and bone tumours. In *WHO Classification of Tumours Soft Tissue and Bone Toumors*; International Agency for Research on Cancer: Lyon, France, 2020.
15. Coffin, C.M.; A Humphrey, P.; Dehner, L.P. Extrapulmonary inflammatory myofibroblastic tumor: A clinical and pathological survey. *Semin. Diagn. Pathol.* **1998**, *15*, 85–101.
16. Shapiro, A.J.; Adams, E.D. Inflammatory Pseudotumor of the Spleen Managed Laparoscopically. Can Preoperative Imaging Establish the Diagnosis? *Surg. Laparosc. Endosc. Percutaneous Tech.* **2006**, *16*, 357–361. [CrossRef]
17. Kalaivani, V.; Vijayakumar, H.M.; Girish, K.S.; Hegde, N. Inflammatory Pseudotumour of the Spleen: A Diagnostic Dilemma. *J. Clin. Diagn. Res.* **2013**, *7*, 1460–1462. [CrossRef]
18. Warshauer, D.M. Splenic Sarcoidosis. *Semin. Ultrasound CT MRI* **2007**, *28*, 21–27. [CrossRef]
19. Jhaveri, K.; Vakil, A.; Surani, S.R. Sarcoidosis and Its Splenic Wonder: A Rare Case of Isolated Splenic Sarcoidosis. *Case Rep. Med.* **2018**, *2018*, 4628439. [CrossRef] [PubMed]
20. Tetikkurt, C.; Yanardag, H.; Pehlivan, M.; Bilir, M. Clinical features and prognostic significance of splenic involvement in sarcoidosis. *Monaldi Arch. Chest Dis.* **2017**, *87*, 893. [CrossRef] [PubMed]
21. Thipphavong, S.; Duigenan, S.; Schindera, S.T.; Gee, M.S.; Philips, S. Nonneoplastic, Benign, and Malignant Splenic Diseases: Cross-Sectional Imaging Findings and Rare Disease Entities. *Am. J. Roentgenol.* **2014**, *203*, 315–322. [CrossRef] [PubMed]
22. Palmucci, S.; Torrisi, S.E.; Caltabiano, D.C.; Puglisi, S.; Lentini, V.; Grassedonio, E.; Vindigni, V.; Reggio, E.; Giuliano, R.; Micali, G.; et al. Clinical and radiological features of extra-pulmonary sarcoidosis: A pictorial essay. *Insights Into Imaging* **2016**, *7*, 571–587. [CrossRef]
23. Sève, P.; Pacheco, Y.; Durupt, F.; Jamilloux, Y.; Gerfaud-Valentin, M.; Isaac, S.; Boussel, L.; Calender, A.; Androdias, G.; Valeyre, D.; et al. Sarcoidosis: A Clinical Overview from Symptoms to Diagnosis. *Cells* **2021**, *10*, 766. [CrossRef]
24. Ioannidis, I.; Kahn, A.G. Splenic Lymphangioma. *Arch. Pathol. Lab. Med.* **2015**, *139*, 278–282. [CrossRef]
25. Urrutia, M.; Mergo, P.J.; Ros, L.H.; Torres, G.M.; Ros, P.R. Cystic masses of the spleen: Radiologic-pathologic correlation. *RadioGraphics* **1996**, *16*, 107–129. [CrossRef] [PubMed]
26. Lee, H.-J.; Kim, J.W.; Hong, J.H.; Kim, G.S.; Shin, S.S.; Heo, S.H.; Lim, H.S.; Hur, Y.H.; Seon, H.J.; Jeong, Y.Y. Cross-sectional Imaging of Splenic Lesions: RadioGraphics fundamentals/online presentation. *RadioGraphics* **2018**, *38*, 435–436. [CrossRef] [PubMed]
27. Dachman, A.; Ros, P.R.; Murari, P.; Olmsted, W.; Lichtenstein, J.; Dachman, P.R.A.; Franquet, T.; Montes, M.; Lecumberri, F.J.; Esparza, J.; et al. Nonparasitic splenic cysts: A report of 52 cases with radiologic-pathologic correlation. *Am. J. Roentgenol.* **1986**, *147*, 537–542. [CrossRef] [PubMed]
28. Robbins, F.G.; Yellin, A.E.; Lingua, R.W.; Craig, J.R.; Turrill, F.L.; Mikkelsen, W.P. Splenic Epidermoid Cysts. *Ann. Surg.* **1978**, *187*, 231–235. [CrossRef]
29. Ingle, S.B.; Ingle, C.R.H.I.; Patrike, S. Epithelial cysts of the spleen: A minireview. *World J. Gastroenterol.* **2014**, *20*, 13899–13903. [CrossRef] [PubMed]
30. Macheras, A.; Misiako, E.P.; Liakakos, T.; Mpistarakis, D.; Fotiadis, C.; Karatza's, G. Non-parasitic splenic cysts: A report of three cases. *World J. Gastroenterol.* **2005**, *11*, 6884–6887. [CrossRef] [PubMed]
31. Schattner, A.; Meital, A.; Ella, K.; Abraham, K. Acute splenic infarction at an academic general hospital over 10 years: Presentation, etiology, and outcome. *Medicine* **2015**, *94*, e1363. [CrossRef] [PubMed]
32. Abbott, R.M.; Levy, A.D.; Aguilera, N.S.; Gorospe, L.; Thompson, W.M. From the Archives of the AFIP: Primary vascular neoplasms of the spleen: Radiologic-pathologic correlation. *RadioGraphics* **2004**, *24*, 1137–1163. [CrossRef] [PubMed]
33. Willcox, T.M.; Speer, R.W.; Schlinkert, R.T.; Sarr, M.G. Hemangioma of the spleen: Presentation, diagnosis, and management. *J. Gastrointest. Surg.* **2000**, *4*, 611–613. [CrossRef]
34. Obeidat, K.A.; Afaneh, M.W.; Al-Domaidat, H.M.; Al-Qazakzeh, H.I.; AlQaisi, F.J. Splenic Hamartoma: A Case Report and Literature Review. *Am. J. Case Rep.* **2022**, *23*, e937195-1. [CrossRef] [PubMed]
35. Karlo, C.A.; Stolzmann, P.; Do, R.K.; Alkadhi, H. Computed tomography of the spleen: How to interpret the hypodense lesion. *Insights Into Imaging* **2013**, *4*, 65–76. [CrossRef]

36. Wang, J.-H.; Ma, X.-L.; Ren, F.-Y.; Zuo, C.-J.; Tian, J.-M.; Wang, Z.-F.; Zheng, J.-M. Multi-modality imaging findings of splenic hamartoma: A report of nine cases and review of the literature. *Abdom. Imaging* **2013**, *38*, 154–162. [CrossRef] [PubMed]
37. Namikawa, T.; Kitagawa, H.; Iwabu, J.; Kobayashi, M.; Matsumoto, M.; Hanazaki, K. Laparoscopic splenectomy for splenic hamartoma: Case management and clinical consequences. *World J. Gastrointest. Surg.* **2010**, *2*, 147–152. [CrossRef] [PubMed]
38. Vancauwenberghe, T.; Snoeckx, A.; Vanbeckevoort, D.; Dymarkowski, S.; Vanhoenacker, F. Imaging of the spleen: What the clinician needs to know. *Singap. Med. J.* **2015**, *56*, 133–144. [CrossRef] [PubMed]
39. Wang, W.; Qi, G.; Zhao, X.; Zhang, Y.; Zhu, R.; Liang, R.; Sun, Y. Clinical Landscape of Littoral Cell Angioma in the Spleen Based on a Comprehensive Analysis. *Front. Oncol.* **2022**, *12*, 175. [CrossRef]
40. Arcuri, P.P.; Taglianetti, S.; Vavalà, B.; Battaglia, C.; Laganà, D.; Manti, F. Incidental littoral cell angioma of the spleen: Cross-sectional imaging findings and review of the literature. *Radiol. Case Rep.* **2022**, *17*, 3545–3550. [CrossRef]
41. Eede, S.V.D.; Van de Voorde, N.; Vanhoenacker, F.; de Beeck, B.O. Sclerosing Angiomatoid Nodular Transformation of the Spleen: A Diagnostic Conundrum. *J. Belg. Soc. Radiol.* **2022**, *106*, 12. [CrossRef] [PubMed]
42. Pradhan, D.; Mohanty, S.K. Sclerosing Angiomatoid Nodular Transformation of the Spleen. *Arch. Pathol. Lab. Med.* **2013**, *137*, 1309–1312. [CrossRef]
43. Chen, N.-X.; Wang, M.-L.; Wang, H.-X.; Zeng, M.-S. Sclerosing angiomatoid nodular transformation of the spleen: Multimodality imaging features and literature review. *BMC Med. Imaging* **2023**, *23*, 50. [CrossRef] [PubMed]
44. Karaosmanoglu, A.D.; Uysal, A.; Onder, O.; Hahn, P.F.; Akata, D.; Ozmen, M.N.; Karcaaltıncaba, M. Cross-sectional imaging findings of splenic infections: Is differential diagnosis possible? *Abdom. Imaging* **2021**, *46*, 4828–4852. [CrossRef] [PubMed]
45. Gaetke-Udager, K.; Wasnik, A.P.; Kaza, R.K.; Al-Hawary, M.M.; Maturen, K.E.; Udager, A.M.; Azar, S.F.; Francis, I.R. Multimodality imaging of splenic lesions and the role of non-vascular, image-guided intervention. *Abdom. Imaging* **2014**, *39*, 570–587. [CrossRef]
46. Elsayes, K.M.; Narra, V.R.; Mukundan, G.; Lewis, J.S.; Menias, C.O.; Heiken, J.P. MR Imaging of the Spleen: Spectrum of Abnormalities. *RadioGraphics* **2005**, *25*, 967–982. [CrossRef]
47. Gupta, A. Splenic tuberculosis: A comprehensive review of literature. *Pol. J. Surg.* **2018**, *90*, 49–51. [CrossRef]
48. Lin, S.-F.; Zheng, L.; Zhou, L. Solitary splenic tuberculosis: A case report and review of the literature. *World J. Surg. Oncol.* **2016**, *14*, 154. [CrossRef]
49. Tojo, Y.; Yanagisawa, S.; Miyauchi, E.; Ichinose, M. Splenic tuberculosis. *Int. J. Infect. Dis.* **2018**, *67*, 41–42. [CrossRef]
50. Higuita, N.I.A.; Brunetti, E.; McCloskey, C. Cystic Echinococcosis. *J. Clin. Microbiol.* **2016**, *54*, 518–523. [CrossRef] [PubMed]
51. Al-Hakkak, S.M.M.; Muhammad, A.S.; Mijbas, S.A.-R. Splenic-preserving surgery in hydatid spleen: A single institutional experience. *J. Med. Life* **2022**, *15*, 15–19. [CrossRef] [PubMed]
52. Gharbi, H.A.; Hassine, W.; Brauner, M.W.; Dupuch, K. Ultrasound examination of the hydatic liver. *Radiology* **1981**, *139*, 459–463. [CrossRef] [PubMed]

Disclaimer/Publisher's Note: The statements, opinions and data contained in all publications are solely those of the individual author(s) and contributor(s) and not of MDPI and/or the editor(s). MDPI and/or the editor(s) disclaim responsibility for any injury to people or property resulting from any ideas, methods, instructions or products referred to in the content.

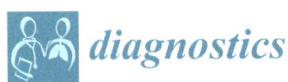

Review

Unravelling Peritoneal Carcinomatosis Using Cross-Sectional Imaging Modalities

Ana Veron Sanchez [1,*], Ilias Bennouna [1], Nicolas Coquelet [1], Jorge Cabo Bolado [2], Inmaculada Pinilla Fernandez [3], Luis A. Mullor Delgado [4], Martina Pezzullo [5], Gabriel Liberale [1], Maria Gomez Galdon [1] and Maria A. Bali [1]

1. Hospital Universitaire de Bruxelles, Institut Jules Bordet, 1070 Brussels, Belgium
2. Teleconsult, Milton Keynes MK12 5NE, UK
3. Hospital Universitario La Paz, 28046 Madrid, Spain
4. Hospital Universitario Gregorio Marañon, 28009 Madrid, Spain
5. Hôpital Universitaire de Bruxelles, Hôpital Erasme, 1070 Brussels, Belgium
* Correspondence: ana.veron@hubruxelles.be

Abstract: Peritoneal carcinomatosis (PC) refers to malignant epithelial cells that spread to the peritoneum, principally from abdominal malignancies. Until recently, PC prognosis has been considered ill-fated, with palliative therapies serving as the only treatment option. New locoregional treatments are changing the outcome of PC, and imaging modalities have a critical role in early diagnosis and disease staging, determining treatment decision making strategies. The aim of this review is to provide a practical approach for detecting and characterizing peritoneal deposits in cross-sectional imaging modalities, taking into account their appearances, including the secondary complications, the anatomical characteristics of the peritoneal cavity, together with the differential diagnosis with other benign and malignant peritoneal conditions. Among the cross-sectional imaging modalities, computed tomography (CT) is widely available and fast; however, magnetic resonance (MR) performs better in terms of sensitivity (92% vs. 68%), due to its higher contrast resolution. The appearance of peritoneal deposits on CT and MR mainly depends on the primary tumour histology; in case of unknown primary tumour (3–5% of cases), their behaviour at imaging may provide insights into the tumour origin. The timepoint of tumour evolution, previous or ongoing treatments, and the peritoneal spaces in which they occur also play an important role in determining the appearance of peritoneal deposits. Thus, knowledge of peritoneal anatomy and fluid circulation is essential in the detection and characterisation of peritoneal deposits. Several benign and malignant conditions show similar imaging features that overlap those of PC, making differential diagnosis challenging. Knowledge of peritoneal anatomy and primary tumour histology is crucial, but one must also consider clinical history, laboratory findings, and previous imaging examinations to achieve a correct diagnosis. In conclusion, to correctly diagnose PC in cross-sectional imaging modalities, knowledge of peritoneal anatomy and peritoneal fluid flow characteristics are mandatory. Peritoneal deposit features reflect the primary tumour characteristics, and this specificity may be helpful in its identification when it is unknown. Moreover, several benign and malignant peritoneal conditions may mimic PC, which need to be considered even in oncologic patients.

Keywords: peritoneum; carcinomatosis; deposits

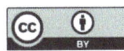

1. Introduction

The peritoneum is the second most common metastatic location for abdominal tumours, only surpassed by the liver.

Only 10% of the cases of peritoneal carcinomatosis (PC) are related to extra abdominal tumours [1], with breast (41%) and lung cancers (21%) and malignant melanoma (9%) being the most frequent causes [2].

Traditionally, PC implied an ill-fated prognosis and only palliative treatments were applied. However, the introduction of new surgical techniques and regional therapies have changed this scenario, and palliative systemic treatment is no longer the only therapeutic option. A combination of systemic chemotherapy, cytoreductive surgery (CRS), and hyperthermic intraperitoneal chemotherapy (HIPEC) achieves promising results in selected PC cases from colorectal, ovarian, and gastric cancers [3–5]. The main purpose of CRS is to remove all visible deposits with curative intent, which may require peritonectomy and visceral resections. Intraperitoneal chemotherapy, its effect enhanced by hyperthermia, is then administered to intensify the dose of chemotherapy delivered to the tumour while controlling systemic toxicity.

Thus, despite its difficulty, the early diagnosis of PC based on imaging findings is essential for disease staging, for the subsequent management of primary tumours and for patient prognosis. Given the aggressiveness of cytoreductive surgery, it is mandatory to adequately select patients in whom the potential benefits will prevail as surgical candidates, distinguishing them from those who should be treated with systemic chemotherapy, either neoadjuvant or palliative. The peritoneal carcinomatosis index (PCI) serves to quantify the extent of the peritoneal involvement and serves as a predictor of incomplete CRS [6].

The aim of this review is to provide a practical approach when encountering a peritoneal carcinomatosis case using cross-sectional imaging, and to establish where to look for deposits, the possible appearances they may show, and the main complications. In the event of no prior known primary tumour, this review also aims to depict the deposits characteristics that may be helpful in suggesting the origin and to describe differential diagnosis.

2. Diagnostic Modalities

The gold standard for the assessment of PC is explorative laparoscopy, which is a minimally invasive procedure that allows for direct visualization and biopsy. However, as an initial approach, cross-sectional imaging modalities are preferred, and the most common and widespread imaging technique used is intravenous contrast-enhanced (CE) computed tomography (CT) thanks to its availability, fast acquisition time, and the possibility of multiplanar reconstructions [7,8]. The administration of water density oral contrast may improve the detection of peritoneal deposits, especially those adjacent to the bowel [9]. CE-CT has demonstrated 68% sensitivity and 88% specificity for peritoneal deposits, although their size and location can undermine this performance [10,11]. When the deposit size is less than 10 mm, the sensitivity dramatically descends to 7–28% [6]. Location, especially in the absence of ascites, has an important impact on sensitivity: metastases within the lesser omentum, left subphrenic space, the root of the mesentery, and small bowel serosa are often missed.

Magnetic resonance (MR), including diffusion-weighted imaging (DWI) and contrast-enhanced T1-weighted sequences, is a promising diagnostic modality, as it provides a higher sensitivity (91%) and similar specificity (85%) to CE-CT [9] due to its high contrast resolution, which allows for tumours to be distinguished from surrounding non-tumour tissues.

Several studies have proven that adding DWI to conventional MR increases the detection of peritoneal deposits [10,12,13], even of small size [14]. Tumoral deposits, due to their high cellular content, restrict the diffusion of water and are displayed as high signal intensity lesions [15], which increases their conspicuity. The diffusion properties of tissues can be quantified by calculating the apparent diffusion coefficient (ADC) maps, where low ADC values correspond to restricted diffusion. ADC values of peritoneal metastasis from ovarian tumours have been measured and found to be comparable to ADC values of the primary tumour [16]. Some studies suggest there is a relation between the ADC values of peritoneal deposits and treatment response [17]. If chemotherapy were successful, deposits would show an increase in their ADC value, even before they would decrease in size.

MR may be preferable to CT in the detection of lesions of less than 10 mm, especially within the subphrenic spaces and bowel serosa. Moreover, in the presence of moderate to substantial ascites, MR still performs better than CT [10]; however, on the other hand, the presence of ascites may lead to dielectric artifacts and false positives [18]. The artifacts caused by respiratory and cardiac motion may impair the detection of deposits within subphrenic and perihepatic spaces. Mucinous and deposits with cystic and necrotic changes may increase the ADC value and cause a false negative result [8]. One final limitation is the insufficient experience with MR interpretation among radiologists [19].

A third non-invasive imaging modality available to assess peritoneal carcinomatosis is positron emission tomography fused with CT images (PET-CT), which provides metabolic information of the lesions, based on the measurement of the increased uptake of a radiotracer, mostly a glucose analogue (FDG [18F]-2-deoxy-2-fluoro-D-glucose). It improves the diagnostic performance of CT but shows slightly lower sensitivity (87%) than MR, probably due to its lower spatial resolution, with limited depiction of small nodules. On the other hand, its specificity is slightly higher (92%) [18]. Moreover, FDG-PET-CT provides a whole-body assessment, which is a major advantage in detecting extra-abdominal metastases. However, in addition to the high costs, PET-CT is less available, and it may provide false-negative findings, such as for mucinous tumours [7], and false-positive findings, such as for postoperative abnormalities or infectious or inflammatory conditions. False-negative interpretations may be also due to deposits being obscured by normal bladder or bowel activity.

Radiologists need to be aware of clinical and laboratory findings.

The clinical presentation of PC is variable, nonspecific, and depends on its extension. Patients may present with characteristic symptoms of the primary tumour and nonspecific symptoms. Abdominal pain and ascites occur in 85% of patients [19]. Complications due to PC, such as ureterohydronephrosis, bowel obstruction, and ischemia, could present as acute abdominal pain.

Serum tumour markers are measurable indicators associated with malignancy, produced either by the tumour or by the body in response to the tumour. They do not serve as a main tool for cancer diagnosis but are useful in supporting diagnosis and treatment response [20]. For instance, high carcinoembryonic antigen (CEA) serum levels are found in 60–90% of colorectal carcinoma, 50–80% of pancreatic carcinoma, and 25–50% of gastric and breast carcinoma, and CA-125 is associated with ovarian cancer [21]. Rising levels of tumour markers should raise concerns, as recurrence may form a miliary pattern that is difficult to spot using imaging [22]. Thus, a combination of imaging findings and tumour markers serum levels is used to determine the response to chemotherapy and to detect recurrence if the levels are elevated upon tumour presentation. However, it should be noted that non-malignant entities may show high tumour marker levels and that patients with extensive peritoneal malignant disease recurrence may have normal tumour markers.

How to proceed? CT is a very useful first-line modality [23]. However, in potential candidates for CRS and HIPEC, where imaging assessment regarding patient selection is critical, CT has been found to underestimate the volume of peritoneal disease [24], while MRI-PCI has shown a stronger correlation with surgical PCI [9]. After peritoneal surgery, it is essential to obtain a baseline MR to determine postsurgical appearance in order to avoid overcalling postsurgical changes for recurrence. Postoperative changes will resolve upon following studies and relapse-related findings will progress [25]. Surveillance should also be performed when using MR.

PET-CT should be considered when encountering equivocal imaging findings, when tumour marker levels rise with no identifiable cause upon imaging, and to detect nodal or extra-abdominal metastases.

In our clinical practice, CT images are acquired on the axial plane at the portal venous after intravenous administration of iodine contrast medium, with a flow rate of 3 mL/s. Multiplane reconstruction can be obtained on coronal and sagittal planes. No oral contrast is required. When using a dual-source scanner, virtual, unenhanced images can be generated.

MR images can be obtained using 1.5 T or 3.0 T field-strength MR scanners with a surface-phased array coil covering the abdomen and the pelvis. The acquisition protocol includes coronal and axial T2-weighted images and diffusion-weighted imaging (respiratory-triggered for the upper abdomen and on breath hold for the inferior abdomen) with 3 b values of 0, 150, and 800 s/mm^2. Following intravenous injection of 0.2 mmol/kg of gadolinium-based contrast agents, fat-suppressed 3D T1-weighted sequences are obtained upon breath hold at the arterial and portal phases covering the upper abdomen and after a 3 min late phase of the whole abdomen.

3. Many Places and Many Faces

The term peritoneal carcinomatosis refers to the spread of malignant epithelial cells as tumour deposits to the peritoneum [26].

PC represents a very complex condition at imaging, more than any other metastatic site.

The appearance of the peritoneal deposits is determined not only by the histological characteristics of the primary tumour, the timepoint of the tumour's evolution, and the treatment [27] but also, and more interestingly, by the peritoneal space in which they occur. Complications secondary to deposits also vary according to the location, depending on the organs involved.

Some anatomic knowledge is required in the quest for deposits. The aim of this review is not to offer a comprehensive description of peritoneal anatomy but to establish sufficient certainty that all locations are thoroughly investigated.

The peritoneal cavity is the virtual space that exists between the parietal and visceral peritoneum [28] and, under normal conditions, contains a small amount of plasma-like fluid.

The parietal peritoneum delineates the periphery of the peritoneal cavity:

- Cranially, it covers the diaphragm (except for the bare area of the liver, the insertion of the ligaments, and along its posterior margin, where it is in contact with retroperitoneal fat) (Figure 1).
- Caudally, it descends into the pelvis. Its complex anatomy in this location is shown in more detail later.
- Anterolaterally, it is separated from the abdominal wall by the fat from the preperitoneal space, that is, the space between the peritoneum and the transversalis fascia (Figure 2).
- Posteriorly, it is distanced from the posterior abdominal wall by the retroperitoneal space. It forms the anterior boundary of the retroperitoneal space (Figure 3).

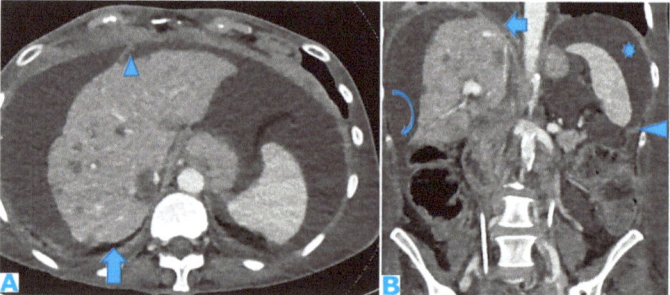

Figure 1. Axial CE-CT (**A**) and coronal MPR (**B**). Massive ascites, helpful to differentiate the peritoneal spaces. (**A**) shows how the posterior margin of the diaphragm (arrow) is not covered by the parietal peritoneum, as it is directly in contact with the retroperitoneal fat. The attachment sites of ligaments on the diaphragmatic surface are not covered by peritoneum; the falciform identified in (**A**) and the phrenicocolic ligaments (arrowhead) in (**B**). Notice in (**B**) how the phrenicocolic ligament partially separates the left parietocolic gutter from the left subphrenic space (*), whereas the right parietocolic gutter fully communicates with the right subphrenic space (curved arrow). The bare area of the liver in (**B**) (arrow) is an area directly attached to the diaphragm by connective tissue and thus not covered by peritoneum, and its diaphragmatic attachment site is not covered either.

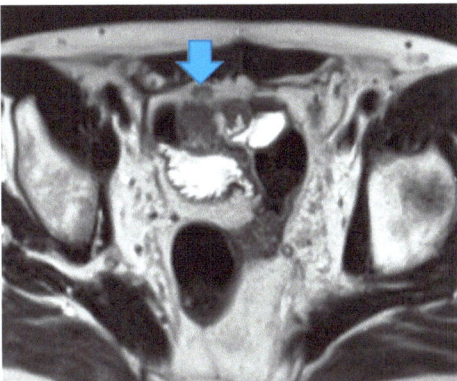

Figure 2. Axial T2WI. PC from neuroendocrine tumour: deposit within the anterior parietal peritoneum (arrow).

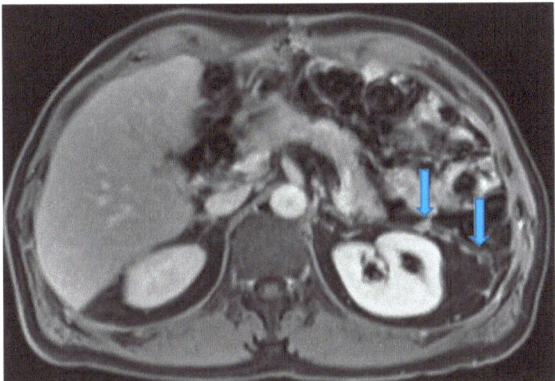

Figure 3. Axial T2WI. PC from neuroendocrine tumour: deposits within the posterior parietal peritoneum (arrows) (which is immediately anterior to the anterior pararenal fascia).

The peritoneum invaginates to fully cover most of the abdominal viscera, anteriorly and posteriorly, becoming the visceral peritoneum. It is organised into a folded disposition as ligaments, folds, and mesenteries to nurture, innervate, and support the intraperitoneal organs, connecting them to the posterior parietal peritoneum.

As a common rule, the abnormal thickening and pathological enhancement of surfaces covered by the peritoneum may be the only initial imaging finding in PC.

It may be difficult, in the absence of ascites, to differentiate parietal peritoneal deposits from their visceral counterparts at locations where the two leaves are adjacent (e.g., a deposit within the parietal peritoneum covering the lateral abdominal wall or within the visceral peritoneum covering the liver). For the sake of simplicity, some examples of parietal peritoneal deposits are shown; the rest are included within their peritoneal space (Figure 4).

If the deposit lies within a fat-containing peritoneal space, the spectrum of presentation ranges from nodular focal fat stranding to irregular haziness, evolving towards solid lesions. These solid lesions may initially be millimetric, appearing as either solitary or multiple soft-tissue nodules that eventually grow and merge to form plaques or sheets, and then masses. Most commonly, PC appears as a combination of all these findings.

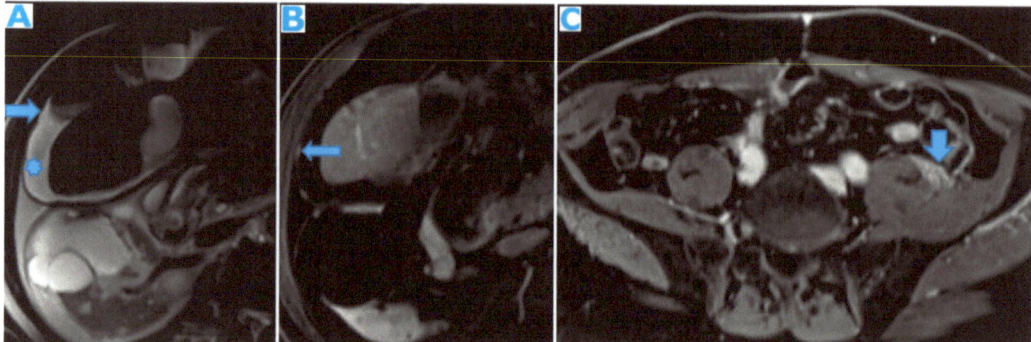

Figure 4. Axial T2WI (**A**) and axial CE portal phase FST1WI (**B**), same patient. PC from colon adenocarcinoma: notice the nodular thickening of the parietal peritoneum due to deposits (arrow). Notice how easy it is to distinguish the parietal peritoneum from the visceral perihepatic peritoneum thanks to the ascites (*). Axial CE portal phase FST1WI (**C**). PC from neuroendocrine tumour: deposits within the posterior parietal peritoneum (arrow). The retroperitoneal space is very thin at this location and the posterior parietal peritoneum is adjacent to the abdominal wall.

Peritoneal spaces are classified as supra- or inframesocolic [29,30]. The anatomic landmark that enables this division is the mesentery of the transverse colon (transverse colon mesocolon). Unfortunately, this is also an easy route for carcinomatosis spread, as it communicates on both sides with other ligaments and centrally with the small bowel mesentery.

Deposits within the transverse mesocolon appear either on its mesentery (Figure 5) or/and on the serosa (visceral peritoneum) covering the transverse colon [30]. Differentiation between them may not always be feasible. Deposits may cause different degrees of luminal stenosis with or without signs of bowel obstruction.

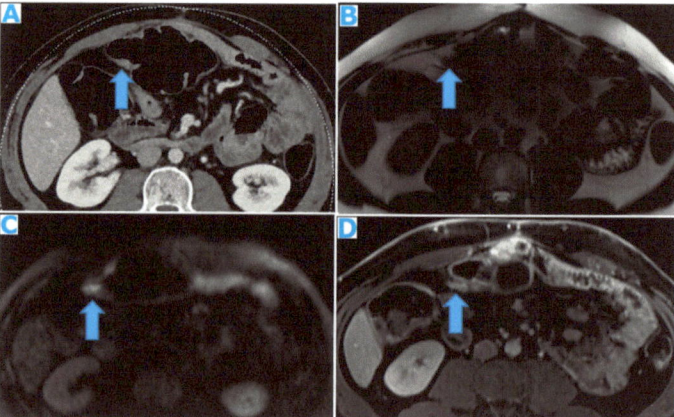

Figure 5. Axial CE-CT (**A**), axial T2WI (**B**), DWI (**C**), axial CE portal phase FST1WI (**D**). PC from gastric adenocarcinoma: subtle deposit within the transverse mesocolon (arrow) using CT; more conspicuous using MR.

Imaging features of serosal bowel deposits include nodular lesions, segmental parietal thickening, and diffuse infiltration. Their detection may be an arduous task, more so if bowel is not sufficiently distended. In addition, it is important to note that layered implants blend in with the bowel contour, whereas nodular deposits alter it and are thus easier to detect (Figure 6).

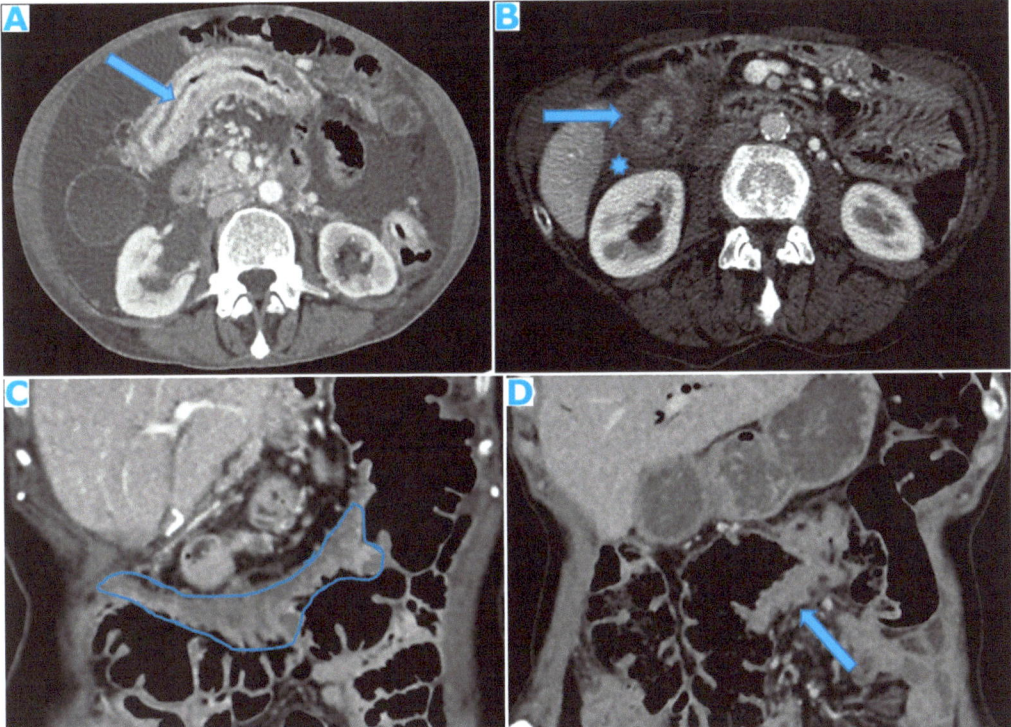

Figure 6. Axial CE-CT (**A**). PC from breast carcinoma: deposits within the transverse colon serosa (arrows), causing luminal stenosis. Axial CE-CT (**B**). PC from breast carcinoma: layered deposits within the transverse colon serosa (arrow); notice the concentric pattern and the luminal stenosis. Ascites (*). Coronal CE-CT MPR (**C,D**). (**C**): PC from signet ring cell gastric carcinoma. Diffuse serosal infiltration of the transverse colon. (**D**): PC from breast carcinoma: segmental parietal thickening of the transverse colon due to nodular deposits within the serosa (arrow). Observe how layered deposits in (**C**) blend in with the bowel contour and may be more difficult to detect than nodular deposits in (**D**).

This description of serosal bowel deposits has the same validity for the rest of the gastrointestinal tract.

Next, we use a cranial-to-caudal and lateral-to-medial approach to review the peritoneal spaces.

3.1. Supramesocolic Spaces

Supramesocolic cavity comprehends the subphrenic, perihepatic, and perisplenic spaces; periportal space, lesser omentum, lesser sac, and right subhepatic space. These locations need to be carefully assessed using multiplanar reconstructions, as deposits within them may require complex surgery or, in some cases, may be considered unresectable.

3.1.1. Subphrenic Spaces

Imaging features include the thickening and pathological enhancement of the diaphragm, nodules, and masses (Figures 7 and 8).

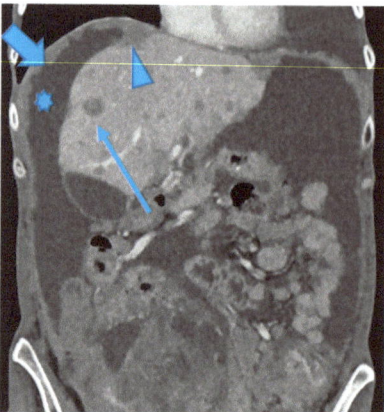

Figure 7. CE-CT coronal MPR. PC from ovarian carcinoma: multiple bilateral diaphragmatic nodular deposits (arrows). Notice how useful ascites (*) is when distinguishing peritoneal deposits within the parietal peritoneum from deposits within the visceral (hepatic) peritoneum (arrowhead). Hepatic metastases (thin arrow).

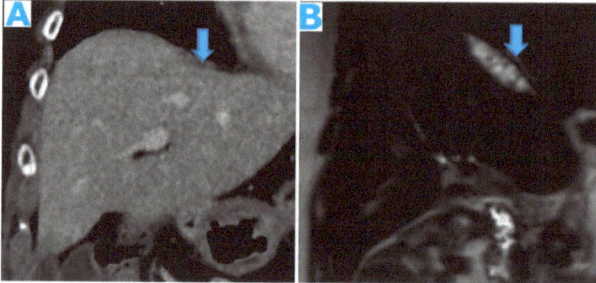

Figure 8. Coronal T2WI ((**A**), from five years prior) and CE-CT coronal MPR ((**B**), current follow-up). PC from ovarian granulosa cell tumour: Notice, in (**B**), a deposit within the right subphrenic space, bulging into the hepatic capsule (arrow). See how subtle it originally was in (**A**) (arrow); it could easily be overlooked upon axial imaging.

3.1.2. Perihepatic and Perisplenic Spaces

Deposits can be identified as a continuum from abnormal peritoneal enhancement to subtle nodularity and well-defined nodules, often showing a biconvex morphology.

Perihepatic deposits may occur on the superficial visceral peritoneum that surrounds most of the liver surface (except for the liver bare area, the porta hepatis, and the attachment site of the gallbladder to the liver) and/or underneath the Glisson capsule, within the subcapsular space. Glisson's capsule is a thick fibrous membrane that lies deep in the visceral peritoneum. It is assumed that deposits infiltrate the liver capsule upon deposition on the visceral peritoneum. The liver capsule covers the entire hepatic surface, including the periportal space, and is in communication with the lesser omentum, thus becoming another route for deposits to reach the subcapsular space. Both the periportal space and the lesser omentum are reviewed next.

In the event of subcapsular deposits, secondary parenchymal invasion may occur, resulting in a characteristic scalloping of the underlying parenchyma (Figure 9). Despite this sign, it may be difficult to distinguish between solely subcapsular deposits and those with parenchymal invasion. A sign that has been found to be highly sensitive to rule out secondary hepatic invasion is the presence of a well-defined interface between the lesion and the liver and/or a clear plane, either fatty or from ascites [31] (Figure 10).

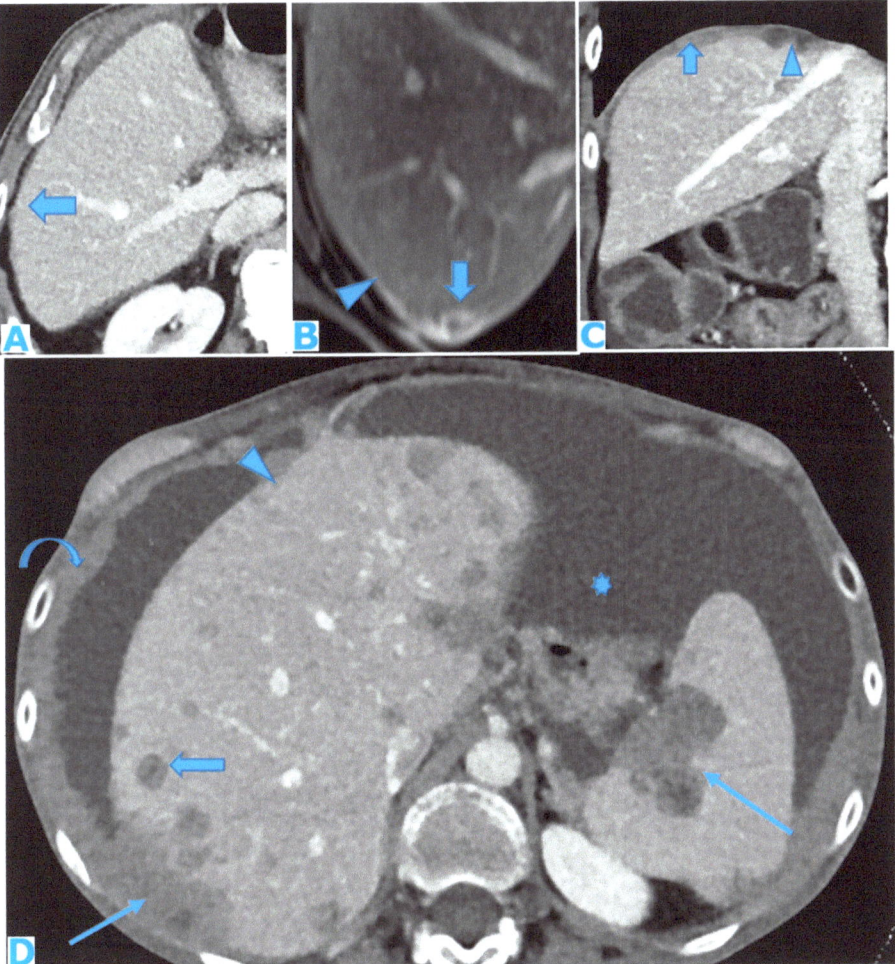

Figure 9. Axial CE-CT (**A**): PC from colon carcinoma: note the subtle irregularities in the liver contour caused by the deposit seeding within the peritoneum covering the hepatic surface. CE portal phase FST1WI (**B**): PC from cervical carcinoma: notice the difference between the linear subcapsular deposits (arrowhead) and the biconvex subcapsular deposit with parenchymal invasion (arrow): observe the scalloped appearance of the underlying parenchyma. CE-CT coronal MPR (**C**): PC from colon carcinoma: thickening of the right diaphragm caused by deposit seeding (arrow). Notice the difference with the subcapsular deposits that scallop the liver contour (arrowhead). Axial CE-CT (**D**): PC from ovarian carcinoma: subcapsular deposits with parenchymal invasion (thin arrows), both hepatic and splenic. Observe how they differ from hepatic metastases, which are well defined and completely surrounded by parenchyma (arrow). Note also the perihepatic (arrowhead) and right subphrenic deposits (curved arrow). Ascites (*).

3.1.3. Periportal Space

Periportal deposits need to be differentiated from parenchymal metastases. Deposits within the periportal space appear as nodular or plaque-like lesions, predominantly at the porta hepatis and along the left branch of the portal vein; they are usually ill defined and not circumferentially surrounded by hepatic parenchyma, unlike their intraparenchymal counterparts (Figure 11).

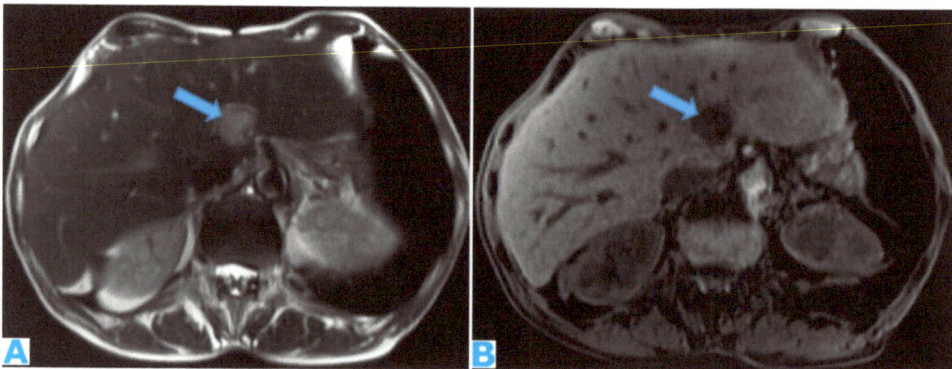

Figure 10. Axial T2WI (**A**); axial NE FST1WI (**B**). PC from ovarian serous carcinoma: subcapsular hepatic deposit, presenting a fatty surrounding plane (arrow) that excludes secondary hepatic invasion.

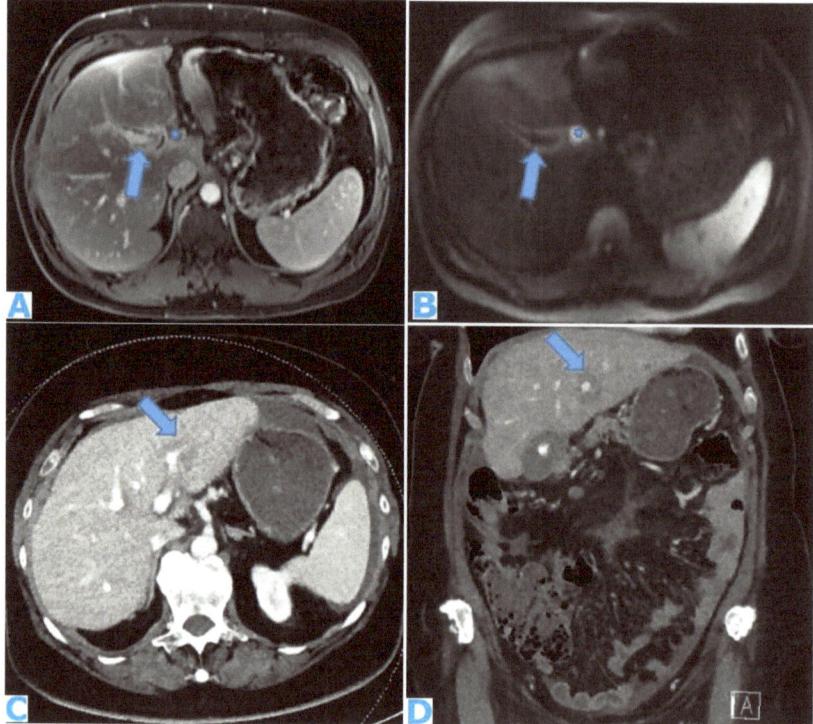

Figure 11. DWI (**A**); axial CE portal phase FST1WI (**B**). PC from colon carcinoma: deposits within the periportal space. Observe the diffusion restriction and enhancement around the periportal space (arrows); also note the nodular deposit (*). Axial CE-CT (**C**) and coronal MPR (**D**). PC from ovarian carcinoma: note the periportal deposit as a soft tissue mass around the left portal branch, which is more conspicuous in the MPR.

A proven useful tip is the distention of the periportal space over time due to the presence of deposits. As with any radiological examination, comparison with prior images in the setting of peritoneal carcinomatosis is mandatory (Figure 12).

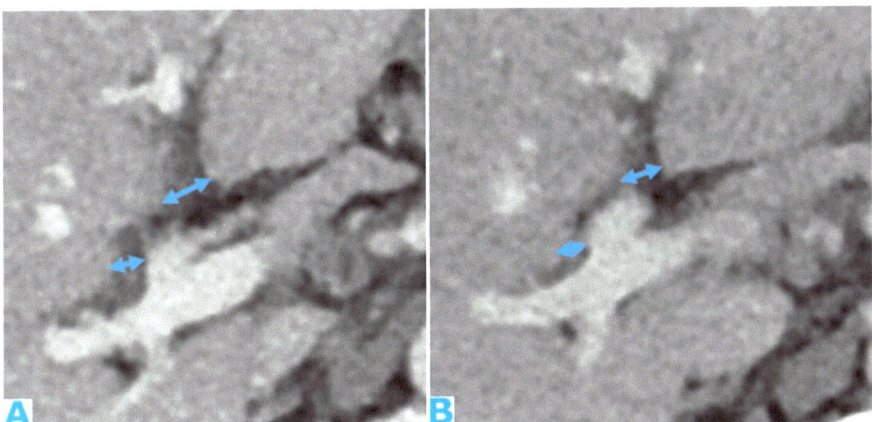

Figure 12. Axial CE-CT ((**A**), current study, and (**B**), from one year prior). PC from gastric adenocarcinoma: subtle soft tissue mass occupying the periportal space. Observe the periportal space enlargement (arrows), which is more conspicuous if compared to the previous CT.

Deposits within this location may cause biliary obstruction, which usually presents at a late stage. Dilatation of the intrahepatic biliary ducts (usually segmentary) with no identifiable cause should raise the possibility of deposits within the periportal spaces. Another secondary finding may be a progressive compressive effect on the portal vein over time (Figure 13).

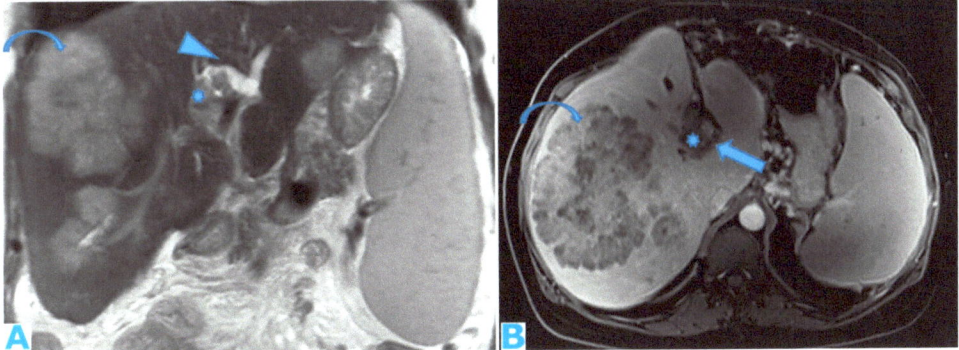

Figure 13. Coronal T2WI (**A**); axial CE portal phase FST1WI (**B**). PC from colon adenocarcinoma: periportal deposit (*) that causes segmental intrahepatic biliary dilatation (arrowhead) and portal vein compression (arrow). The patient had a known portal hypertension due to massive hepatic metastases (curved arrow) and splenomegaly.

3.1.4. Lesser Omentum

This portion of the peritoneum suspends the liver and the lesser curvature of the stomach and separates the first two centimetres of the duodenum from the liver. It is formed by the gastrohepatic and hepatoduodenal ligaments.

Deposits within this space show features that are common to any fat-containing space. Furthermore, since the porta hepatis runs in the hepatoduodenal ligament, biliary obstruction or portal vein compression may be found to be indirect signs of PC (Figure 14).

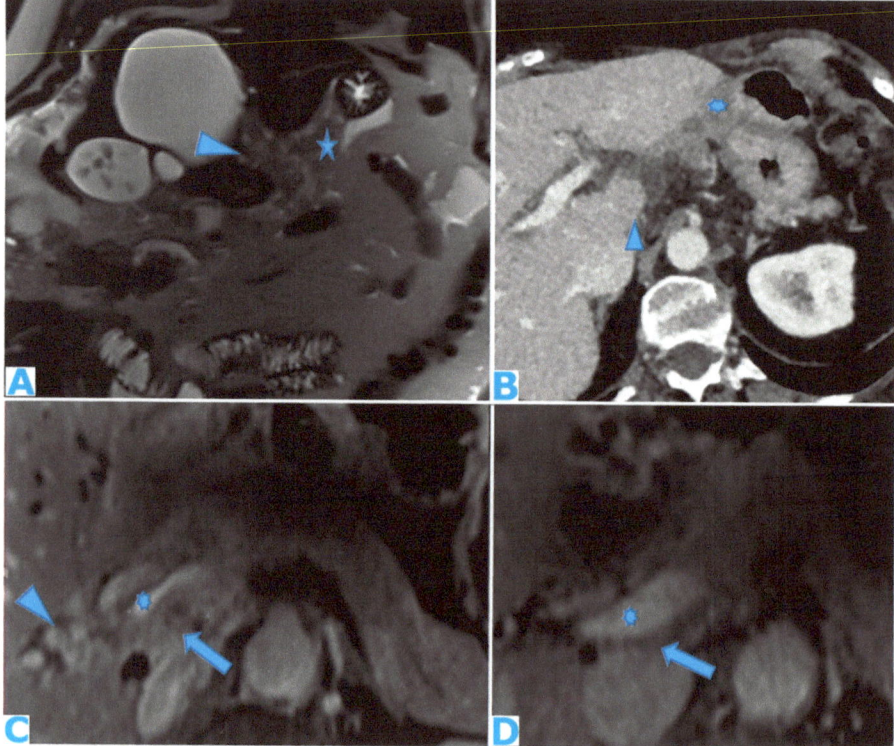

Figure 14. Axial CE-CT (**A**). PC from ovarian carcinoma: deposits within the gastrohepatic (*) and hepatoduodenal ligaments (arrowheads). Coronal T2WI (**B**). PC from ovarian carcinoma: deposits within the lesser omentum: its two components are identified—the gastrohepatic (*) and the hepatoduodenal (arrowhead) ligaments. Axial CE portal phase FST1W1 (**C,D**): the current study (**C**) and from one year prior (**D**), for comparison. PC from colon adenocarcinoma: deposits within the gastrohepatic ligament (lesser omentum) (arrows). Note the compression of the portal vein (*) in (**C**) and the development of collateral vessels (arrowheads).

As previously seen, once the disease is in the lesser omentum it can easily spread to the periportal space thanks to the surrounding connective tissue of the Glisson sheath, which makes them continuous. This is a particularly important route for the spread of pancreatic and gastrointestinal tumours.

3.1.5. Lesser Sac

Potential space between the pancreas and the stomach. Its distention, either by a solid lesion or by ascites, as is reviewed later, is a sign of its involvement by PC (Figure 15). It communicates with the rest of the peritoneal cavity (greater sac) through an opening immediately posterior to the lesser omentum, the foramen of Winslow.

3.1.6. Right Subhepatic Space

Pouch inferior to segment VI of the liver. It communicates with the right subphrenic space, the right paracolic gutter and the lesser sac. Deposits within this space tend to be more subtle, partly due to small size of this space, and range from an ill-defined outer hepatic contour to focal fat stranding and nodules (Figure 16).

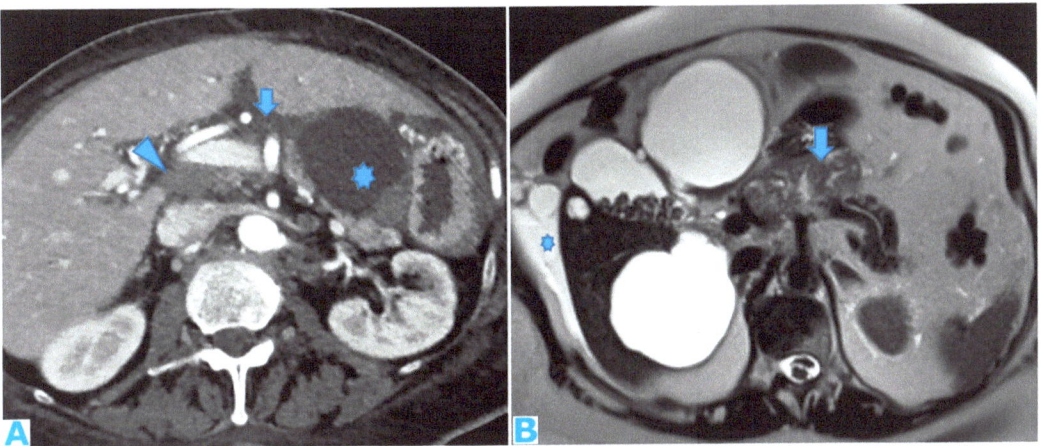

Figure 15. Axial CE-CT (**A**). PC from ovarian carcinoma: mass-like deposit within the lesser sac (*). Also, note the seeding within the lesser omentum (arrow). Portacaval lymph node (arrowhead). Axial T2WI (**B**). PC from ovarian carcinoma: mass-like deposit within the lesser sac (arrow). Ascites (*).

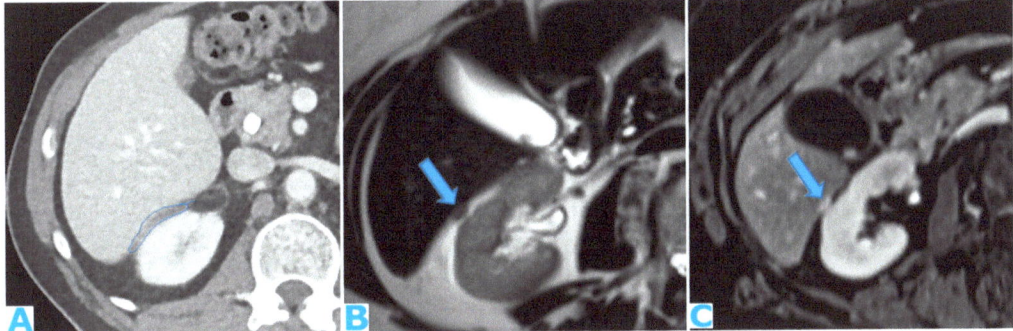

Figure 16. Axial CE-CT (**A**): PC from breast carcinoma: deposits within the subhepatic space as reticulation of its fatty content. Axial T2WI CE-CT (**B**); CE portal phase FST1WI (**C**): PC from colon carcinoma: nodular deposit within the subhepatic space (arrow).

3.2. Inframesocolic Spaces

Inframesocolic spaces are also described using the same cranial-to-caudal and lateral-to-medial approach: greater omentum, paracolic gutters, small bowel mesentery, sigmoid mesocolon, and pelvis recesses.

3.2.1. Greater Omentum

The greater omentum is the main peritoneal fold. It connects the stomach to the anterior surface of the transverse colon and then extends caudally into the pelvis covering the small bowel loops. It lies mainly inferior to the transverse colon mesocolon, although its smaller cranial portion (the gastrocolic ligament) is within the supramesocolic space.

The uniqueness of the imaging features of deposits in this location is the omental cake, which occurs when nodular deposits collide (Figure 17) and blend with one another, boosting a fibrotic response and replacing the omental fat (Figure 18).

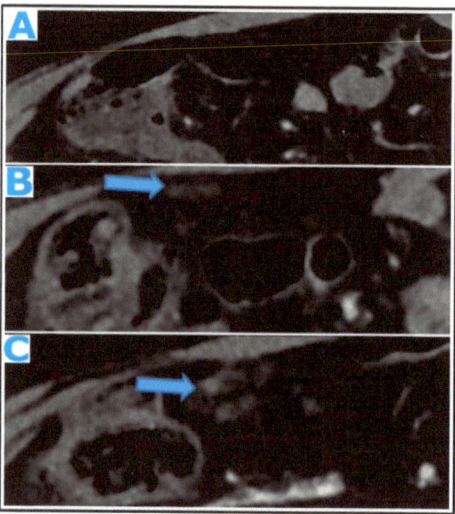

Figure 17. Axial CE-CT (**A**) from one year prior (disease-free peritoneum); (**B**) from four months prior; (**C**) current follow-up. Note the early stages and evolution of omental deposits (arrows).

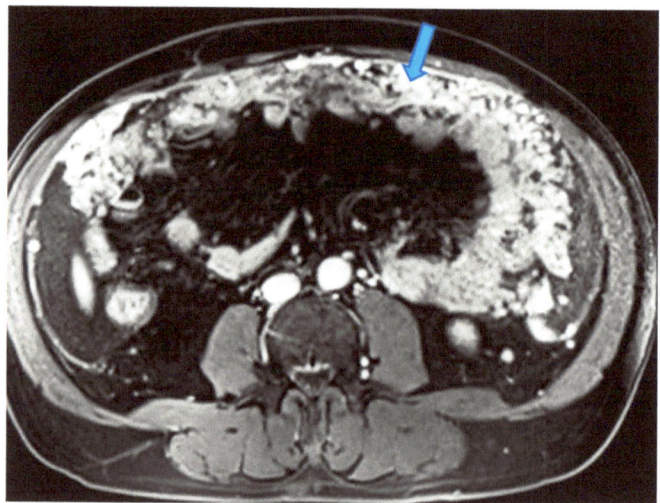

Figure 18. Axial CE portal phase FST1W. PC from melanoma: omental cake (arrow) replacing the omental fat.

A helpful diagnostic sign as the infiltration progresses is the subsequent displacement of the bowel loops. Enlargement of the fatty content and mass effect due to omental seeding may be more apparent than the actual deposits (Figure 19).

Omental deposits are more easily detected using MR. However, in the early stages and especially in thin patients, CT appears to perform better, although the scarce fatty content in thin patients may negatively contribute to the identification of peritoneal deposits (Figure 20).

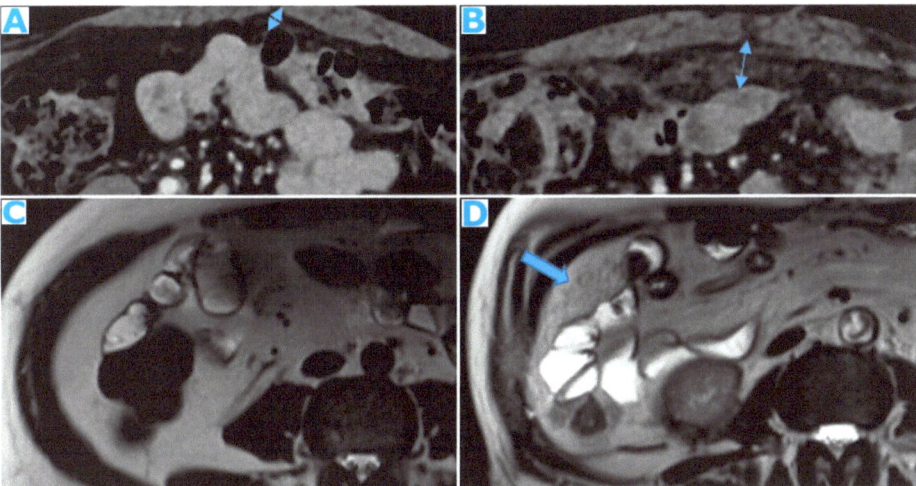

Figure 19. Axial CE-CT ((**A**) from one-year prior; (**B**) current follow-up). PC from breast carcinoma: note the omental infiltration on (**B**) associated with a posterior displacement of the small bowel loops (arrows). Axial T2WI ((**C**) peritoneal disease-free study from two years prior; (**D**) current follow-up). PC from renal cell carcinoma: enlargement of the fatty content and mass effect due to omental seeding (arrow) that may be more conspicuous than the actual deposits.

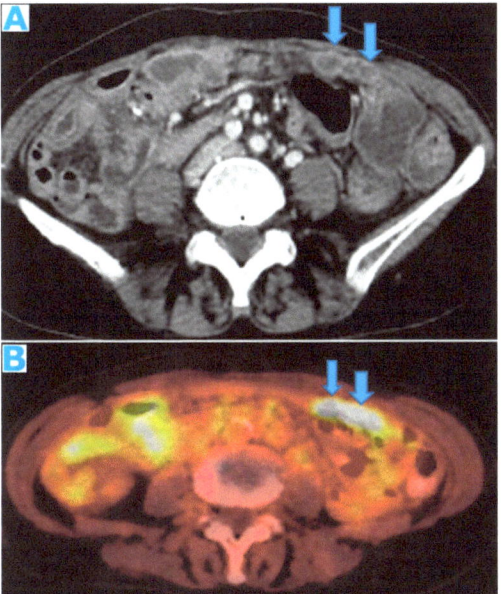

Figure 20. Axial CE-CT (**A**); FDG-PET-CT (**B**). PC from colon adenocarcinoma: nodular deposits within the omentum (arrows) that were originally mistaken for SB loops upon CT due to the scarce intrabdominal fat.

3.2.2. Small Bowel Mesentery

The small-bowel mesentery is a fan-shaped peritoneal double layer that surrounds the small bowel and then extends diagonally from the ligament of Treitz in the left upper quadrant to the ileocecal junction, anchoring at these two locations and at the posterior parietal peritoneum.

Mesenteric deposits show a rather unique and more complex appearance when compared to deposits elsewhere in the abdominal cavity. Deposits may be found in the following locations:

- Within the mesenteric fat: as in the rest of the fat-containing peritoneal spaces, they may range from focal nodular fat stranding to irregular haziness to nodules and masses (Figure 21).

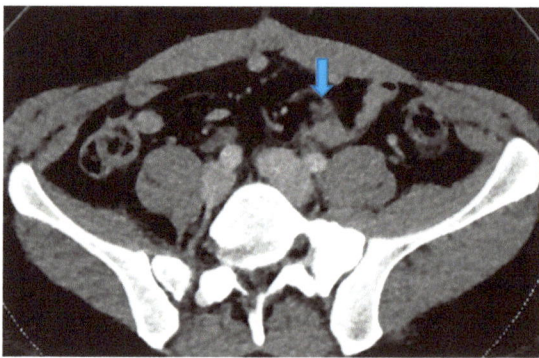

Figure 21. Axial CE-CT. PC from colon adenocarcinoma: nodular deposit within the mesentery (arrow).

- Within the SB and caecal serosa: deposits may also lie within the serosa covering the small bowel and the caecum (Figure 22).

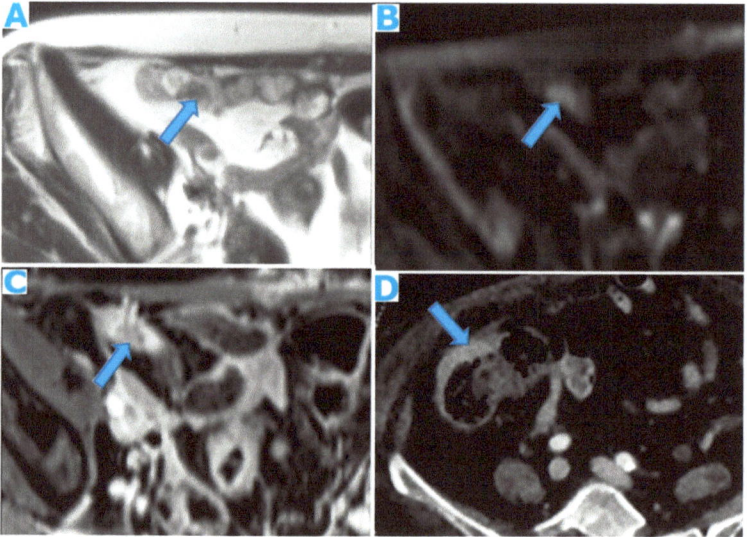

Figure 22. Axial T2WI (**A**); axial DWI (**B**); CE portal phase FST1WI (**C**). PC from duodenal adenocarcinoma: deposits within the distal ileum serosa (arrow). Axial CE-CT (**D**). PC from breast carcinoma: deposits within the caecal serosa (arrow).

- Involving both the mesentery and the serosa: as in the transverse mesocolon, deposits may appear both within the mesentery and the serosa covering the small bowel loops and the caecum (Figure 23).

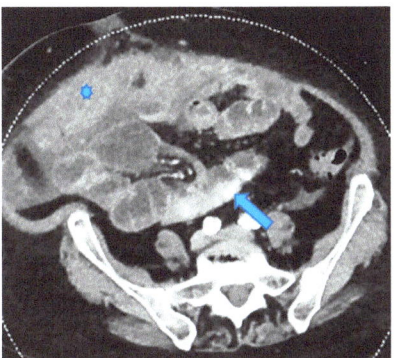

Figure 23. Axial CE-CT. PC from ovarian carcinoma: mesenteric seeding. Mesenteric involvement may occur as a combination of deposits involving both the mesentery and the bowel serosa, as in this case. Observe the clustered SB loops' appearance. The calcified content of some of the deposits enhances their presence (arrow). Omental deposits (*).

- Within the mesenteric leaves: Deposits within the mesenteric leaves may go unperceived. The nodular thickening and enhancement of the mesenteric leaves is usually more conspicuous using MR but can be also spotted using CT and becomes more noticeable when accompanied by ascites (Figures 24 and 25).

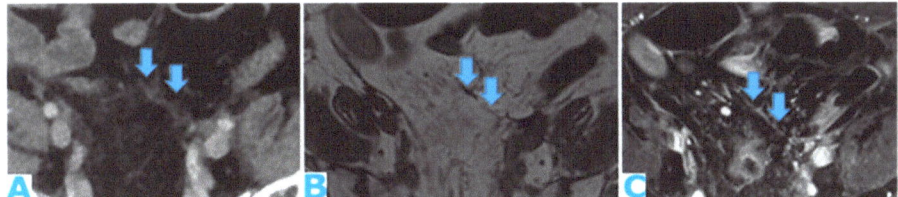

Figure 24. Axial CE-CT (**A**); axial T2WI (**B**); axial CE portal phase FS T1WI (**C**). PC from endometrial carcinoma: deposits seeding within the mesenteric leaves (arrows).

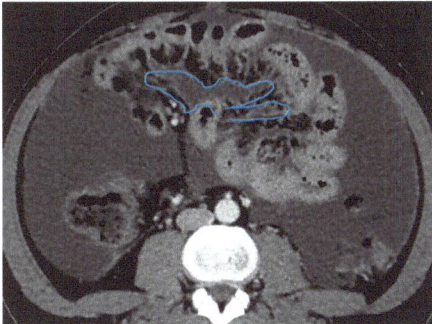

Figure 25. Axial CE-CT. PC from colon adenocarcinoma: involvement of the mesenteric leaves (note the nodular thickening and enhancement, highlighted in blue) that becomes more apparent with ascites.

- Stellate mesentery: Diffuse mesenteric infiltration leads to a stellate appearance, which is commonly associated with breast (especially lobular carcinoma) [32], gastric, pancreatic, and ovarian tumours [33]. This deposition pattern follows the distribution of the mesenteric vessels, causing the thickening and rigidity of perivascular bundles (Figure 26).

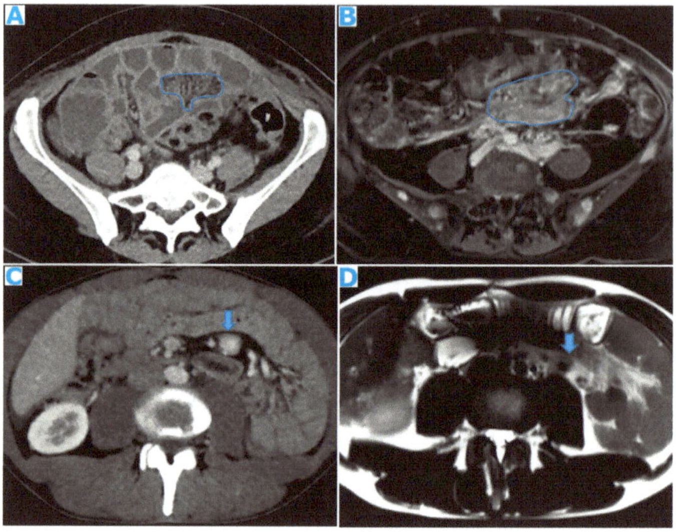

Figure 26. Axial CE-CT (**A**). PC from stomach adenocarcinoma: stellate mesentery. Axial CE portal phase FST1WI (**B**). PC from lobular breast adenocarcinoma: stellate mesentery; note the perivascular distribution. Axial CE-CT (**C**); axial T2WI (**D**). PC from stomach adenocarcinoma: isolated perivascular deposit within the mesentery as a soft-tissue mass surrounding a branch of the SMV (arrow).

As a result of tumour infiltration, the mesentery becomes rigid and loses its usual free wavering. SB loops appear thickened, with restricted distensibility, looking initially separated and angulated and, finally, clustered (Figure 27). Over time, the retraction caused by the deposits causes a decrease in the size of the mesenteric fat (Figure 28). These effects on the SB loops and the mesenteric fat may be more conspicuous than the actual deposits.

The main complication of deposits lying within this space is bowel obstruction, which usually occurs at a late stage, and its diagnosis is not challenging. However, it may also be the presenting sign. It typically involves more than one small bowel loop, and the degree of occlusion may vary. Another, less frequent, complication is bowel ischaemia due to perivascular infiltration (Figure 29).

3.2.3. Paracolic Gutters

Peritoneal recesses occur between the colon, partially covered by the posterior parietal peritoneum (on its anterior, medial, and lateral walls) and the lateral parietal peritoneum on each side. They constitute the attachments of the ascending and descending colon to the posterior parietal peritoneum.

Both are in continuity with the peritoneal spaces in the pelvis. Superiorly, the right paracolic gutter communicates with the right subphrenic and right subhepatic spaces, whereas the left paracolic gutter, which is much smaller, is partially separated from the left subphrenic space by the phrenicocolic ligament (Figure 1b).

The infiltrated peritoneum typically appears to be nodularly thickened, showing pathological enhancement (Figure 30).

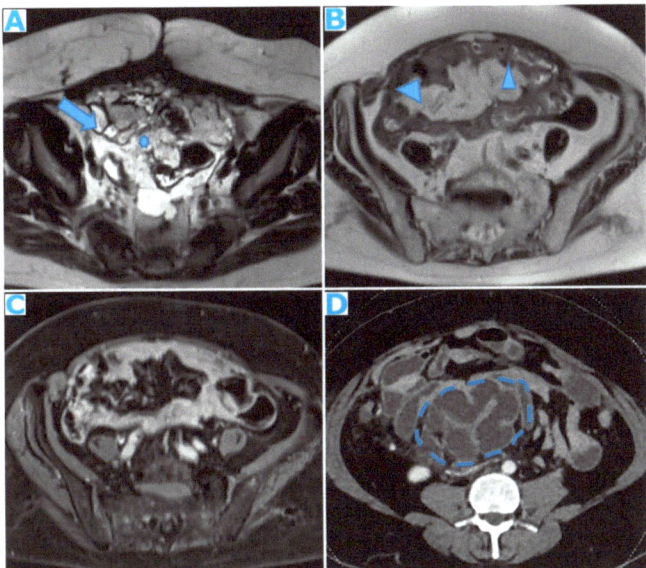

Figure 27. Axial T2WI (**A**). PC from mucinous adenocarcinoma of the urachus: notice the hyperintense mesenteric deposits (*) (signal due to mucin content) and how the SB loops appear separated and angulated (arrow). Axial T2WI (**B**); axial CE portal phase FST1WI (**C**). PC from breast carcinoma: mesenteric deposits (arrowheads on (**B**)) make SB loops appear thickened and separated. Notice how deposits are more conspicuous in T2WI due to its high tissue contrast. Axial CE-CT (**D**). PC from ovarian carcinoma: clustered small bowel loops as the end point of mesenteric seeding.

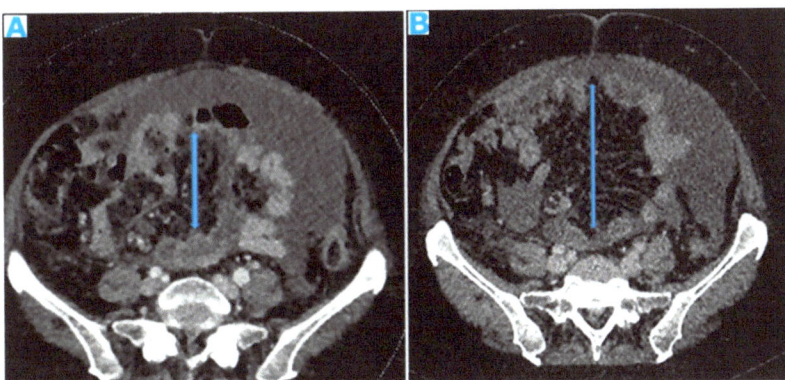

Figure 28. Axial CE-CT: current study (**A**) and from six months prior (**B**). PC from colon carcinoma: the mesentery becomes fibrotic as the seeding evolves and, secondary to the retraction effect, a decrease in the size of the mesenteric fat occurs (arrows). This effect may be more conspicuous than the actual deposits.

The oblique orientation of the small bowel mesentery described earlier divides the inframesocolic compartment into two compartments, right and left, with the latter being larger. The only structure standing in the way of free communication between the left inframesocolic space and the pelvis is the sigmoid mesocolon, thus the reason why it constitutes a common site of deposits, as it is an area of arrested flow. Deposits within the sigmoid mesocolon lie on its fat and/or on the serosa, and differentiation between them may not always be feasible. Sigmoid luminal stenosis with/without signs of obstruction is a frequent consequence of the seeding (Figure 31).

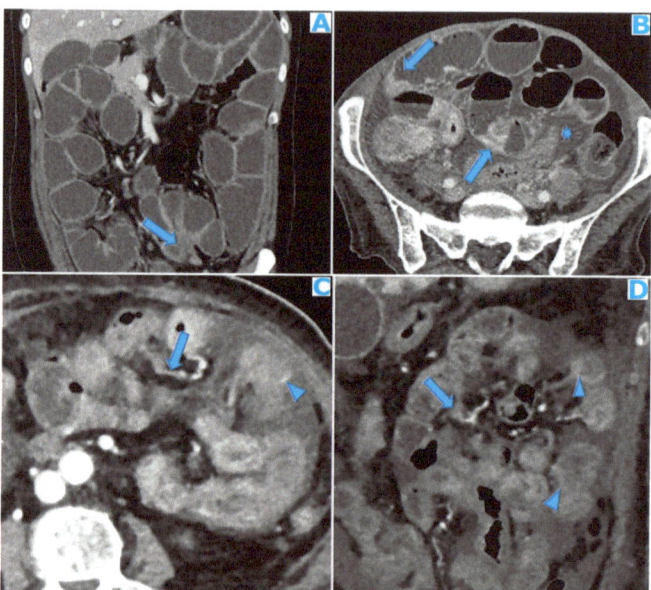

Figure 29. Coronal MPR (**A**). PC from mucinous colon adenocarcinoma: solitary mesenteric deposit (arrow) as the cause of an SB obstruction, involving several loops. Axial CE-CT (**B**). PC from breast carcinoma: SB multifocal obstruction due to several deposits within the SB serosa (arrows). Ascites (*). Axial CE-CT (**C**) and coronal MPR (**D**). PC from adenocarcinoma of the urachus: severe mesenteric infiltration causing SB ischemia as distal SMA and SMV branches are compressed and infiltrated by deposits (arrows). Observe the SB loops thickening and the heterogenous and patchy bowel wall enhancement (arrowheads) due to the ischemia.

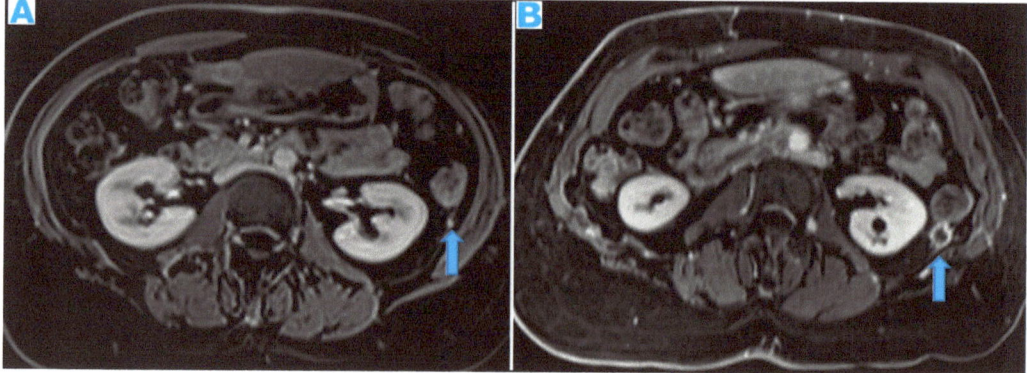

Figure 30. CE portal phase FST1WI ((**A**), from four months prior; (**B**), current study). PC from colon adenocarcinoma: Nodular deposit within the left paracolic gutter that was undercalled (arrow). See the growth in (**B**) (arrow).

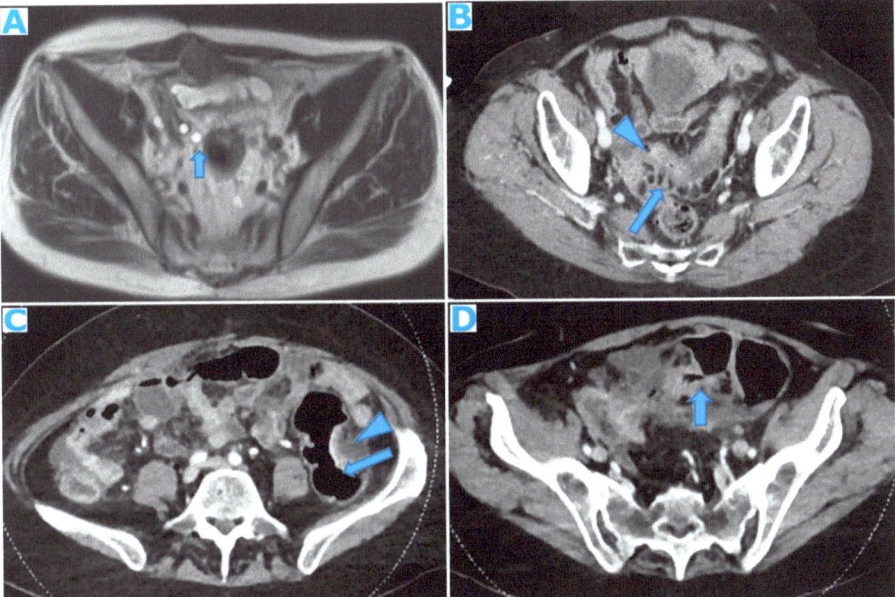

Figure 31. Axial T2WI (**A**). PC from mucinous adenocarcinoma of the terminal ileum: hyperintense nodular deposits (due to mucin content) within the sigmoid mesocolon. Axial CE-CT (**B**). PC from undifferentiated carcinoma of unknown origin: deposits within both the sigmoid mesocolon (arrows), outlining the epiploic appendices, and within the sigmoid serosa, making the sigmoid colon appear thickened (arrowheads). Axial CE-CT (**C,D**). PC from colon adenocarcinoma: (**A**). Observe in (**C**) the seeding involving the sigmoid mesocolon (arrowhead) and the serous layer of the bowel (arrow), partially obstructing the sigmoid lumen. In (**B**), the two components cannot be differentiated but luminal stenosis is clearly identified (arrow).

The mesentery of the appendix is anchored to the lower end of the small bowel mesentery, close to the ileocecal junction and the tip of the appendix. Despite its small size, it may be an important site in appendiceal neoplasms: in case of rupture, deposits will likely appear there first.

3.2.4. Peritoneal Recesses of the Pelvis–Ovarian Metastases

Deposits within the pelvis may be quite tricky to find, as the anatomy is rather complex and there are several structures that fit in a small cavity; therefore, careful exploration using multiplanar reconstructions is recommended.

The parietal peritoneum that covers the abdominal wall goes down to the pelvis, where it does not reach the pelvis floor, as it reflects on the pelvis organs (peritoneal reflexion). The peritoneal reflexion covers the dome of the urinary bladder, then descends along its posterior wall and laterally forms paravesical spaces, a fold over the ureters; in men, it also covers the deferent ducts and the seminal vesicles. It continues towards the rectum and then ascends, partially cloaking the upper and middle rectum (thus subperitoneal; the rest is extraperitoneal) and the lateral pelvic walls (Figure 32). In women, it also coats the uterine fundus and body and the posterior part of the vagina and extends laterally (broad ligament), wrapping up the tubes and suspending the ovaries.

Two blind-end pouches are found in women—the uterovesical, anteriorly, and the rectouterine, posteriorly—while there is only one in men, the rectovesical [7].

Pelvic organs, except for the tubes, which are intraperitoneal, are only superiorly and laterally covered by the peritoneum. Thus, deposits can be identified as enhancing nodular peritoneal thickenings on the pelvic walls (Figure 33) or within the peritoneal reflexion, either surrounded by fat or on the partially peritonealised organ surfaces (Figure 34).

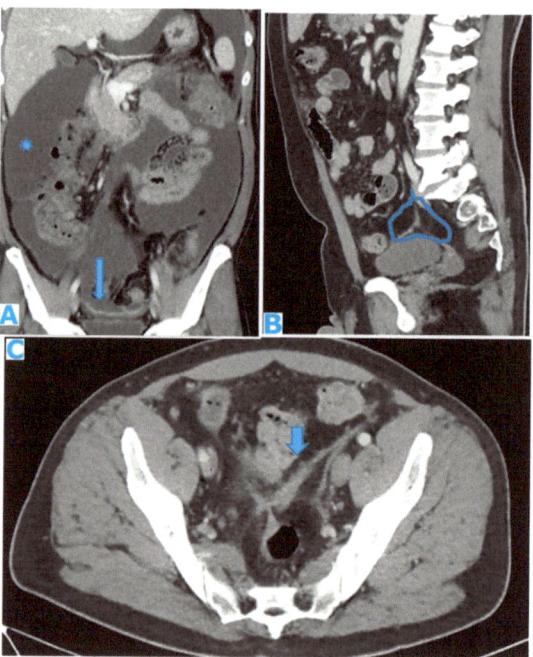

Figure 32. CE-CT coronal MPR (**A**). PC from colon carcinoma: observe how the parietal peritoneum does not reach the pelvis floor. Ascites (*). Deposits within the pelvic reflexion (arrow). Sagittal MPR (**B**); axial CE-CT (**C**). PC from adenocarcinoma of the appendix: irregularly thickened peritoneal reflexion due to seeding. Observe in the sagittal MPR how the peritoneal reflexion covers the dome of the urinary bladder and then descends, following its posterior wall.

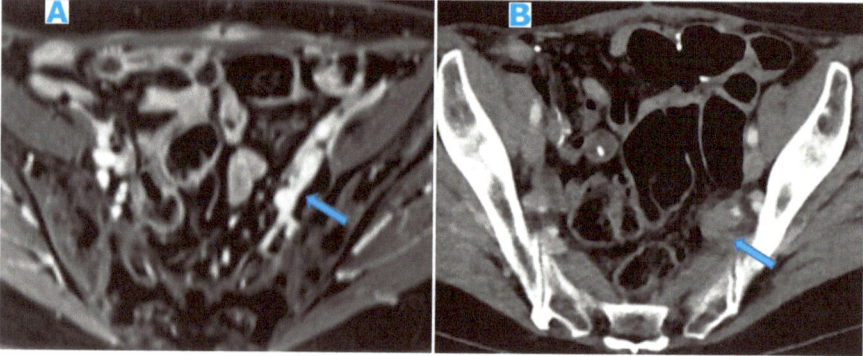

Figure 33. Axial CE portal phase FST1WI (**A**). PC from duodenal adenocarcinoma: deposits seeding within the peritoneum that covers the left pelvic wall, which looks diffusely thickened (arrow). Axial CE-CT (**B**). PC from undifferentiated caecal adenocarcinoma: nodular deposits within the peritoneum that covers the left pelvic wall (arrow).

As ureters are in close contact with the peritoneum at the paravesical spaces, pelvis deposits may be the cause of ureterohydronephrosis, and this is frequently overlooked, especially as the only sign of PC. Any deposit along the posterior parietal peritoneum in the proximity of the course of the ureter may also be the cause of a urinary obstruction, but the pelvis is a very frequent location (Figure 35).

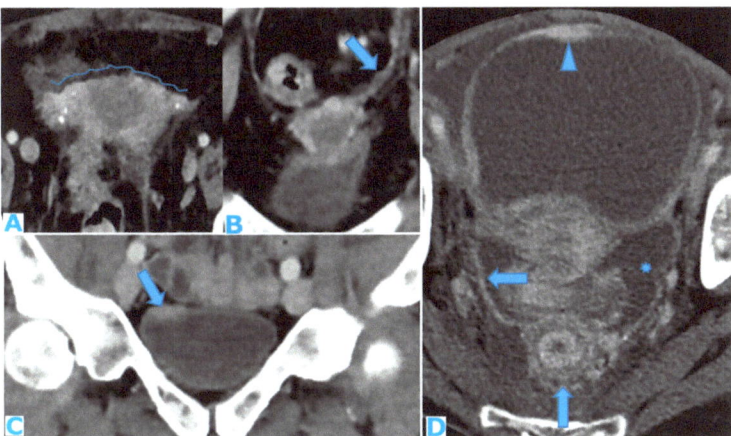

Figure 34. Axial CE-CT (**A**); CE-CT coronal MPR (**B**). PC from breast carcinoma: the peritoneal reflexion covers the uterine fundus and body and the posterior part of the vagina and extends laterally (broad ligament, arrow in (**B**)). Note the nodular appearance of the peritonealised uterine surface and the broad ligaments (arrow in (**B**)) due to deposit seeding. CE-CT coronal MPR (**C**). PC from cardia adenocarcinoma: deposits within the peritoneal reflexion covering the vesical dome (arrow). Axial CE-CT (**D**). PC from breast carcinoma: notice the peritoneal seeding on the peritonealised surfaces of the bladder (arrowhead), rectum (vertical arrow) and within the peritoneum that covers the pelvic walls (horizontal arrow). Ascites (*).

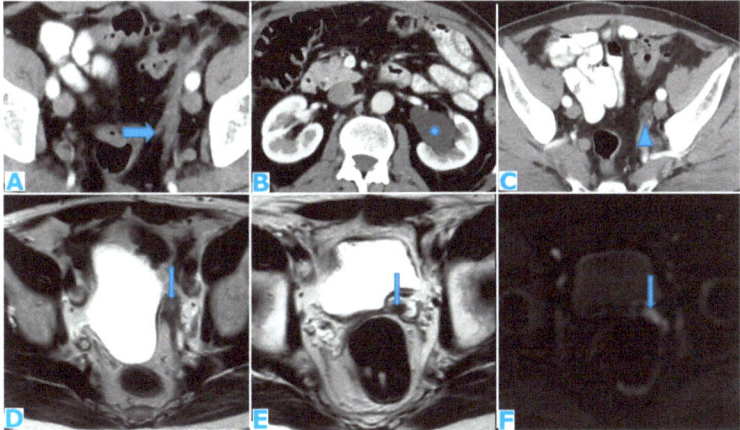

Figure 35. Axial CE-CT (**A**–**C**). Axial T2WI (**D**,**E**); DWI (**F**). PC from mucinous adenocarcinoma of the appendix: Notice the peritoneal deposit within the left lateral pelvis (arrow in (**A**)) as an elongated soft tissue mass. The patient presented with a left ureterohydronephrosis (* in (**B**)) due to the pelvic deposit, which obstructed the ureter (arrowhead in (**C**)). Paravesical spaces are peritoneal recesses that cover, on each side, the distal ureter, the seminal vesicle, and the deferent duct. Note the deposit within the left paravesical space and how it obstructs the left ureter (arrow in (**C**)). The deposit also follows the course of the left deferent duct (arrow in (**E**,**F**)).

Occlusion may occur as a result of pelvis deposits within the peritonealised portion of the rectum.

Another common site of PC in the pelvis is the ovaries. As seen previously, these are extraperitoneal organs, but are considered intraperitoneal, as they communicate with the peritoneal cavity. This is the reason why ovaries are included among the PC locations.

Compared to primary ovarian tumours, ovarian metastases seem to be smaller and more frequently bilateral, showing more uniform cysts and more moderate enhancement of the solid portions [34]. However, a solid appearance may also be found, or even characteristics resembling the primary tumour (Figure 36).

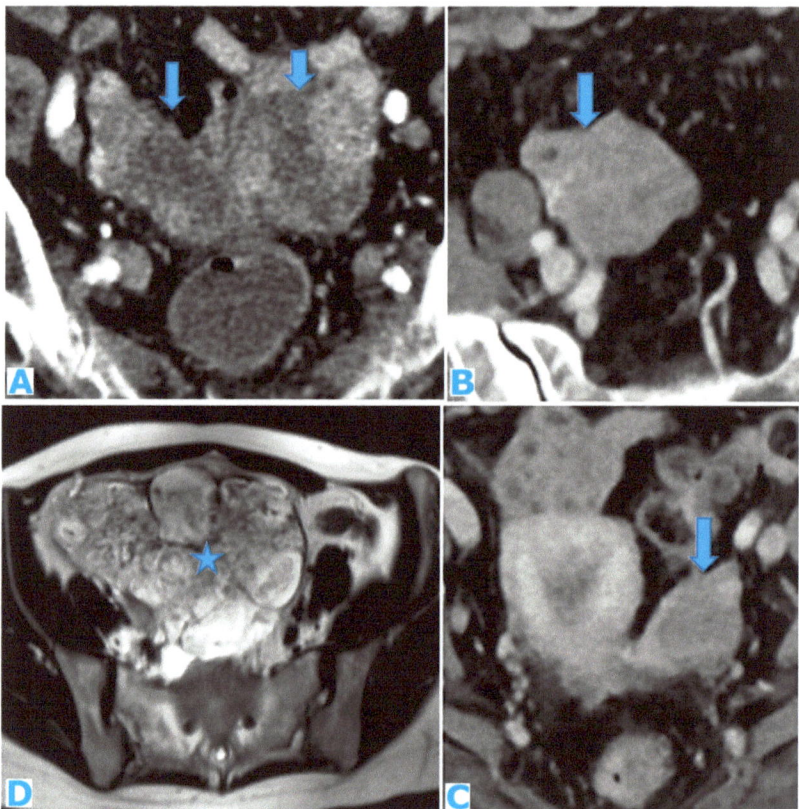

Figure 36. Axial CE-CT (**A**). PC from sigmoid adenocarcinoma: bilateral ovarian metastases as complex cystic masses with solid poles (arrows). Axial CE-CT (**B**,**D**). PC from colon adenocarcinoma: bilateral ovarian metastases as solid masses (arrow). Axial T2WI (**C**). PC from mucinous tumour of the appendix: left ovarian metastases (*) presenting as a predominantly hyperintense mass due to the mucin content.

The term Krukenberg tumour is sometimes misused in the setting of ovarian metastases from a gastrointestinal tumour, as its use should be limited to ovarian metastasis from a poorly differentiated adenocarcinoma with signet ring cell features [35]. Krukenberg tumour should be considered in the differential diagnosis when solid bilateral ovarian masses containing intratumoural cystic components are detected, even in the absence of a primary malignancy [36].

4. Peritoneal Fluid Circulation–Ascites

Now that the peritoneal anatomy has been revised, the focus is placed on the fluid contained in the peritoneal cavity, as it plays a determinant role in the seeding of the deposits.

Peritoneal fluid circulates following the path determined by ligaments and mesenteries, under the influence of the abdominal pressure fluctuations caused by respiration and intestinal peristalsis.

In the case of tumour spread to the peritoneum, the quantity of the peritoneal liquid rises due to two conditions: the obstruction of the lymphatics in charge of the resorption and the overproduction of fluid caused by the vascular permeability factor secreted by the tumour cells [37,38].

Fluid in the inframesocolic space naturally goes down on the right of the small bowel mesentery [39] through the mesenteric leaves, and on the left through the medial mesosigmoid, thus forming an area of arrested flow. It then reaches the pelvic recesses, the most gravity-dependent spaces. After filling the pelvis, it goes up the paracolic gutters: preferentially on the right, as the left gutter is shallower, and the flow is cranially limited by the phrenicocolic ligament [40] (Figure 1b). On the right, it reaches the subhepatic space and, finally, the right subphrenic space, where most of the peritoneal lymphatic clearance takes place, along with the omentum [40]. Therefore, places that normally constitute a free route or barrier for the flow or where most of the resorption takes place need to be particularly scrutinised.

Table 1 summarises the favoured locations for peritoneal seeding and the underlying reasons for this.

Table 1. Favoured PC sites and underlying reasons.

Favoured PC Sites	Underlying Reason
Ileocecal region	Anchor of the small bowel mesentery
Sigmoid mesocolon	Area of arrested flow
Right paracolic gutter	Major gravity dependent pathway
Subhepatic space	Gravity dependence
Right subphrenic space and omentum	Resorption sites

Ascites may be one of the first signs of PC. Its appearance correlates closely with its volume: if minimal, is only be found in the pelvic recesses, surrounding the liver and the spleen, or between the small bowel loops, in a triangle-shaped fashion (Figure 37). If quantity increases, it fills up the gutters, the omentum, and the mesentery leaves.

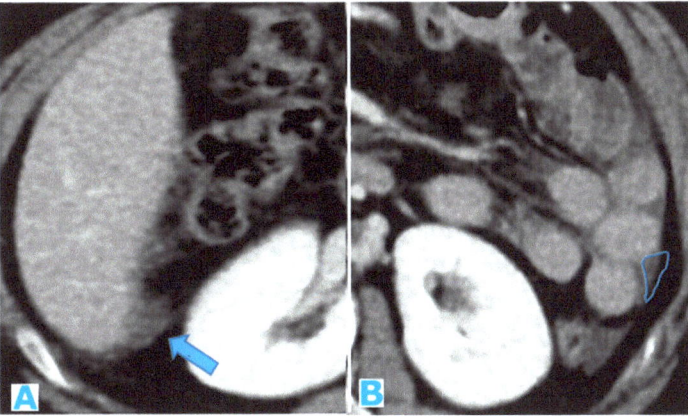

Figure 37. Axial CE-CT (**A**,**B**). PC from ovarian carcinoma: minimal ascites within the subhepatic space (arrow in (**A**)) and between the SB loops, triangle-shaped (**B**).

Suspicious signs may be ascites with rounded or bulging contours, or concomitantly present in the greater and lesser sacs (Figure 38).

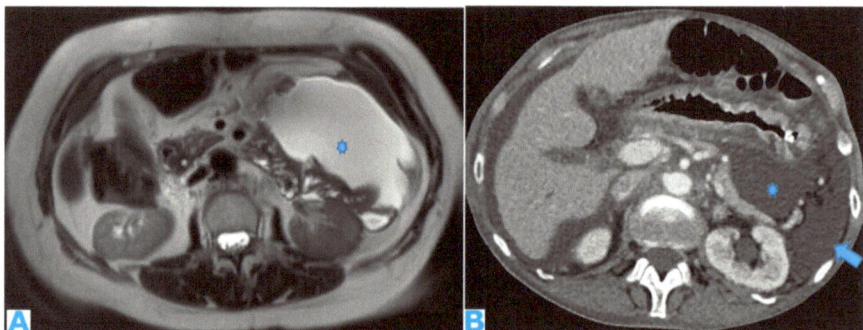

Figure 38. Axial T2WI (**A**). PC from ovarian adenocarcinoma: loculated ascites within the mesentery (*). Axial CE-CT (**B**). PC from breast carcinoma: concomitant ascites within greater (arrow) and lesser (*) sacs.

Another important clue is how SB loops behave in peritoneal liquid: in nonneoplastic ascites or in the early stages of PC, they float freely, with an anterior location, whereas in advanced PC, as the mesentery becomes fibrotic and rigid, SB loops are pulled back centrally and posteriorly (the tethered bowel sign) [41]. Characteristically, there is little fluid between these rigid infiltrated mesenteric leaves, while fluid is predominant elsewhere in the peritoneal cavity (Figure 39).

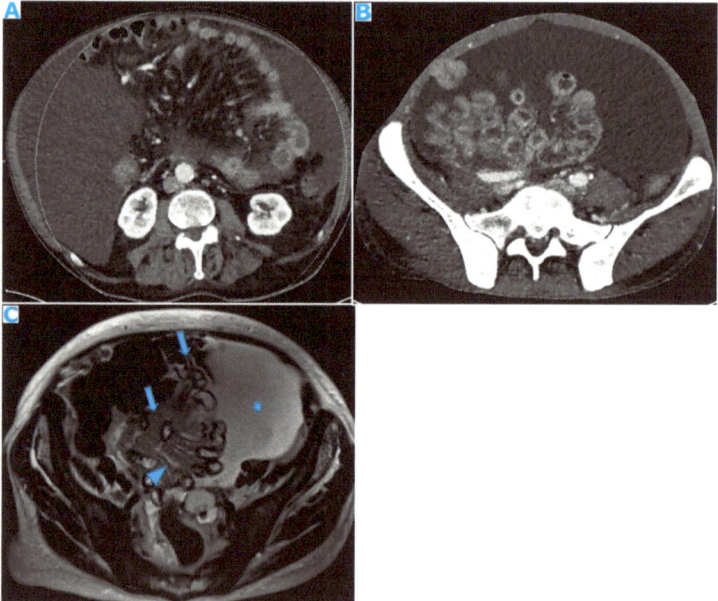

Figure 39. Axial CE-CT (**A**,**B**). (**A**): non-malignant ascites; (**B**): malignant ascites from colon adenocarcinoma. Observe how SB loops float freely in (**A**), with an anterior disposition. In a malignant ascites (**B**), SB loops are drawn posteriorly and lose contact with the anterior abdominal wall (tethered bowel sign) due to the rigid infiltrated mesenteric leaves. Axial T2WI (**C**). PC from endometrial carcinoma: diffuse mesenteric deposit seeding (arrow) that causes SB retraction (tethered bowel sign). Notice that, despite the massive ascites (*), there is little liquid between the rigid infiltrated mesenteric leaves (arrowhead).

In the setting of portal hypertension and non-malignant ascites, collateral vessels within the parietal peritoneum should be cautiously noted, so as not to misdiagnose them as deposits (Figure 40).

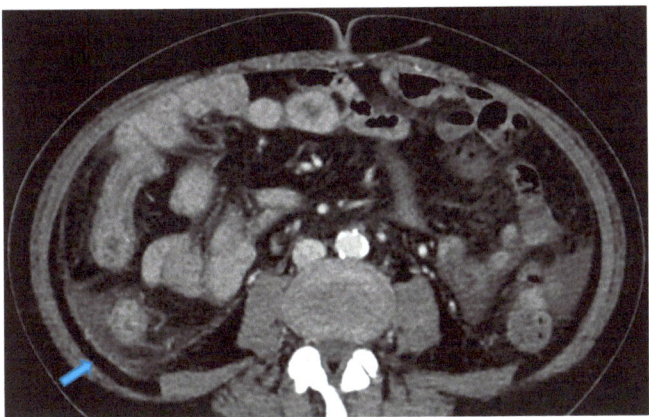

Figure 40. Axial CE-CT. Observe the enhancing pseudonodular parietal peritoneum (arrows), which corresponds to collaterals vessels, and is not to be mistaken for peritoneal deposits.

5. Deposit Behaviour in Cross-Sectional Images

With regard to signal, the deposit does not fall far from the primary tumour; that is, deposits will usually show a density/signal intensity and enhancement pattern resembling the primary tumour, as extraperitoneal metastases do.

Thus, one should always bear in mind the underlying histology and imaging features of the primary tumour and contemplate the possibility of a second primary tumour if a discrepancy is found.

In addition, in the event of no known primary tumour, which occurs in about 3–5% of cases of PC [2], the behaviour in the different MR sequences and, to a lesser degree, in CT, may suggest the origin, despite the non-specificity of the imaging findings.

Indeed, knowledge of the underlying deposit content responsible for the appearance of high signal intensity in T1- and T2-weighted images of peritoneal deposits is an important diagnostic criterion that can contribute to the diagnosis of the primary tumour.

Table 2 summarises the behaviour of the peritoneal deposits according to their appearance on MR and CT, their content, and the corresponding primary tumour, regardless of cell line.

Table 2. Behaviour of peritoneal deposits according to their appearance on MR and CT, their content and the corresponding primary tumour, regardless of the cell line.

Content	T1	T2	CT	Primary Tumour
Melanin	↑	↓	↓	Melanoma
Calcium	↑=	↓=	↑	Mucinous tumors (ovary, stomach, colon, pancreas, appendix, gallbladder, urachus) Serous papillary ovarian tumour
Blood	↑ ↑	↓ ↑	↑	Hypervascular tumours. High-grade ovarian tumours (serous and endometrioid adenocarcinoma). Clear cell ovarian carcinoma Granulosa cell tumour. In the subacute stage of a haematoma, the methemoglobin causes a high SI on T1WI, and a variable SI on T2WI (low in early subacute stage, high in late subacute stage).
Myxoid	↓	↑	↓	Myxoid tumours
Non mineralized cartilage	↓	↑	↓	Condrosarcoma

Table 2. *Cont.*

Content	T1	T2	CT	Primary Tumour
Mucin	↓	↑	↓	Mucinous tumours (ovary, stomach, colon, pancreas, appendix, gallbladder, urachus)
Keratin	↓	↑	↓	Squamous differentiation

↑: High signal intensity (SI)/attenuation, ↓: Low SI/attenuation, =: Isointense

T1 hyperintensity may be observed within a deposit due to three contents: melanin, blood, and calcium.

- Melanin-containing deposits: from melanoma (Figure 41).

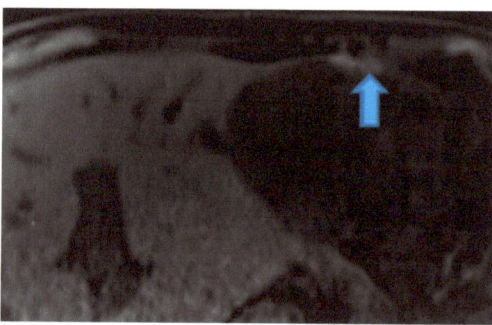

Figure 41. Axial NE FST1WI. PC from melanoma: Note the hyperintense melanin-containing perihepatic deposits (arrow).

- Calcium-containing deposits: mucinous tumours of different origins (ovary, stomach, colon, pancreas, appendix, gallbladder, urachus) may calcify (Figure 42).

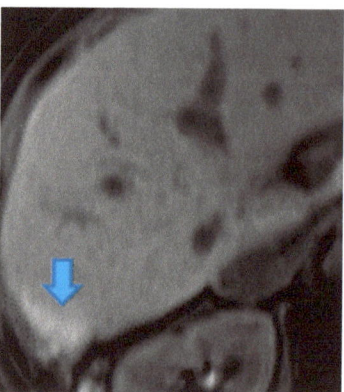

Figure 42. Axial NE FST1WI.PC from serous ovarian adenocarcinoma: Hyperintense perihepatic deposits (due to calcified content) (arrow).

- Blood-containing deposits: blood content is frequently found in peritoneal deposits from hypervascular tumours of different origins (for instance, clear-cell and granulosa ovarian tumours) (Figure 43).

T2 hyperintensity can reflect different contents within deposits: myxoid, non-mineralised cartilage, or mucin. This may also be due to keratin in the setting of a squamous differentiation.

- Myxoid-containing deposits: as in myxoid liposarcoma (Figure 44).

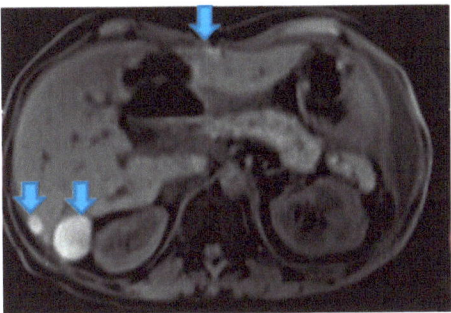

Figure 43. Axial NE FST1WI PC from serous ovarian adenocarcinoma: Blood-containing peri and subhepatic deposits (arrows).

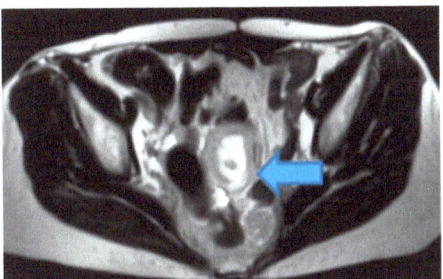

Figure 44. Axial T2WI. Myxoid leiomyosarcoma of the uterus: patient with pelvic deposits in the setting of a relapse (arrow). Observe the deposit central high SI on T2WI due to the myxoid content.

- Non-mineralised cartilage-containing deposits: from chondrosarcoma (Figure 45).

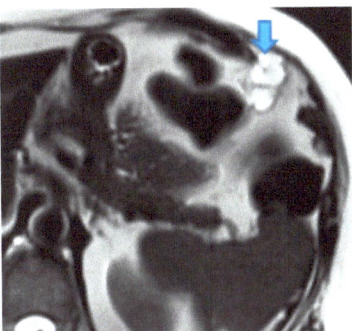

Figure 45. Axial T2WI. Peritoneal deposit from rib condrosarcoma: Omental deposit showing high SI on T2WI, due to the non-mineralized cartilage content (arrow).

- Mucin-containing deposits: from mucinous tumours arising on different organs, namely ovary, stomach, colon, pancreas, appendix, gallbladder, and the urachus (Figure 46).
- Keratin-containing deposits: from tumours showing squamous differentiation (Figure 47).

CT hyperdensity can be due to calcium (Figure 48) or blood content. Calcification may occur secondary to treatment.

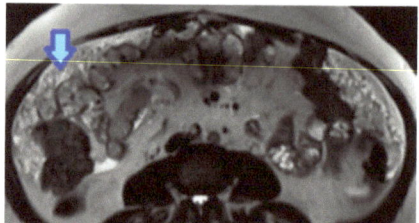

Figure 46. Axial T2WI. PC from mucinous adenocarcinoma of the urachus: Hyperintense omental-cake due to mucinous content (arrow).

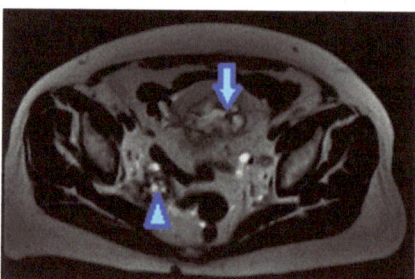

Figure 47. Axial T2WI. Bladder adenocarcinoma with a squamous differentiation. Observe the locally advanced vesical tumor (arrow). Note the right pelvic peritoneal deposit (arrowhead), showing the same imaging features as the tumour. The high signal on T2WI may be due to the keratin formed by the squamous differentiation.

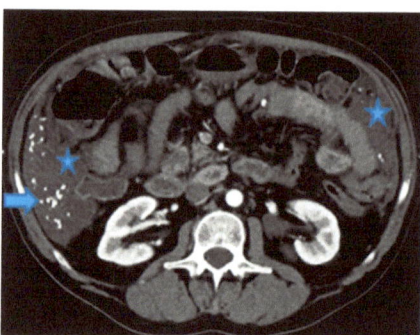

Figure 48. Axial CE CT. PC from colloid adenocarcinoma of the caecum: Observe the specks of calcification (arrows) scattered throughout the deposits (*).

The vascular pattern of deposits also correlates with the characteristics of the primary tumour and may impact the differential diagnosis (Table 3) depending on whether deposits are hyper- (Figure 49) or hypovascular (Figure 50).

Table 3. Relation between vascular pattern of the deposits and differential diagnosis of possible primary tumours.

Hypervascular Deposits	Hypovascular Deposits
Ovarian (clear cell, granulosa)	Mucinous tumours (ovary, stomach, colon, pancreas, appendix, gallbladder, urachus)
Breast carcinoma	Pancreas adenocarcinoma

Table 3. *Cont.*

Hypervascular Deposits	Hypovascular Deposits
Lung carcinoma	Liposarcoma (myxoid or undifferentiated)
Melanoma	
Sarcoma: - GIST - Leiomyosarcoma - Fibrous solitary tumour	
Renal cell carcinoma	
Neuroendocrine tumours	
Hepatocellular carcinoma	
Thyroid carcinoma	
Paraganglioma	
Choriocarcinoma	

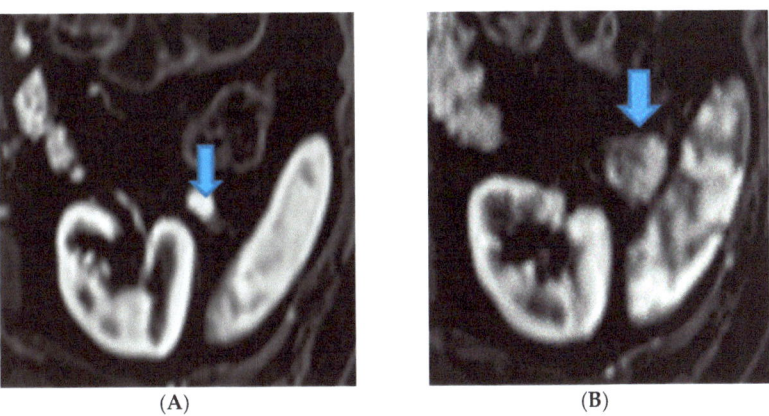

Figure 49. Axial CE portal phase FST1WI. PC from clear cell renal carcinoma: Note the hypervascular deposit adjacent to the spleen that was mistaken for an accessory spleen (arrow in (**A**)). Observe the growth on the follow-up CT (arrow in (**B**)).

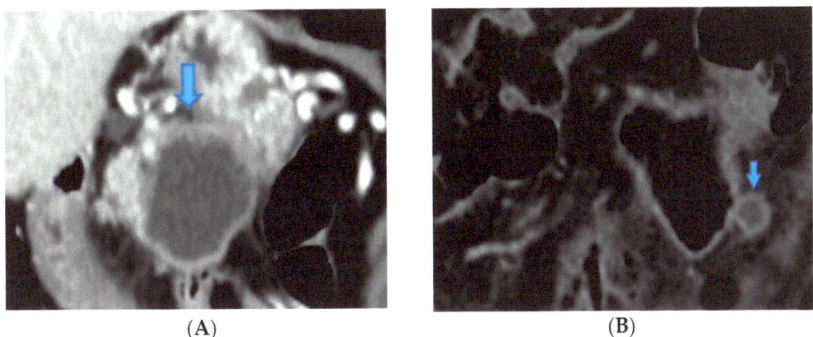

Figure 50. Coronal MPR CE CT PC from pancreatic cystoadenocarcinoma: Observe the primary tumour (arrow in (**A**)) and its deposit within the sigmoid mesocolon (arrow in (**B**)). Notice the hypovascular resemblance between them.

6. Differential Diagnosis

It is worth underlining that, in oncologic patients, not all peritoneal abnormalities correspond to carcinomatosis; hence, PC needs to be differentiated from other neoplastic and nonneoplastic conditions (inflammatory, infectious, and other types of benign causes, noninflammatory and noninfectious) (Table 4). This may be a challenging task as imaging features often overlap.

Table 4. Differential diagnosis.

Inflammatory	Infectious	Benign Noninflammatory Noninfectious	Malignant
Omental infarction	Peritoneal tuberculosis	Splenosis Accessory spleen	Primary peritoneal serous carcinoma
Peritoneal amyloidosis	Peritoneal echinococcosis	Bowel perforation	Pseudomyxoma peritonei
Peritoneal sarcoidosis		Encapsulated omental fat necrosis	Peritoneal malignant mesothelioma
Familial Mediterranean fever		Endometriosis	Desmoplastic small round cell tumour
Encapsulated sclerosing peritonitis		Leiomyomatosis peritonealis	Peritoneal lymphomatosis
		Desmoid tumours	Peritoneal sarcomatosis

6.1. Inflammatory

6.1.1. Omental Infarction—Figure S1

Omental infarction is a rare cause of acute abdomen, usually self-limiting, that presents with nonspecific symptoms. The right omentum is more commonly affected, as it moves more freely, and its vascularization is longer and more tortuous. It can be primary or secondary to other processes such as tumour, hernia, or postoperative adhesions [42].

It is usually a straightforward diagnosis of CT: striking fat stranding of the infarcted omentum with minimal or no involvement of the adjacent bowel (this is the reason why the fat stranding is usually described as disproportionate) [43].

Omental infarction may mimic PC at first glance, but the clinical setting and the inflamed aspect of the omental fat usually reveal the diagnosis. The importance of the correct diagnosis upon imaging relies on its conservative management unless superinfection occurs.

6.1.2. Peritoneal Amyloidosis—Figure S2

Amyloidosis is a rare disease consisting of abnormal protein deposition throughout the body, which more frequently occurs in the gastrointestinal tract, kidneys, and heart. Peritoneal deposition is very rare and can mimic PC [44].

Two forms of peritoneal involvement have been described [45]: diffuse, in which the peritoneum is diffusely thickened, and nodular, where mesenteric masses are the key finding. Calcifications may be found within the deposits.

6.1.3. Peritoneal Sarcoidosis—Figure S3

Sarcoidosis is a systemic granulomatous disease of unknown aetiology. The most common location is the lung [46]. Extrapulmonary involvement is found in 30% of all cases, with the abdomen being the most frequent site, and patients typically present with hepatosplenomegaly. Peritoneal involvement is a rare presentation, and the most frequent findings are ascites and peritoneal nodules. Peritoneal involvement is most frequently accompanied by a generalised disease that reveals the diagnosis, but a histological exam is necessary to confirm it [47].

6.1.4. Familial Mediterranean Fever—Figure S4

This is a hereditary condition characterised by recurrent episodes of fever and systemic serosal inflammation, which mainly occurs in the abdomen. It especially affects patients of Mediterranean heritage. Imaging features are nonspecific; if it presents with ascites and peritonitis, it may strongly mimic PC [48]. The most fatal complication of FMF is amyloidosis and the chances of developing it are higher if left untreated [49].

6.1.5. Encapsulating Sclerosing Peritonitis—Figure S5

This is a rare but serious condition. It can be idiopathic or secondary, either to peritoneal dialysis or other causes, benign (such as surgery, peritonitis, cirrhosis, and enteritis) and malignant (such as pancreatic and renal adenocarcinoma) [50]. It presents with recurrent episodes of bowel obstruction caused by a thickened and calcified peritoneal membrane that encircles the bowel [50].

6.2. Infectious

6.2.1. Peritoneal Tuberculosis—Figure S6

Peritoneal tuberculosis may be a challenging entity to diagnose, given its insidious onset, its vague clinical presentation (abdominal pain and distention, weight loss, and fever), and the difficult isolation of the agents (*M. tuberculosis* complex) [51].

It is important to achieve a prompt diagnosis, as a delay in treatment may cause a worse outcome.

Imaging classification includes three main types [52]:

- Wet (the most common), where the salient feature is ascites, either free or loculated, which may show high attenuation on CT due to the high protein contents.
- Dry, where cellular content is predominant.
- Fibrotic fixed, where the main features are fibrotic changes, causing clustered SB loops.
- An in-between state may also be found (fibrotic mixed).

The findings may overlap with PC but the presence of a smooth peritoneum with minimal thickening and pronounced enhancement suggests PT, whereas nodular implants and irregular peritoneal thickening suggest PC. Prominent mesenteric and retroperitoneal adenopathies may be seen in PT, which may present with a necrotic centre and rim enhancement.

6.2.2. Peritoneal Echinococcosis—Figures S7 and S8

This is a parasitic condition secondary to the peritoneal seeding of Equinococcus larvae. The two main species of the Echinococcus tapeworm are *E. granulosus*, the causal agent in cystic echinococcosis, also known as hydatid disease hosts, and *E. multilocularis*, in alveolar echinococcosis [53]. Both domestic and wild canines are the definite hosts and humans are potentially involved as intermediate hosts [54]. In both entities, the initial infestation is localised to the liver.

E. granulosus hydatid cysts appear as well-defined, thick-walled cystic lesions, with mural calcifications as a characteristic feature [55]. Peritoneal involvement generally results from the rupture of hepatic or splenic cysts, with ascites and peritoneal enhancement as the main imaging features. Daughter cysts scattered throughout the peritoneal cavity may also be found.

Hepatic alveolar echinococcosis usually appears as a tumour-like infiltrative and partially calcified heterogeneous mass, with cystic and necrotic components. It may spread directly to the peritoneum, resulting in peritoneal lesions presenting the same imaging characteristics that inevitably mimic features of peritoneal carcinomatosis. The most salient feature is the infiltrative behaviour, with a tendency to invade adjacent structures. It is important to achieve an early diagnosis, as complete surgical excision is the only curative treatment [56].

6.3. Benign Noninflammatory/Noninfectious

6.3.1. Splenosis/Accessory Spleen—Figure S9

These terms comprehend ectopic foci of splenic tissue that may be found throughout the abdominal cavity, differing in whether the cause is acquired (splenosis) or congenital (accessory spleen).

Splenosis is usually a consequence of spleen injury, either from trauma or surgery, resulting in splenic fragments that acquire a vascular supply and may grow. They may seed on the liver, as in the case shown in the figure, although they most frequently seed in the left lobe, with a subcapsular location. Intrahepatic splenosis usually shows increased enhancement on the arterial phase and may be a potential pitfall for hepatocarcinoma, neuroendocrine metastases, or adenoma [57–59]. Definitive diagnosis is confirmed using heat denaturation red blood cell scintigraphy.

Accessory spleens enhance similar to the spleen, although this may be difficult to evaluate due to their small size. As a rule, these nodules are well-defined and homogeneous, whereas peritoneal deposits may tend to be more irregular and heterogeneous.

6.3.2. Foreign Body Bowel Perforation—Figure S10

Inflammatory–phlegmonous changes secondary to bowel perforation caused by a foreign body may mimic peritoneal carcinomatosis in oncologic patients.

6.3.3. Encapsulated Omental Fat Necrosis—Figure S11

Either spontaneous or secondary to inflammation or trauma, it is usually asymptomatic and its presentation on imaging depends on the time of evolution. Using CT, if acute, it appears as an omental or mesenteric focal fat stranding that may have a discrete mass effect on the adjacent organs; over time, it shrinks and becomes well-defined and peripherally calcified. Initially, it may mimic a liposarcoma and, when it becomes fibrotic (usually, it shows heterogeneous low signal intensity in T1 and T2WI and may slightly enhance), it can be misdiagnosed as a deposit, especially in oncologic patients. Clinical history and previous imaging examinations are essential to achieve a correct diagnosis.

6.3.4. Endometriosis—Figure S12

This is a benign condition characterised by the implantation of endometrial tissue outside the uterine cavity. Peritoneal endometriosis is usually accompanied by other imaging findings that suggest the diagnosis; however, peritoneal involvement may appear as the sole finding. Endometriotic deposits will likely show areas of high signal intensity in T1WI due to blood content and/or low signal intensity in T2WI due to fibrosis.

6.3.5. Leiomyomatosis Peritonealis—Figure S13

This is a rare condition that occurs in women of reproductive age, characterised by the development of multiple leiomyomas within the peritoneum. Potential risk factors are increased levels of endogenous/exogenous oestrogens [60] and prior laparoscopic myomectomy [61].

Malignant transformation is a rare complication [62]. Peritoneal leiomyomas are observed as iso-hypodense nodules using CT with a muscle-like signal intensity using MR and strong homogeneous enhancement, which becomes heterogeneous (due to necrosis and haemorrhage) in the event of malignant transformation. This entity may mimic a PC of unknown origin. Definitive diagnosis is made histopathologically.

6.3.6. Desmoid Tumours—Figure S14

Desmoid tumours (DT) belong to a heterogeneous group of locally aggressive fibromatosis, although non-metastasising, that may arise throughout the body, most commonly extra-abdominally. In 30% of patients, there is an association with familial adenomatous polyposis and, in this setting, tumours are most frequently multiple and intra-abdominal (80% compared to 5% of intra-abdominal sporadic DT) [63].

There is also an association with pregnancy and prior trauma and surgery have been described as possible risk factors [64]. In the abdomen, they are mostly mesenteric, although pregnancy-associated DTs usually occur within the abdominal wall [65].

DTs are soft-tissue masses that may show either well-demarcated or ill-defined margins that extend into the adjacent mesenteric fat. They are usually isodense to muscle; their signal intensity on MR depends on the predominant content (myxoid, cellular, or fibrosis). Enhancement ranges from moderate to intense. As infiltrating mesenteric soft-tissue masses, they can mimic PC.

6.4. Malignant

6.4.1. Primary Peritoneal Serous Carcinoma—Figure S15

It occurs in women, predominantly postmenopausal, and is challenging to diagnose as it resembles advanced epithelial ovarian carcinoma (AEOC), both in imaging and in the histological exam. It occurs less frequently than AEOC and has a worse prognosis [66]. The distinguishing features are the sparing of the ovaries or the disproportionate burden of extra-ovarian disease compared to the ovarian involvement [67].

6.4.2. Pseudomyxoma Peritonei (PMP)—Figure S16

This clinical term refers to a syndrome characterised by the presence of mucinous loculated ascites within the peritoneum [68].

These mucinous septated collections disseminate along the peritoneal surface and their mass effect causes a scalloped appearance of adjacent organs. Pseudomyxoma cells lack adherence molecules on their surface, so they spread by a redistribution phenomenon, which means they follow the current of the intraperitoneal fluid and tend to accumulate at the gravity-dependent and resorption sites described at the beginning of this review [69]. Thus, the mobile small bowel is initially spared thanks to its continuous peristaltic movement.

This entity has been classically associated with a perforated epithelial neoplasm of the appendix; although less frequently, it can originate from mucinous tumours arising from other organs [70]. It should be distinguished from mucinous peritoneal carcinomatosis—as these conditions differ histologically—upon imaging findings and prognosis [71].

6.4.3. Peritoneal Malignant Mesothelioma (PMM)—Figure S17

This very rare and fatal primary malignancy of the peritoneum shows features that overlap those of PC; thus, it is difficult to distinguish these entities using imaging alone. The link with asbestos exposure is weaker than in pleural mesothelioma but remains its best-defined risk factor [72]: a history of asbestos exposure or the presence of pleural plaques can be helpful in differentiating PMM from PC.

6.4.4. Desmoplastic Small Round Cell Tumour—Figure S18

A rare mesenchymal malignancy that arises from peritoneal surfaces as multiple soft-tissue masses. This occurs most frequently in young male patients. Imaging features overlap with other peritoneal malignant tumours. Calcification may occur on 30% of the cases [73].

6.4.5. Peritoneal Lymphomatosis and Peritoneal Sarcomatosis—Figures S19 and S20

As described at the beginning of this review, the term peritoneal carcinomatosis is used when the disease is caused by epithelial cells. The peritoneum may also be the soil of malignant nonepithelial cellular lines, mesenchymal or lymphoid, and thus refer to sarcomatosis and lymphomatosis, respectively [26].

In the setting of an unknown primary tumour, the differential diagnosis should always include the possibility of another cell line being the origin of the peritoneal deposits.

Peritoneal lymphomatosis (PL) is a rare condition but important to suspect, as it responds favourably to chemotherapy. It is uncommon, as the peritoneum lacks lymphoid tissue, and the underlying mechanism is unknown. It is associated most frequently with diffuse large B-cell lymphoma, although it can occur in many subtypes [74].

Imaging features include homogeneous soft-tissue diffuse infiltration of peritoneal leaves [26], associated with prominent retroperitoneal lymph nodes [75] and bulky mesenteric lymph nodes that surround the mesenteric vessels and the perivascular fat on both sides (sandwich sign) [76]. In the presence of lymph nodes, diagnosis is easier, as the burden of the nodal disease is usually disproportionate to the peritoneal disease and its distribution is more diffuse than in PC, where lymph nodes are usually located adjacent to the primary tumour [77].

Ascites, which can be massive in PC, is rather mild in PL, and hepatosplenomegaly occurs more frequently.

Isolated peritoneal disease with no bowel or lymph node involvement is rare [78].

Bowel obstruction is uncommon, even in extensive lymphomatous infiltration of small bowel, due to its lack of desmoplastic reaction [79].

Peritoneal sarcomatosis (PS) is defined as a disseminated intraperitoneal spread either from an intra-abdominal primary sarcoma or from extremity sarcomas [80]. Sarcomatous peritoneal deposits tend to be larger, more hypervascular and heterogeneous (Table 2) than in PC. In addition, lymph node involvement is rare. Ascites is variable [80] and hemoperitoneum may occur more frequently than in PC [81].

Bowel obstruction and hydronephrosis tend to be more common in PC [80].

Despite these differences, the diagnosis of PL/PS based on imaging can be difficult to achieve as PC is much more frequent; thus, the diagnosis should be confirmed using histology.

7. Conclusions

To correctly diagnose PC, a systematic approach to the abdominal cavity is highly recommended. The knowledge of peritoneal anatomy and peritoneal fluid flow characteristics substantially contribute to an understanding of where to look for deposits and their appearance on cross-sectional imaging.

Indeed, in CT and MR, features of peritoneal deposits and their behaviour on contrast-enhanced cross-sectional images are related to the histologic characteristics of the primary tumour. Therefore, in the event of peritoneal carcinomatosis with unknown primary tumour, signal intensity/density characteristics of the peritoneal deposits, together with their vascular properties, may be helpful in the identification of the primary tumour.

Moreover, it can occur that the sole presenting sign of peritoneal carcinomatosis is intra-abdominal complications, such as bowel obstruction or ureterohydronephrosis, which should be considered suspicious in oncologic patients, even in the absence of clear radiological evidence of peritoneal deposits.

Furthermore, there are several benign and malignant peritoneal conditions that may mimic peritoneal carcinomatosis. Thus, even in oncologic patients, it is important to consider these conditions in the differential diagnosis with peritoneal carcinomatosis. However, when relying solely on imaging, it remains difficult to conduct a differential diagnosis, since the imaging features overlap between benign/other malignant conditions.

Supplementary Materials: The following supporting information can be downloaded at: https://www.mdpi.com/article/10.3390/diagnostics13132253/s1. Figure S1. Omental infarction. Figure S2. Peritoneal amyloidosis. Figure S3. Peritoneal sarcoidosis. Figure S4. Familial Mediterranean fever. Figure S5. Encapsulated sclerosing peritonitis. Figure S6. Peritoneal tuberculosis. Figure S7. Peritoneal echinococcosis (same patient as Figure S58). Figure S8. Peritoneal echinococcosis. Figure S9. Accessory spleen. Figure S10. Bowel perforation. Figure S11. Encapsulated omental fat necrosis. Figure S12. Endometriosis. Figure S13. Leiomyomatosis peritonealis. Figure S14. Desmoid tumours. Figure S15. Primary peritoneal serous carcinoma. Figure S16. Pseudomyxoma peritonei. Figure S17. Peritoneal mesothelioma. Figure S18. Desmoplastic small round cell tumour. Figure S19. Peritoneal lymphomatosis. Figure S20. Peritoneal sarcomatosis.

Funding: This research received no external funding.

Institutional Review Board Statement: Not applicable.

Informed Consent Statement: Not applicable.

Data Availability Statement: Not applicable.

Conflicts of Interest: The authors declare no conflict of interest.

References

1. Flanagan, M.; Solon, J. Peritoneal metastases from extra-abdominal cancer—A population-based study. *Eur. J. Surg. Oncol.* **2018**, *44*, 1811–1817. [CrossRef] [PubMed]
2. Desai, J.P.; Moustarah, F. Peritoneal Metastasis. In *StatPearls [Internet]*; StatPearls Publishing: Treasure Island, FL, USA, 2022.
3. Pereira, F.; Serrano, A.; Manzanedo, I.; Pérez-Viejo, E.; González-Moreno, S.; González-Bayón, L.; Arjona-Sánchez, A.; Torres, J.; Ramos, I.; Barrios, M.E.; et al. GECOP-MMC: Phase IV randomized clinical trial to evaluate the efficacy of hyperthermic intraperitoneal chemotherapy (HIPEC) with mytomicin-C after complete surgical cytoreduction in patients with colon cancer peritoneal metastases. *BMC Cancer* **2022**, *22*, 536. [CrossRef] [PubMed]
4. van Driel, W.J.; Koole, S.N.; Sikorska, K.; Schagen van Leeuwen, J.H.; Schreuder, H.W.R.; Hermans, R.H.M.; de Hingh, I.H.J.T.; van der Velden, J.; Arts, H.J.; Massuger, L.F.A.G.; et al. Hyperthermic Intraperitoneal Chemotherapy in Ovarian Cancer. *N. Engl. J. Med.* **2018**, *378*, 230–240. [CrossRef]
5. Yang, X.-J.; Huang, C.-Q.; Suo, T.; Mei, L.-J.; Yang, G.-L.; Cheng, F.-L.; Zhou, Y.-F.; Xiong, B.; Yonemura, Y.; Li, Y. Cytoreductive surgery and hyperthermic intraperitoneal chemotherapy improves survival of patients with peritoneal carcinomatosis from gastric cancer: Final results of a phase III randomized clinical trial. *Ann. Surg. Oncol.* **2011**, *18*, 1575–1581. [CrossRef] [PubMed]
6. Szadkowska, M.A.; Pałucki, J.; Cieszanowski, A. Diagnosis and treatment of peritoneal carcinomatosis—A comprehensive overview. *Pol. J. Radiol.* **2023**, *88*, e89–e97. [CrossRef]
7. González-Moreno, S.; González-Bayón, L. Imaging of peritoneal carcinomatosis. *Cancer J. Sudbury Mass* **2009**, *15*, 184–189. [CrossRef]
8. Patel, C.M.; Sahdev, A. CT, MRI and PET imaging in peritoneal malignancy. *Cancer Imaging* **2011**, *11*, 123–139. [CrossRef]
9. Van 't Sant, I.; Engbersen, M.P. Diagnostic performance of imaging for the detection of peritoneal metastases: A meta-analysis. *Eur. Radiol.* **2020**, *30*, 3101–3112. [CrossRef]
10. Cianci, R.; Delli Pizzi, A. Magnetic Resonance Assessment of Peritoneal Carcinomatosis: Is There a True Benefit from Diffusion-Weighted Imaging? *Curr. Probl. Diagn. Radiol.* **2020**, *49*, 392–397. [CrossRef]
11. Low, R.N. Magnetic Resonance Imaging in the Oncology Patient: Evaluation of the Extrahepatic Abdomen. *Semin. Ultrasound CT MRI* **2005**, *26*, 224–236. [CrossRef]
12. Satoh, Y.; Ichikawa, T.; Motosugi, U.; Kimura, K.; Sou, H.; Sano, K.; Araki, T. Diagnosis of peritoneal dissemination: Comparison of 18F-FDG PET/CT, diffusion-weighted MRI, and contrast-enhanced MDCT. *AJR Am. J. Roentgenol.* **2011**, *196*, 447–453. [CrossRef] [PubMed]
13. Low, R.N.; Sebrechts, C.P.; Barone, R.M.; Muller, W. Diffusion-weighted MRI of peritoneal tumors: Comparison with conventional MRI and surgical and histopathologic findings—A feasibility study. *AJR Am. J. Roentgenol.* **2009**, *193*, 461–970. [CrossRef] [PubMed]
14. Dong, L.; Li, K.; Peng, T. Diagnostic value of diffusion-weighted imaging/magnetic resonance imaging for peritoneal metastasis from malignant tumor: A systematic review and meta-analysis. *Medicine* **2021**, *100*, e24251. [CrossRef] [PubMed]
15. Koh, D.M.; Collins, D.J. Diffusion-weighted MRI in the body: Applications and challenges in oncology. *AJR Am. J. Roentgenol.* **2007**, *188*, 1622–1635. [CrossRef]
16. Sala, E.; Priest, A.N.; Kataoka, M.; Graves, M.J.; McLean, M.A.; Joubert, I.; Lomas, D.J. Apparent diffusion coefficient and vascular signal fraction measurements with magnetic resonance imaging: Feasibility in metastatic ovarian cancer at 3 Tesla: Technical development. *Eur. Radiol* **2010**, *20*, 491–496. [CrossRef]
17. Kyriazi, S.; Collins, D.J.; Messiou, C.; Pennert, K.; Davidson, R.L.; Giles, S.L.; Kaye, S.B.; Desouza, N.M. Metastatic ovarian and primary peritoneal cancer: Assessing chemotherapy response with diffusion-weighted MR imaging--value of histogram analysis of apparent diffusion coefficients. *Radiology* **2011**, *261*, 182–192. [CrossRef]
18. Kim, S.J.; Lee, S.W. Diagnostic accuracy of (18)F-FDG PET/CT for detection of peritoneal carcinomatosis; a systematic review and meta-analysis. *Br. J. Radiol.* **2018**, *91*, 20170519. [CrossRef]
19. Bhuyan, P.; Mahapatra, S.; Mahapatra, S.; Sethy, S.; Parida, P.; Satpathy, S. Extraovarian primary peritoneal papillary serous carcinoma. *Arch. Gynecol. Obstet.* **2010**, *281*, 561–564. [CrossRef]
20. Bhatt, A.N.; Mathur, R.; Farooque, A.; Verma, A.; Dwarakanath, B.S. Cancer biomarkers—Current perspectives. *Indian J. Med. Res.* **2010**, *132*, 129–149.
21. Nagpal, M.; Singh, S.; Singh, P.; Chauhan, P.; Zaidi, M.A. Tumor markers: A diagnostic tool. *Natl. J. Maxillofac. Surg.* **2016**, *7*, 17–20.
22. Nougaret, S.; Addley, H.C. Ovarian carcinomatosis: How the radiologist can help plan the surgical approach. *Radiographics* **2012**, *32*, 1775–1800. [CrossRef] [PubMed]

23. Laghi, A.; Bellini, D.; Rengo, M.; Accarpio, F.; Caruso, D.; Biacchi, D.; Di Giorgio, A.; Sammartino, P. Diagnostic performance of computed tomography and magnetic resonance imaging for detecting peritoneal metastases: Systematic review and meta-analysis. *Radiol. Med.* **2017**, *122*, 1–15. [CrossRef] [PubMed]
24. Rivard, J.D.; Temple, W.J.; McConnell, Y.J.; Sultan, H.; Mack, L.A. Preoperative computed tomography does not predict resectability in peritoneal carcinomatosis. *Am. J. Surg.* **2014**, *207*, 760–765. [CrossRef] [PubMed]
25. Low, R.N.; Barone, R.M.; Rousset, P. Peritoneal MRI in patients undergoing cytoreductive surgery and HIPEC: History, clinical applications, and implementation. *Eur. J. Surg. Oncol.* **2021**, *47*, 65–74. [CrossRef]
26. Cabral, F.C.; Krajewski, K.M. Peritoneal lymphomatosis: CT and PET/CT findings and how to differentiate between carcinomatosis and sarcomatosis. *Cancer Imaging* **2013**, *13*, 162–170. [CrossRef]
27. Low, R.N. MR imaging of the peritoneal spread of malignancy. *Abdom. Imaging* **2007**, *32*, 267–283. [CrossRef]
28. Tirkes, T.; Sandrasegaran, K. Peritoneal and retroperitoneal anatomy and its relevance for cross-sectional imaging. *Radiographics* **2012**, *32*, 437–451. [CrossRef]
29. Gore, R.M.; Levine, L.S. *Textbook of Gastrointestinal Radiology*, 3rd ed.; Saunders: Philadelphia, PA, USA, 2007; pp. 2071–2097.
30. Meyers, M.A.; Oliphant, M. The peritoneal ligaments and mesenteries: Pathways of intraabdominal spread of disease. *Radiology* **1987**, *163*, 593–604. [CrossRef]
31. Akin, O.; Sala, E. Perihepatic metastases from ovarian cancer: Sensitivity and specificity of CT for the detection of metastases with and those without liver parenchymal invasion. *Radiology* **2008**, *248*, 511–517. [CrossRef]
32. Winston, C.B.; Hadar, O. Metastatic lobular carcinoma of the breast: Patterns of spread in the chest, abdomen, and pelvis on CT. *AJR Am. J. Roentgenol.* **2000**, *175*, 795–800. [CrossRef]
33. Healy, J.C.; Reznek, R.H. The peritoneum, mesenteries and omenta: Normal anatomy and pathological processes. *Eur. Radiol.* **1998**, *8*, 886–900. [CrossRef] [PubMed]
34. Xu, Y.; Yang, J. MRI for discriminating metastatic ovarian tumors from primary epithelial ovarian cancers. *J. Ovarian Res.* **2015**, *8*, 61. [CrossRef] [PubMed]
35. Zulfiqar, M.; Koen, J. Krukenberg Tumors: Update on Imaging and Clinical Features. *AJR Am. J. Roentgenol.* **2020**, *215*, 1020–1029. [CrossRef] [PubMed]
36. Kim, S.H.; Kim, W.H. CT and MR findings of Krukenberg tumors: Comparison with primary ovarian tumors. *J. Comput. Assist. Tomogr.* **1996**, *20*, 393–398. [CrossRef] [PubMed]
37. Saif, M.W.; Siddiqui, I.A. Management of ascites due to gastrointestinal malignancy. *Ann. Saudi Med.* **2009**, *29*, 369–377. [CrossRef]
38. Chang, D.K.; Kim, J.W. Clinical significance of CT-defined minimal ascites in patients with gastric cancer. *World J. Gastroenterol.* **2005**, *11*, 6587. [CrossRef]
39. Meyers, M.A. Intraperitoneal seeding: Pathways of spread and localization. In *Meyers' Dynamic Radiology of the Abdomen*, 6th ed.; Meyers, M.A., Charnsangavej, C., Eds.; Springer: New York, NY, USA, 2000; pp. 69–105.
40. Feldman, G.B.; Knapp, R.C. Lymphatic drainage of the peritoneal cavity and its significance in ovarian cancer. *Am. J. Obstet. Gynecol.* **1974**, *119*, 991–994. [CrossRef]
41. Seltzer, S.E. Analysis of the tethered-bowel sign on abdominal CT as a predictor of malignant ascites. *Gastrointest. Radiol.* **1987**, *12*, 245–249. [CrossRef]
42. Leitner, M.J.; Jordan, C.G. Torsion, infarction and hemorrhage of the omentum as a cause of acute abdominal distress. *Ann. Surg.* **1952**, *135*, 103–110. [CrossRef]
43. Pereira, J.M.; Sirlin, C.B. Disproportionate fat stranding: A helpful CT sign in patients with acute abdominal pain. *Radiographics* **2004**, *24*, 703–715. [CrossRef]
44. Pickhardt, P.J.; Bhalla, S. Unusual nonneoplastic peritoneal and subperitoneal conditions: CT findings. *Radiographics* **2005**, *25*, 719–730. [CrossRef] [PubMed]
45. Kim, M.S.; Ryu, J.A. Amyloidosis of the mesentery and small intestine presenting as a mesenteric haematoma. *Br. J. Radiol.* **2008**, *81*, e1–e3. [CrossRef] [PubMed]
46. Iannuzzi, M.C.; Rybicki, B.A. Sarcoidosis. *N. Engl. J. Med.* **2007**, *357*, 2153–2165. [CrossRef] [PubMed]
47. Gezer, N.S.; Basara, I. Abdominal sarcoidosis: Cross-sectional imaging findings. *Diagn. Interv. Radiol.* **2015**, *21*, 111–117. [CrossRef]
48. Zissin, R.; Rathaus, V. CT findings in patients with familial Mediterranean fever during an acute abdominal attack. *Br. J. Radiol.* **2003**, *76*, 22–25. [CrossRef] [PubMed]
49. Bhatt, H.; Cascella, M. Familial Mediterranean Fever. In *StatPearls [Internet]*; StatPearls Publishing: Treasure Island, FL, USA, 2022.
50. Manphool, S.; Satheesh, K. Encapsulating peritoneal sclerosis: The abdominal cocoon. *Radiographics* **2019**, *39*, 62–77.
51. Uygur-Bayramicli, O.; Dabak, G. A clinical dilemma: Abdominal tuberculosis. *World J. Gastroenterol.* **2003**, *9*, 1098–1101. [CrossRef]
52. Burrill, J.; Williams, C.J. Tuberculosis: A radiologic review. *Radiographics* **2007**, *27*, 1255–1273. [CrossRef]
53. Pedrosa, I.; Saíz, A. Hydatid disease: Radiologic and pathologic features and complications. *Radiographics* **2000**, *20*, 795–817. [CrossRef]
54. Moro, P.; Schantz, P.M. Echinococcosis: A review. *Int. J. Infect. Dis.* **2009**, *13*, 125–133. [CrossRef]
55. Zalaquett, E.; Menias, C. Imaging of hydatid disease with a focus on extrahepatic involvement. *Radiographics* **2007**, *37*, 901–923. [CrossRef] [PubMed]
56. McManus, D.P.; Zhang, W. Echinococcosis. *Lancet* **2003**, *362*, 1295–1304. [CrossRef] [PubMed]

57. Sato, N.; Abe, T. Intrahepatic splenosis in a chronic hepatitis C patient with no history of splenic trauma mimicking hepatocellular carcinoma. *Am. J. Case Rep.* **2014**, *15*, 416–420.
58. Leong, C.W.; Menon, T. Post-Traumatic Intrahepatic Splenosis Mimicking a Neuroendocrine Tumour. *BMJ Case Rep.* **2013**, *2013*, bcr2012007885. [CrossRef] [PubMed]
59. Gruen, D.R.; Gollub, M. Intrahepatic splenosis mimicking hepatic adenoma. *AJR Am. J. Roentgenol.* **1997**, *168*, 725–726. [CrossRef]
60. Drake, A.; Dhundee, J. Disseminated leiomyomatosis peritonealis in association with oestrogen secreting ovarian fibrothecoma. *BJOG* **2001**, *108*, 661–664.
61. Kumar, S.; Sharma, J.B. Disseminated peritoneal leiomyomatosis: An unusual complication of laparoscopic myomectomy. *Arch. Gynecol. Obstet.* **2008**, *278*, 93–95. [CrossRef]
62. Surmacki, P.; Sporny, S. Disseminated peritoneal leiomyomatosis coexisting with leiomyoma of the uterine body. *Arch. Gynecol. Obstet.* **2006**, *273*, 301–303. [CrossRef]
63. Sinha, A.; Hansmann, A. Imaging assessment of desmoid tumours in familial adenomatous polyposis: Is state-of-the-art 1.5 T MRI better than 64-MDCT? *Br. J. Radiol.* **2012**, *85*, e254–e261. [CrossRef]
64. Brooks, A.P.; Reznek, R.H. CT appearances of desmoid tumours in familial adenomatous polyposis: Further observations. *Clin. Radiol.* **1994**, *49*, 601–607. [CrossRef]
65. Robinson, W.A.; McMillan, C. Desmoid tumors in pregnant and postpartum women. *Cancers* **2012**, *4*, 184–192. [CrossRef] [PubMed]
66. Li, X.; Yang, Q. Differences between primary peritoneal serous carcinoma and advanced serous ovarian carcinoma: A study based on the SEER database. *J. Ovarian Res.* **2021**, *14*, 40. [CrossRef] [PubMed]
67. Morita, H.; Aoki, J. Serous surface papillary carcinoma of the peritoneum: Clinical, radiologic, and pathologic findings in 11 patients. *Am. J. Roentgenol.* **2004**, *183*, 923–928. [CrossRef] [PubMed]
68. Diop, A.D.; Fontarensky, M. CT imaging of peritoneal carcinomatosis and its mimics. *Diagn. Interv. Imaging* **2014**, *95*, 861–872. [CrossRef] [PubMed]
69. Sugarbaker, P.H. Pseudomyxoma peritonei. A cancer whose biology is characterized by a redistribution phenomenon. *Ann. Surg.* **1994**, *219*, 109–111.
70. Mittal, R.; Chandramohan, A. Pseudomyxoma peritonei: Natural history and treatment. *Int. J. Hyperthermia.* **2017**, *33*, 511–519. [CrossRef]
71. Ronnett, B.M.; Yan, H. Patients with pseudomyxoma peritonei associated with disseminated peritoneal adenomucinosis have a significantly more favorable prognosis than patients with peritoneal mucinous carcinomatosis. *Cancer* **2001**, *92*, 85–91. [CrossRef]
72. Broeckx, G.; Pauwels, P. Malignant peritoneal mesothelioma: A review. *Transl. Lung Cancer Res.* **2018**, *7*, 537–542. [CrossRef]
73. Chen, J.; Wu, Z. Intra-abdominal desmoplastic small round cell tumors: CT and FDG-PET/CT findings with histopathological association. *Oncol. Lett.* **2016**, *11*, 3298–3302. [CrossRef]
74. Yoo, E.; Kim, J.H. Greater and lesser omenta: Normal anatomy and pathologic processes. *Radiographics* **2007**, *27*, 707–720. [CrossRef]
75. Karaosmanoglu, D.; Karcaaltincaba, M.; Oguz, B.; Akata, D.; Ozmen, M.; Akhan, O. CT findings of lymphoma with peritoneal, omental and mesenteric involvement: Peritoneal lymphomatosis. *Eur. J. Radiol.* **2009**, *71*, 313–317. [CrossRef] [PubMed]
76. Hardy, S.M. Signs in imaging: The sandwich sign. *Radiology* **2003**, *226*, 651–652. [CrossRef]
77. Kim, Y.; Cho, O. Peritoneal lymphomatosis: CT findings. *Abdom. Imaging* **1998**, *23*, 87–90. [CrossRef] [PubMed]
78. Wong, S.; Sanchez, T.R.S. Diffuse peritoneal lymphomatosis: Atypical presentation of Burkitt lymphoma. *Pediatr. Radiol.* **2009**, *39*, 274–276. [CrossRef] [PubMed]
79. Balthazar, E.J.; Noordhoorn, M. CT of small-bowel lymphoma in immunocompetent patients and patients with AIDS: Comparison of findings. *AJR Am. J. Roentgenol.* **1997**, *168*, 675–680. [CrossRef] [PubMed]
80. Tamara, N.O.; Jyothi, P. Peritoneal sarcomatosis versus peritoneal carcinomatosis: Imaging findings at MDCT. *AJR Am. J. Roentgenol.* **2010**, *195*, W229–W235.
81. Bilimoria, M.M.; Holtz, D.J. Tumor volume as a prognostic factor for sarcomatosis. *Cancer* **2002**, *94*, 2441–2446. [CrossRef]

Disclaimer/Publisher's Note: The statements, opinions and data contained in all publications are solely those of the individual author(s) and contributor(s) and not of MDPI and/or the editor(s). MDPI and/or the editor(s) disclaim responsibility for any injury to people or property resulting from any ideas, methods, instructions or products referred to in the content.

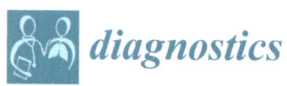 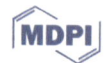

Review

Immunotherapy Assessment: A New Paradigm for Radiologists

Vincenza Granata [1,*], Roberta Fusco [2,3], Sergio Venanzio Setola [1], Igino Simonetti [1], Carmine Picone [1], Ester Simeone [4], Lucia Festino [4], Vito Vanella [4], Maria Grazia Vitale [4], Agnese Montanino [5], Alessandro Morabito [5], Francesco Izzo [6], Paolo Antonio Ascierto [3] and Antonella Petrillo [1]

1. Division of Radiology, Istituto Nazionale Tumori IRCCS Fondazione Pascale—IRCCS di Napoli, 80131 Naples, Italy
2. Medical Oncology Division, Igea SpA, 80013 Naples, Italy
3. Italian Society of Medical and Interventional Radiology (SIRM), SIRM Foundation, 20122 Milan, Italy
4. Melanoma, Cancer Immunotherapy and Development Therapeutics Unit, Istituto Nazionale Tumori IRCCS Fondazione G. Pascale, 80131 Naples, Italy
5. Thoracic Medical Oncology, Istituto Nazionale Tumori IRCCS Fondazione Pascale—IRCCS di Napoli, 80131 Naples, Italy
6. Division of Epatobiliary Surgical Oncology, Istituto Nazionale Tumori IRCCS Fondazione Pascale—IRCCS di Napoli, 80131 Naples, Italy
* Correspondence: v.granata@istitutotumori.na.it

Abstract: Immunotherapy denotes an exemplar change in an oncological setting. Despite the effective application of these treatments across a broad range of tumors, only a minority of patients have beneficial effects. The efficacy of immunotherapy is affected by several factors, including human immunity, which is strongly correlated to genetic features, such as intra-tumor heterogeneity. Classic imaging assessment, based on computed tomography (CT) or magnetic resonance imaging (MRI), which is useful for conventional treatments, has a limited role in immunotherapy. The reason is due to different patterns of response and/or progression during this kind of treatment which differs from those seen during other treatments, such as the possibility to assess the wide spectrum of immunotherapy-correlated toxic effects (ir-AEs) as soon as possible. In addition, considering the unusual response patterns, the limits of conventional response criteria and the necessity of using related immune-response criteria are clear. Radiomics analysis is a recent field of great interest in a radiological setting and recently it has grown the idea that we could identify patients who will be fit for this treatment or who will develop ir-AEs.

Keywords: immunotherapy; radiological response assessment; Recist 1.1; i-Recist; immuno-related adverse events

1. Background

Immunotherapy denotes an exemplar change in an oncological setting [1–6]. In fact, different to other therapies as conventional chemotherapy [7–13], such as radiation [14–20] or targeted therapies [21–27] which target the cancer, these treatments work by stimulating the patient's immune system to obtain an immune reaction against the tumor [2,3].

Immunotherapy can be categorized as passive or active, according to the action mechanism [28–34]. In passive treatment [28–30], immunoglobulins can be administered and attached to tumor-related antigens. Otherwise, in the active treatment, there is a stimulation of the immune system to recognize antigens of the tumor and act against them [30–34]. Although several approaches are presently utilized in clinical and pre-clinical settings, the main means are centered on the so-called checkpoint inhibitors (ICI), that include programmed cell death–1 (PD-1) protein, PD-1′s main ligand (PD-L1), and cytotoxic T-lymphocyte–associated protein 4 (CTLA-4) [35–43].

In 2011, the U.S. Food and Drug Administration (FDA) approved the first agent, ipilimumab, a CTLA-4 inhibitor, for metastatic and unresectable melanoma [44]. Subsequently, different FDA approved agents, have been introduced in both routine and experimental studies to treat different categories of solid and hematologic tumors as after failure of conventional therapies or as first-line therapies [39,45–69]. Moreover, these treatments may be combined with conventional treatments since they can increase the cytotoxic effect of chemotherapy [70–72].

Although the effective utility of these treatments is within a wide range of tumors, only a sub-group of patients show real benefits [73]. The efficacy of immunotherapy is affected by several factors, including human immunity, which is strongly correlated to genetic features [74–77], such as intra-tumor heterogeneity [78–86]. In fact, cancer is complex, flexible, and heterogeneous, representing the result of an innumerable number of genetic mutations that affect the regular cell functionality. However, these mutations allow the cancer cell to appear as foreign to the immune system, offering an opportunity for this treatment [78–86]. Clinical studies have demonstrated that even when several patients are well qualified as immunotherapy responders (e.g., high tumor PD-L1 expression), a large percentage of them (>50%) do not respond to this [87]. In addition, during treatment, some patients can have a clinical and/or radiological disease progression [88]; these events are known as "primary immune escape" and "secondary immune escape", respectively [89]. The mechanisms implicated in these two phenomena (also known as resistance) can overlap. Multi-omics analyses obtained from immunotherapy-treated patient tissues showed as several features are correlated to immune resistance [90–92].

In addition, while immunotherapy has increased patient outcomes, it can cause several immune-related adverse events (ir-AEs), which can be transitory or chronic, life-threatening or mild, and could affect several organ systems, sometimes numerous organs at the same time [93–108].

Classic imaging assessment, based on computed tomography (CT) [109–116] or magnetic resonance imaging (MRI) [117–127], which is useful for conventional treatment, has a limited role in immunotherapy. The reason is due to different patterns of response and/or progression during this kind of treatment which differs from those seen during other treatments, such as the possibility to assess the wide spectrum of immunotherapy-related toxic effects as soon as possible [128–139]. Thus, the introduction of robust noninvasive imaging biomarkers that can allow the immunotherapy-response prediction and prognosis is crucial.

The aim of this article is to (a) explain the response pattern and response criteria utilized during immunotherapy assessments, (b) explain the wide spectrum of toxic effects due to immunotherapy, and (c) explain the potential role of radiomics features as imaging biomarkers for immunotherapy.

2. Treatment Assessment and Pattern Response

The frequently employed radiological response criteria have been introduced considering the chemotherapeutic agents' cytotoxic results, which caused a decrease in target size when the treatment has been effective [132,133,140]. The World Health Organization (WHO) criteria assessed the tumor burden considering the sum of the products of orthogonal largest diameters of the target lesions [141], while the response evaluation criteria in solid tumors (RECIST) criteria [142] assessed the tumor burden considering a one-dimensional (the largest diameter of target lesions). These criteria are not able to evaluate functional or metabolic status, such as necrosis, that causes morphological changes on CT (density decrease) or MRI (inhomogeneous signal on conventional sequences and different pattern on functional ones) [130,143–146]. The CHOI criteria [143] were introduced to assess target therapy in gastrointestinal stromal tumors, such as the PET response criteria in solid tumors (PERCIST) to evaluate FDG uptake reduction [147,148].

In contrast to conventional treatments, immunotherapy involves a complex process that includes different phases and during each one, the immune system is activated. Such as, a number of immune cells move to the target with increasing in target volume and/or new lesion growth [139,149,150]. This process can cause an unusual response pattern known as pseudoprogression [139]. Although, it is possible to obtain conventional response patterns as a complete response (Figure 1) or a partial response (Figure 2), pseudoprogression (Figure 3), characterized by an increment in volume target, can occur in 4–10% of immunotherapy-treated patients [128]. Divergent to pseudoprogression, in which treatment is preserved, a true severe progression is hyperprogression (Figures 4 and 5) [128]. During an imaging study assessment, it could be complicated differ pseudoprogression to hyperprogression [128], so a multidisciplinary team should assess complete patient status [128].

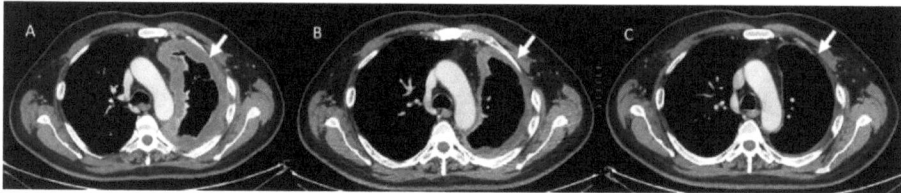

Figure 1. Complete response pattern in a mesothelioma patient treated with immunotherapy. CT scan assessment in pre-treatment phase (**A**) of lesion (arrow), at 3 months (**B**), and after 6 months (**C**).

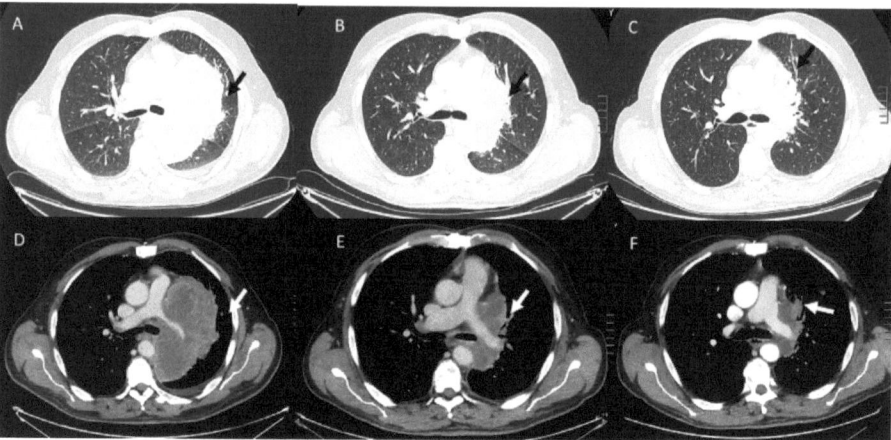

Figure 2. Partial response pattern in non small lung cancer (NSLC) treated with immunotherapy (arrows). CT scan assessment in pre-treatment phase (**A,D**), at 3 months (**B,E**), and after 6 months (**C,F**).

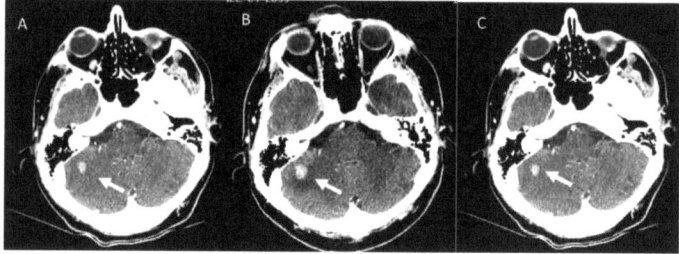

Figure 3. Pseudoprogression of brain metastasis (arrows) in an NSLC patient treated with immunotherapy. CT evaluation (**A**) in pre-treatment phase, after 1 month (**B**), and after 12 weeks of the first CT evaluation (**C**).

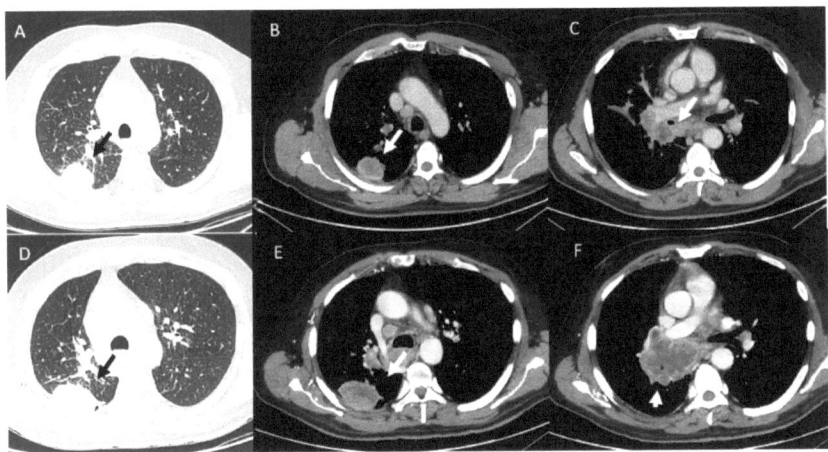

Figure 4. Iperprogression in an NSLC (arrows) patient treated with immunotherapy. CT assessment in pre-treatment phase (**A**–**C**) and after 3 months (**D**–**F**).

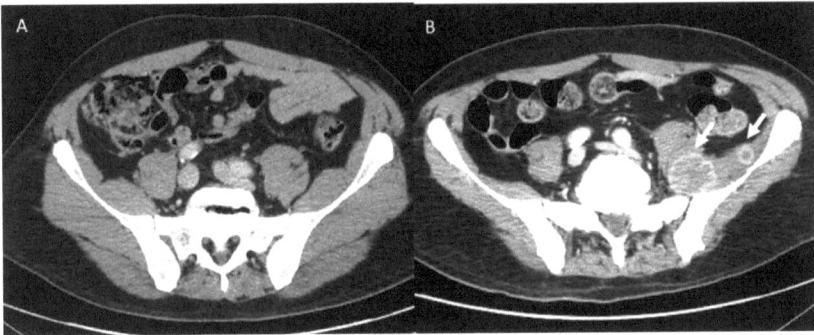

Figure 5. The same patient in Figure 4 (**A**). New lesions (arrows) in ileo-psoas muscle (**B**) due to iperprogression during immunotherapy.

Another atypical response pattern are dissociated responses (Figure 6) [128]. In this pattern, several lesions show dimension increase and others show regression. This pattern is associated with a better survival compared to true progressions [128].

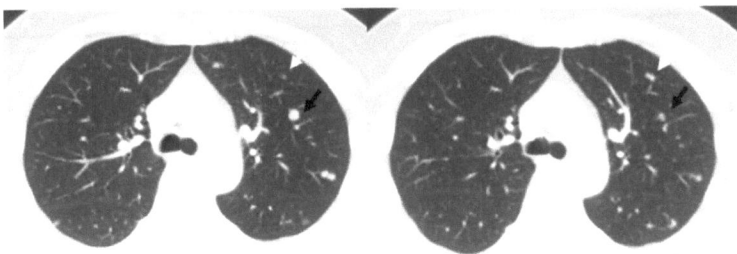

Figure 6. Dissociated responses in a melanoma patient during immunotherapy. CT assessment in pre-treatment phase (**A**) and at 3 months (**B**) follow-up: black arrows show the regression of the lesion while white arrows show the increase in lesion dimensions.

Considering these response patterns, the limits of conventional response criteria are clear. So, to overcome these limits, new criteria have been proposed. The first criteria were the immune-related response criteria (irRC), based on the WHO criteria [136]. In these criteria, two main features were introduced: (*a*) the first radiological progression may be confirmed after 4 weeks, so in this phase, the patient can be treated; (*b*) the development of new lesions is not assessed as a disease progression, but these may be included in the total tumor burden [136]. The main limit of irRC is due to the bi-dimensional measurement of target lesions. In addition, since the greater part of immunotherapy trials in development at that time have been assessed according to RECIST, the obtained results could be difficult to compare according to the new criteria [137]. Subsequently, the immune-related RECIST (irRECIST), established on the unidimensional evaluation [138], have been proposed. According to irRECIST, an increase of 20% in the total tumor burden from nadir with a minimum of 5 mm, such as the progression of non-target lesions or the appearance of a new lesion, has been defined as immune-related progression disease (irPD). Moreover, in this case, the irPD must been verified after 4 weeks, and if there is also a new unequivocal progression (UEP) in this phase, the patient is defined in disease progression [138].

To homogenize results between different trials, the RECIST working group proposed an adaptation to the immunotherapy version of RECIST1.1, the immune RECIST (iRECIST) [139]. The iRECIST identified a standard lexicon including immune complete response (iCR), immune stable disease (iSD), immune PR (iPR), and immune unconfirmed PD (iUPD) or confirmed PD (iCPD). The key element in iRECIST is that iUPD must be confirmed by imaging at least 4 weeks after the first evaluation, but no more than 8 weeks from iUPD, and that a patient may be classified as iUPD more times until there is an iCPD [139]. Regarding new lesions, these must not be involved in the sum of total tumor burden, but the patient can be classified as an iUPD. After an iUPD, the appearance of another new lesion, increase in size of target or non-target lesions, an increase in the sum of measurement of new target lesions >5 mm, or any progression of new non-target lesions can cause an iCPD [139].

Although these immunotherapy-response evaluation criteria have been proposed to allow the comparison of different clinical trial results, at the present, these are not utilized in clinical settings, such as none of these takes into account the atypical response patterns as hyperprogression or dissociated responses.

3. Immune-Related Adverse Events Assessment

If on the one hand, immunotherapy has improved oncological patient outcomes, on the other, these treatments have caused a rise in adverse events, called ir-AEs, which can involve several tissues and organs, from head to toe [93,95,96,151–153]. The ir-AEs are classified according to the Common Terminology Criteria for Adverse Events (CTCAE v 5.0) [94], which; moreover, permits to assess these events throughout several clinical trials. A systematic review showed that about 74% of patients treated with anti-PD-L-1 inhibitors developed ir-AEs, and among them, 14% had a grade ≥ 3, while the rate increased in anti-CTLA-4 inhibitors treated patients (about 89% and in this group, about 34% had a grade ≥ 3). When the authors evaluated patients treated with a combination of ICIs, the rate was 90%, and among them, 55% had a grade ≥ 3 [95].

The ir-AEs are relatively new conditions, so very little is known about them. The enhancement of the immune system is probably also responsible for an accidental autoimmune response [97–102,154–160]. Recombinant cytokines have a high toxicity profile, with low possibility either in terms of the target population either duration time. Toxic effects can involve several organs, as gastrointestinal tract, liver, lungs, heart, skin, endocrine, and hematologic systems [161–164]. The ir-AEs can appear early, even after the first dose. During ipilimumab treatment, the majority of ir-AEs appeared around 12 weeks, although the appearance time is due to the target: for skin, around 3 weeks; for the liver, around 3–9 weeks; for the gastrointestinal-tract, around 8 weeks; and for the endocrine system, around 7–20 weeks [165]. The majority of ir-AEs are mild or moderate, and readily reversed by stopping the treatment and starting corticosteroid therapy [128]. Otherwise, endocrinopathy related events are usually irreversible [128]. Life-threatening ir-AEs necessitate hospitalization and, in higher grade, intensive care unit admission [128]. To prevent the risk of milder forms becoming life threatening, radiologists should recognize ir-AEs and should inform the clinical team as soon as possible. Consequently, there is a rising request for radiologists to recognize ir-AEs imaging features to permit proper patient management [97–102,154,155].

Regarding ir-endocrinopathies, hypophysitis, occurring in 10–13% of ipilimumab patients, is the most frequent [99–101,166,167]. The typical symptoms are headache and fatigue with anterior hypopituitarism and multiple hormonal deficiencies. At MR assessment, the patient shows diffuse enlargement of the pituitary with no optic chiasm compression. It is possible to find pituitary stalk thickening, such as during post-contrast assessment pituitary enhancement [128].

With regard to gastrointestinal ir-AEs, the main symptom is diarrhea in a colitis setting [128]. A study of 162 melanoma ipilimumab treated patients showed colitis in 28 (19%) of them [168]. On CT evaluation, typical colitis features include bowel wall thickening with increased enhancement and mesenteric hyperemia, such as a fluid-filled colon. Considering the extension of the colitis, two patterns have been reported: the diffuse and segmental.

In the diffuse pattern, we find a fluid-filled distended colon with mild diffuse wall thickening and mesenteric vessel engorgement. In the segmental pattern, colitis is associated with pre-existing diverticulosis (SCAD), so that we find a moderate segmental wall thickening and pericolic fat stranding [128].

Pneumonia (Figure 7) is an ir-AE characterized by a focal or diffuse inflammation of the pulmonary parenchyma, and its incidence in immunotherapy-treated patients ranges from 0 to 10% [43]. Compared to pneumonia due to conventional chemotherapy, immunotherapy treated patients showed a greater susceptibility to develop this adverse event, showing an increased risk of high-grade pneumonia, which could cause significant morbidity, possible discontinuation of treatment, and a significant rate of mortality. However, according to previous authors, clinical and radiological diagnosis can improve patient outcomes [102,159,169–187]. Imaging has a critical role in pneumonitis detection, and CT is the modality that should been chosen since this tool allows the identification of all little changes in the lung and the characterization of different sub-types [179–187]. Delaunay et al. [159] identified different patterns on CT studies from 64 patients, (*a*) organized pneumonia (OP) (occurred in about the 23% of patients), (*b*) hypersensitivity pneumonitis (HP) (in 16% of patients), (*c*) non-specific interstitial pneumonia (NSIP) (in 8% of patients), and (*d*) bronchiolitis (in 6% of patients), showing as in the same patients was possible to detect different patterns [159].

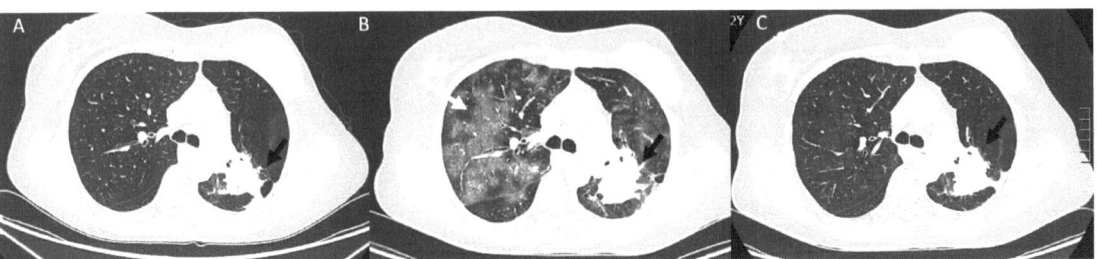

Figure 7. NSLC (black arrows) patient treated with immunotherapy. CT assessment in pre-treatment phase (**A**). During follow-up, in (**B**), appearance of ir-Pneumonitis (white arrow), with disease regression after corticosteroid treatment (**C**).

Usually, in OPs sub-type, the typical features are bilateral peribronchovascular and subpleural ground-glass and air space opacities, with mid- to lower-lung predominance [159].

CT features in HP pattern include diffuse and predominant ground glass centrilobular nodules in the upper lobe [159]. In NSIP pattern, there are ground glass and lattice opacities prevalently in the lower lobe. Sub-pleural sparing of the posterior and inferior lobes is a specific feature [159]. The bronchiolitis pattern is characterized by centrilobular nodularity, with a tree-in-bud pattern [159]. Acute interstitial pneumonia (AIP)–acute respiratory distress syndrome (ARDS) is not a typical pattern of ir-pneumonitis; however, it is possible to find this sub-type in extensive pulmonary involvement [43].

Granulomatosis and sarcoid-like lymphadenopathies involve mediastinal and hilar lymph nodes [128]. On CT, mediastinal and hilar lymphadenopathies have an appearance and distribution similar to sarcoidosis nodes [128], so it is critical to recognize this condition to avoid defining a PD.

Liver involvement is a rare condition (nearby 1–2% of treated patients) [128]; usually only elevated liver function test results are detected, while in severe cases of ir-hepatitis on imaging tools, it is possible to assess periportal edema, hepatomegaly, and periportal lymphadenopathies [128].

4. Radiomics and Immunotherapy

Recently, the idea that imaging studies contain a great amount of data as grey level patterns that usually are imperceptible to the human eyes has become more and more interesting [188–198]. These texture features, when correlated with clinical-pathological data and outcomes [199–211], theoretically allow for diagnostic and prognostic assessments and it could produce evidence-based clinical-decision support systems [212–220]. The assessment of textural characteristics, obtained using radiological images which depend on mathematical analysis as histogram analysis, is called radiomics [221–233]. The main objective is to combine several multimodal quantitative data with mathematical methods to provide clear and robust parameters allowing an outcome prediction. Radiomics offers outstanding benefits over qualitative imaging assessment since this is clearly limited by the subjective evaluation of radiologists. A radiomics information extension can be obtained by adding genomics data (radiogenomics); in fact, genomic markers, such as microRNA expression, have been shown to be associated with treatment response, metastatic spread, and prognosis that could offer personalized and precision medicine. This approach is captivating since it could be used to obtain molecular data from images [229,234–245] with no invasive approach to reduce costs, time, and any risk for the patient. For several tumors, radiomics has already offered a precise molecular assessment, allowing the recognition of biomarkers that are associated with the prognostic assessment [223–240].

Tumor immune phenotypes can be classified by histological and immunohistochemical analysis as immune-inflamed, immune-excluded, and immune-desert types [246]. Dense tumor-infiltrating lymphocytes (TILs) and a high tumor mutational burden characterize immune-inflamed tumors. These elements correlate strongly to favor immunotherapy response [247]. Otherwise, in immune-excluded and immune-desert types, which have low TILs and highly proliferating tumor cells, the probability of primary immune escape is high [89]. New biomarkers are needed to quantify TILs and PD-L1 expression to predict and monitor tumor immunotherapy response [248].

Several authors have assessed the radiomics features in predicting response for this treatment [39,249–256]. Granata et al. [39], in lung adenocarcinoma patients, showed that the shift in the center of mass of the lesion was significant as in prediction of overall survival (OS) as in prediction of progression free survival (PFS). By using univariate analysis, the authors obtained low diagnostic accuracy, while by using multivariate analysis, a support vector machine model showed the best results for stratifying patients based on OS (area under curve (AUC) of 0.89 and an accuracy of 81.6%). In addition, a decision tree model showed the best results for stratifying patients based on PFS time (AUC of 0.96 and an accuracy of 94.7%) [39]. Sun et al. [249], in a retrospective multicohort study, analyzed CT images and CD8 T cell RNA expression data from 135 treated patients with anti-PD-1 and anti-PD-L1 antibodies to identify and validate a radiomics signature to predict treatment response. They showed that a high baseline radiomics score was correlated with a higher objective response rate and OS [249]. Moreover, Tang et al. validated a non-small-cell lung cancer (NSCLC) radiomics signature associated with PD-L1 expression and density of TILs [250]. They showed that the radiomics signature was correlated to OS [250]. Tunali et al. [252] demonstrated that a pretreatment radiomics model was able to predict rapid disease progression phenotypes, including hyperprogression (AUCs ranging 0.804–0.865).

The results of these studies, although still in an embryonic phase, could support the hypothesis that radiomics analysis may represent an effective biomarker to select immunotherapy-responsive patients.

In addition, with great interest, we look at the possibility of applying radiomics to the identification of patients who will develop ir-AEs. Colen et al. [253], as the first group, assessed the possibility of radiomics to predict ir-pneumonitis. They obtained radiomics features from a CT study of patients who did ($n = 2$) and did not ($n = 30$) develop this event. However, the major limitation of this study was related to the number of patients and unbalanced groups ($n = 2$ vs. $n = 30$). Larger groups of patients and balanced groups are needed for radiomics analysis.

Thomas et al. [254] assessed 39 patients subjected to chemo-radiation therapy and consolidative ICI therapy for locally advanced NSCLC. They evaluated radiomics data, obtained by pre-treatment [99 mTc] MAA SPECT/CT perfusion images and clinical data. In their study population, 16/39 (41%) patients developed pneumonitis and, with regard to clinical characteristics, only the presence of baseline chronic obstructive pulmonary disease (COPD) was correlated to pneumonitis. Perfused lung radiomics texture features were correlated with lung volume, representing surrogates rather than independent predictors of pneumonitis risk. However, the major limit of this study was related to the number of patients and the lack of external validation group.

Several limitations to the clinical application of radiomics remain. The first key challenge is the use of different imaging techniques by different institutions. To ensure that the academic community can obtain high-quality radiological data resources, it is necessary to establish and promote certain imaging acquisition protocols. Second, the current research uses different software and different feature-selection methods, focuses on different feature sets, and applies different statistical and bioinformatic methods for data analysis and interpretation, which limit the reproducibility of radiomics models. Future research workflows need to be standardized. Third, many relevant radiomics studies employ single-center retrospective datasets. A quality-controlled multicenter prospective study plan is ideal. In addition, the evidence level rating reflects the feasibility of incorporating radiomics research into clinical practice. Recently published guidelines and checklists aiming to improve the quality of radiomics studies, including the radiomics quality score, modified Quality Assessment of Diagnostic Accuracy Studies tool, image biomarker standardization initiative guideline, and Transparent Reporting of a multivariable prediction model for Individual Prognosis or Diagnosis checklist, have been applied to radiomics evaluation [257,258].

5. Conclusions

Immunotherapy has a crucial role in the treatment of several tumors. Radiological assessment is essential for evaluating tumor response such as ir-AEs in immunotherapy-treated patients. Knowledge of the current response criteria and the response patterns, such as the different patterns of ir-AES, is critical for radiologists to offer valuable data for clinical providers to guide patient therapies. Radiomics analysis is a promising tool for the selection of responsive patients to immunotherapy such as in early ir-AES detections in order to avoid unnecessary treatments for unfit patients.

Author Contributions: Conceptualization, V.G., A.P. and R.F.; methodology, V.G. and S.V.S.; software, I.S. and V.V.; validation, C.P. and E.S.; formal analysis, V.G., R.F. and L.F.; investigation, L.F., C.P. and V.V.; resources, E.S., S.V.S. and M.G.V.; data curation, A.M. (Agnese Montanino), I.S. and E.S.; writing—original draft preparation, F.I., M.G.V. and A.M. (Agnese Montanino); writing—review and editing, P.A.A. and A.M. (Alessandro Morabito); visualization, A.P., A.M. (Alessandro Morabito), V.V. and F.I.; supervision, V.G.; project administration, V.G. All authors have read and agreed to the published version of the manuscript.

Funding: Funding by the Ministry of Health—Current Research 2022.

Data Availability Statement: Data are reported in the manuscript and images are reported at link https://zenodo.org/record/7521647#.Y72ceXbMK3A (accessed on 25 October 2022).

Acknowledgments: The authors are grateful to Alessandra Trocino, a librarian at the National Cancer Institute of Naples, Italy.

Conflicts of Interest: The authors declare no conflict of interest.

References

1. Riley, R.S.; June, C.H.; Langer, R.; Mitchell, M.J. Delivery technologies for cancer immunotherapy. *Nat. Rev. Drug Discov.* **2019**, *18*, 175–196. [CrossRef] [PubMed]
2. Abbott, M.; Ustoyev, Y. Cancer and the Immune System: The History and Background of Immunotherapy. *Semin. Oncol. Nurs.* **2019**, *35*, 150923. [CrossRef] [PubMed]
3. O'Donnell, J.S.; Teng, M.W.L.; Smyth, M.J. Cancer immunoediting and resistance to T cell-based immunotherapy. *Nat. Rev. Clin. Oncol.* **2019**, *16*, 151–167. [CrossRef] [PubMed]
4. Zhang, Y.; Zhang, Z. The history and advances in cancer immunotherapy: Understanding the characteristics of tumor-infiltrating immune cells and their therapeutic implications. *Cell. Mol. Immunol.* **2020**, *17*, 807–821. [CrossRef]
5. Merlotti, A.; Bruni, A.; Borghetti, P.; Ramella, S.; Scotti, V.; Trovò, M.; Chiari, R.; Lohr, F.; Ricardi, U.; Bria, E.; et al. Sequential chemo-hypofractionated RT versus concurrent standard CRT for locally advanced NSCLC: GRADE recommendation by the Italian Association of Radiotherapy and Clinical Oncology (AIRO). *Radiol. Med.* **2021**, *126*, 1117–1128. [CrossRef] [PubMed]
6. Lesch, S.; Gill, S. The promise and perils of immunotherapy. *Blood Adv.* **2021**, *5*, 3709–3725. [CrossRef]
7. Avallone, A.; Pecori, B.; Bianco, F.; Aloj, L.; Tatangelo, F.; Romano, C.; Granata, V.; Marone, P.; Leone, A.; Botti, G.; et al. Critical role of bevacizumab scheduling in combination with pre-surgical chemo-radiotherapy in MRI-defined high-risk locally advanced rectal cancer: Results of the BRANCH trial. *Oncotarget* **2015**, *6*, 30394–30407. [CrossRef]
8. Bimonte, S.; Leongito, M.; Barbieri, A.; Del Vecchio, V.; Barbieri, M.; Albino, V.; Piccirillo, M.; Amore, A.; Di Giacomo, R.; Nasto, A.; et al. Inhibitory effect of (-)-epigallocatechin-3-gallate and bleomycin on human pancreatic cancer MiaPaca-2 cell growth. *Infect. Agent Cancer* **2015**, *10*, 22. [CrossRef]
9. Ottaiano, A.; Scala, S.; Santorsola, M.; Trotta, A.M.; D'Alterio, C.; Portella, L.; Clemente, O.; Nappi, A.; Zanaletti, N.; De Stefano, A.; et al. Aflibercept or bevacizumab in combination with FOLFIRI as second-line treatment of mRAS metastatic colorectal cancer patients: The ARBITRATION study protocol. *Ther. Adv. Med. Oncol.* **2021**, *13*, 1758835921989223. [CrossRef]
10. Ottaiano, A.; Caraglia, M.; Di Mauro, A.; Botti, G.; Lombardi, A.; Galon, J.; Luce, A.; D'Amore, L.; Perri, F.; Santorsola, M.; et al. Evolution of Mutational Landscape and Tumor Immune-Microenvironment in Liver Oligo-Metastatic Colorectal Cancer. *Cancers* **2020**, *12*, 3073. [CrossRef]
11. Izzo, F.; Granata, V.; Fusco, R.; D'Alessio, V.; Petrillo, A.; Lastoria, S.; Piccirillo, M.; Albino, V.; Belli, A.; Tafuto, S.; et al. Clinical Phase I/II Study: Local Disease Control and Survival in Locally Advanced Pancreatic Cancer Treated with Electrochemotherapy. *J. Clin. Med.* **2021**, *10*, 1305. [CrossRef]
12. Izzo, F.; Granata, V.; Fusco, R.; D'Alessio, V.; Petrillo, A.; Lastoria, S.; Piccirillo, M.; Albino, V.; Belli, A.; Nasti, G.; et al. A Multicenter Randomized Controlled Prospective Study to Assess Efficacy of Laparoscopic Electrochemotherapy in the Treatment of Locally Advanced Pancreatic Cancer. *J. Clin. Med.* **2021**, *10*, 4011. [CrossRef] [PubMed]
13. Avallone, A.; Piccirillo, M.C.; Nasti, G.; Rosati, G.; Carlomagno, C.; Di Gennaro, E.; Romano, C.; Tatangelo, F.; Granata, V.; Cassata, A.; et al. Effect of Bevacizumab in Combination with Standard Oxaliplatin-Based Regimens in Patients with Metastatic Colorectal Cancer: A Randomized Clinical Trial. *JAMA Netw. Open* **2021**, *4*, e2118475. [CrossRef] [PubMed]
14. Fiore, F.; Somma, F.; D'Angelo, R.; Tarotto, L.; Stoia, V. Cone beam computed tomography (CBCT) guidance is helpful in reducing dose exposure to pediatric patients undergoing radiofrequency ablation of osteoid osteoma. *Radiol Med.* **2022**, *127*, 183–190. [CrossRef] [PubMed]
15. Falcinelli, L.; Mendichi, M.; Chierchini, S.; Tenti, M.V.; Bellavita, R.; Saldi, S.; Ingrosso, G.; Reggioli, V.; Bini, V.; Aristei, C. Pulmonary function in stereotactic body radiotherapy with helical tomotherapy for primary and metastatic lung lesions. *Radiol. Med.* **2021**, *126*, 163–169. [CrossRef] [PubMed]
16. Arslan, A.; Aktas, E.; Sengul, B.; Tekin, B. Dosimetric evaluation of left ventricle and left anterior descending artery in left breast radiotherapy. *Radiol. Med.* **2021**, *126*, 14–21. [CrossRef]

17. Barra, S.; Guarnieri, A.; di Monale EBastia, M.B.; Marcenaro, M.; Tornari, E.; Belgioia, L.; Magrini, S.M.; Ricardi, U.; Corvò, R. Short fractionation radiotherapy for early prostate cancer in the time of COVID-19: Long-term excellent outcomes from a multicenter Italian trial suggest a larger adoption in clinical practice. *Radiol. Med.* **2021**, *126*, 142–146. [CrossRef] [PubMed]
18. Cellini, F.; Di Franco, R.; Manfrida, S.; Borzillo, V.; Maranzano, E.; Pergolizzi, S.; Morganti, A.G.; Fusco, V.; Deodato, F.; Santarelli, M.; et al. Palliative radiotherapy indications during the COVID-19 pandemic and in future complex logistic settings: The NORMALITY model. *Radiol. Med.* **2021**, *126*, 1619–1656. [CrossRef] [PubMed]
19. Ottaiano, A.; Petito, A.; Santorsola, M.; Gigantino, V.; Capuozzo, M.; Fontanella, D.; Di Franco, R.; Borzillo, V.; Buonopane, S.; Ravo, V.; et al. Prospective Evaluation of Radiotherapy-Induced Immunologic and Genetic Effects in Colorectal Cancer Oligo-Metastatic Patients with Lung-Limited Disease: The PRELUDE-1 Study. *Cancers* **2021**, *13*, 4236. [CrossRef] [PubMed]
20. Lancellotta, V.; Del Regno, L.; Di Stefani, A.; Fionda, B.; Marazzi, F.; Rossi, E.; Balducci, M.; Pampena, R.; Morganti, A.G.; Mangoni, M.; et al. The role of stereotactic radiotherapy in addition to immunotherapy in the management of melanoma brain metastases: Results of a systematic review. *Radiol. Med.* **2022**, *127*, 773–783. [CrossRef]
21. Lev, S. Targeted therapy and drug resistance in triple-negative breast cancer: The EGFR axis. *Biochem. Soc. Trans.* **2020**, *48*, 657–665. [CrossRef]
22. Shariati, M.; Meric-Bernstam, F. Targeting AKT for cancer therapy. *Expert Opin. Investig. Drugs* **2019**, *28*, 977–988. [CrossRef] [PubMed]
23. Hussein, M.A.M.; Cafarelli, F.P.; Paparella, M.T.; Rennie, W.J.; Guglielmi, G. Phosphaturic mesenchymal tumors: Radiological aspects and suggested imaging pathway. *Radiol. Med.* **2021**, *126*, 1609–1618. [CrossRef]
24. Wang, F.H.; Zheng, H.L.; Li, J.T.; Li, P.; Zheng, C.H.; Chen, Q.Y.; Huang, C.M.; Xie, J.W. Prediction of recurrence-free survival and adjuvant therapy benefit in patients with gastrointestinal stromal tumors based on radiomics features. *Radiol Med.* **2022**, *127*, 1085–1097. [CrossRef] [PubMed]
25. Zafar, A.; Wang, W.; Liu, G.; Wang, X.; Xian, W.; McKeon, F.; Foster, J.; Zhou, J.; Zhang, R. Molecular targeting therapies for neuroblastoma: Progress and challenges. *Med. Res. Rev.* **2021**, *41*, 961–1021. [CrossRef] [PubMed]
26. Laurelli, G.; Falcone, F.; Gallo, M.S.; Scala, F.; Losito, S.; Granata, V.; Cascella, M.; Greggi, S. Long-Term Oncologic and Reproductive Outcomes in Young Women with Early Endometrial Cancer Conservatively Treated: A Prospective Study and Literature Update. *Int. J. Gynecol. Cancer* **2016**, *26*, 1650–1657. [CrossRef] [PubMed]
27. Colli, L.M.; Machiela, M.J.; Zhang, H.; Myers, T.A.; Jessop, L.; Delattre, O.; Yu, K.; Chanock, S.J. Landscape of Combination Immunotherapy and Targeted Therapy to Improve Cancer Management. *Cancer Res.* **2017**, *77*, 3666–3671. [CrossRef]
28. Polesel, J.; Talamini, R.; Montella, M.; Maso, L.D.; Crovatto, M.; Parpinel, M.; Izzo, F.; Tommasi, L.G.; Serraino, D.; La Vecchia, C.; et al. Nutrients intake and the risk of hepatocellular carcinoma in Italy. *Eur. J. Cancer* **2007**, *43*, 2381–2387. [CrossRef]
29. Pignata, S.; Gallo, C.; Daniele, B.; Elba, S.; Giorgio, A.; Capuano, G.; Adinolfi, L.E.; De Sio, I.; Izzo, F.; Farinati, F.; et al. Characteristics at presentation and outcome of hepatocellular carcinoma (HCC) in the elderly. A study of the Cancer of the Liver Italian Program (CLIP). *Crit. Rev. Oncol. Hematol.* **2006**, *59*, 243–249. [CrossRef] [PubMed]
30. Baxter, D. Active and passive immunization for cancer. *Hum. Vaccines Immunother.* **2014**, *10*, 2123–2129. [CrossRef]
31. Bregy, A.; Wong, T.M.; Shah, A.H.; Goldberg, J.M.; Komotar, R.J. Active immunotherapy using dendritic cells in the treatment of glioblastoma multiforme. *Cancer Treat. Rev.* **2013**, *39*, 891–907. [CrossRef]
32. Foy, J.P.; Karabajakian, A.; Ortiz-Cuaran, S.; Boussageon, M.; Michon, L.; Bouaoud, J.; Fekiri, D.; Robert, M.; Baffert, K.A.; Hervé, G.; et al. Datasets for gene expression profiles of head and neck squamous cell carcinoma and lung cancer treated or not by PD1/PD-L1 inhibitors. *Data Brief* **2022**, *44*, 108556. [CrossRef]
33. Vavolizza, R.D.; Petroni, G.R.; Mauldin, I.S.; Chianese-Bullock, K.A.; Olson, W.C.; Smith, K.T.; Dengel, L.T.; Haden, K.; Grosh, W.W.; Kaur, V.; et al. Phase I/II clinical trial of a helper peptide vaccine plus PD-1 blockade in PD-1 antibody-naïve and PD-1 antibody-experienced patients with melanoma (MEL64). *J. Immunother. Cancer* **2022**, *10*, e005424. [CrossRef] [PubMed]
34. Yang, M.; Mahanty, A.; Jin, C.; Wong, A.N.N.; Yoo, J.S. Label-free metabolic imaging for sensitive and robust monitoring of anti-CD47 immunotherapy response in triple-negative breast cancer. *J. Immunother. Cancer* **2022**, *10*, e005199. [CrossRef] [PubMed]
35. Gao, T.T.; Shan, J.H.; Yang, Y.X.; Zhang, Z.W.; Liu, S.L.; Xi, M.; Zhao, L. Comparative efficacy and safety of immunotherapy for patients with advanced or metastatic esophageal squamous cell carcinoma: A systematic review and network Meta-analysis. *BMC Cancer* **2022**, *22*, 992. [CrossRef] [PubMed]
36. Wang, Y.; Lai, Y.; Peng, H.; Yan, S.; Liu, Z.; Tong, C.; Huang, X. Multiparametric immune profiling of advanced cervical cancer to predict response to programmed death-1 inhibitor combination therapy: An exploratory study of the CLAP trial. *Clin. Transl. Oncol.* **2022**, *25*, 256–268. [CrossRef] [PubMed]
37. Yuan, Z.G.; Zeng, T.M.; Tao, C.J. Current and emerging immunotherapeutic approaches for biliary tract cancers. *Hepatobiliary Pancreat. Dis. Int.* **2022**, *21*, 440–449. [CrossRef]
38. Taieb, J.; Svrcek, M.; Cohen, R.; Basile, D.; Tougeron, D.; Phelip, J.M. Deficient mismatch repair/microsatellite unstable colorectal cancer: Diagnosis, prognosis and treatment. *Eur. J. Cancer* **2022**, *175*, 136–157. [CrossRef]
39. Granata, V.; Fusco, R.; De Muzio, F.; Cutolo, C.; Setola, S.V.; Dell'Aversana, F.; Grassi, F.; Belli, A.; Silvestro, L.; Ottaiano, A.; et al. Radiomics and machine learning analysis based on magnetic resonance imaging in the assessment of liver mucinous colorectal metastases. *Radiol. Med.* **2022**, *127*, 763–772. [CrossRef]

40. Granata, V.; Grassi, R.; Fusco, R.; Belli, A.; Palaia, R.; Carrafiello, G.; Miele, V.; Grassi, R.; Petrillo, A.; Izzo, F. Local ablation of pancreatic tumors: State of the art and future perspectives. *World J. Gastroenterol.* **2021**, *27*, 3413–3428. [CrossRef]
41. Cholangiocarcinoma Working Group. Italian Clinical Practice Guidelines on Cholangiocarcinoma—Part II: Treatment. *Dig. Liver Dis.* **2020**, *52*, 1430–1442. [CrossRef] [PubMed]
42. Ottaiano, A.; de Vera d'Aragona, R.P.; Trotta, A.M.; Santorsola, M.; Napolitano, M.; Scognamiglio, G.; Tatangelo, F.; Grieco, P.; Zappavigna, S.; Granata, V.; et al. Characterization of KRAS Mutational Regression in Oligometastatic Patients. *Front. Immunol.* **2022**, *13*, 898561. [CrossRef] [PubMed]
43. Fusco, R.; Simonetti, I.; Ianniello, S.; Villanacci, A.; Grassi, F.; Dell'Aversana, F.; Grassi, R.; Cozzi, D.; Bicci, E.; Palumbo, P.; et al. Pulmonary Lymphangitis Poses a Major Challenge for Radiologists in an Oncological Setting during the COVID-19 Pandemic. *J. Pers. Med.* **2022**, *12*, 624. [CrossRef] [PubMed]
44. Hodi, F.S.; O'Day, S.J.; McDermott, D.F.; Weber, R.W.; Sosman, J.A.; Haanen, J.B.; Gonzalez, R.; Robert, C.; Schadendorf, D.; Hassel, J.C.; et al. Improved survival with ipilimumab in patients with metastatic melanoma. *New Engl. J. Med.* **2010**, *363*, 711–723. [CrossRef]
45. Fushimi, Y.; Yoshida, K.; Okawa, M.; Maki, T.; Nakajima, S.; Sakata, A.; Okuchi, S.; Hinoda, T.; Kanagaki, M.; Nakamoto, Y. Vessel wall MR imaging in neuroradiology. *Radiol. Med.* **2022**, *127*, 1032–1045. [CrossRef] [PubMed]
46. Granata, V.; Simonetti, I.; Fusco, R.; Setola, S.V.; Izzo, F.; Scarpato, L.; Vanella, V.; Festino, L.; Simeone, E.; Ascierto, P.A.; et al. Management of cutaneous melanoma: Radiologists challenging and risk assessment. *Radiol. Med.* **2022**, *127*, 899–911. [CrossRef]
47. Michielin, O.; van Akkooi, A.C.J.; Ascierto, P.A.; Dummer, R.; Keilholz, U. Cutaneous melanoma: ESMO Clinical Practice Guidelines for diagnosis, treatment and follow-up. *Ann. Oncol.* **2019**, *30*, 1884–1901. [CrossRef]
48. Keilholz, U.; Ascierto, P.A.; Dummer, R.; Robert, C.; Lorigan, P.; van Akkooi, A.; Arance, A.; Blank, C.U.; Chiarion Sileni, V.; Donia, M.; et al. ESMO consensus conference recommendations on the management of metastatic melanoma: Under the auspices of the ESMO Guidelines Committee. *Ann. Oncol.* **2020**, *31*, 1435–1448. [CrossRef] [PubMed]
49. Cirillo, L.; Rustici, A.; Toni, F.; Zoli, M.; Bartiromo, F.; Gramegna, L.L.; Cicala, D.; Tonon, C.; Caranci, F.; Lodi, R. Vessel Wall MRI: Clinical implementation in cerebrovascular disorders-technical aspects. *Radiol. Med.* **2022**, *127*, 645–651. [CrossRef]
50. Tagliafico, A.S.; Campi, C.; Bianca, B.; Bortolotto, C.; Buccicardi, D.; Francesca, C.; Prost, R.; Rengo, M.; Faggioni, L. Blockchain in radiology research and clinical practice: Current trends and future directions. *Radiol. Med.* **2022**, *127*, 391–397. [CrossRef]
51. Perrone, F.; Gallo, C.; Daniele, B.; Gaeta, G.B.; Izzo, F.; Capuano, G.; Adinolfi, L.E.; Mazzanti, R.; Farinati, F.; Elba, S.; et al. Tamoxifen in the treatment of hepatocellular carcinoma: 5-year results of the CLIP-1 multicentre randomised controlled trial. *Curr. Pharm. Des.* **2002**, *8*, 1013–1019. [CrossRef] [PubMed]
52. Granata, V.; Fusco, R.; Salati, S.; Petrillo, A.; Di Bernardo, E.; Grassi, R.; Palaia, R.; Danti, G.; La Porta, M.; Cadossi, M.; et al. A Systematic Review about Imaging and Histopathological Findings for Detecting and Evaluating Electroporation Based Treatments Response. *Int. J. Environ. Res. Public Health* **2021**, *18*, 5592. [CrossRef]
53. Larkin, J.; Chiarion-Sileni, V.; Gonzalez, R.; Grob, J.J.; Rutkowski, P.; Lao, C.D.; Cowey, C.L.; Schadendorf, D.; Wagstaff, J.; Dummer, R.; et al. Five-Year Survival with Combined Nivolumab and Ipilimumab in Advanced Melanoma. *New Engl. J. Med.* **2019**, *381*, 1535–1546. [CrossRef]
54. Chiti, G.; Grazzini, G.; Flammia, F.; Matteuzzi, B.; Tortoli, P.; Bettarini, S.; Pasqualini, E.; Granata, V.; Busoni, S.; Messserini, L.; et al. Gastroenteropancreatic neuroendocrine neoplasms (GEP-NENs): A radiomic model to predict tumor grade. *Radiol. Med.* **2022**, *127*, 928–938. [CrossRef]
55. Granata, V.; Grassi, R.; Fusco, R.; Setola, S.V.; Belli, A.; Ottaiano, A.; Nasti, G.; La Porta, M.; Danti, G.; Cappabianca, S.; et al. Intrahepatic cholangiocarcinoma and its differential diagnosis at MRI: How radiologist should assess MR features. *Radiol. Med.* **2021**, *126*, 1584–1600. [CrossRef] [PubMed]
56. Cholangiocarcinoma Working Group. Italian Clinical Practice Guidelines on Cholangiocarcinoma—Part I: Classification, diagnosis and staging. *Dig. Liver Dis.* **2020**, *52*, 1282–1293. [CrossRef]
57. Granata, V.; Fusco, R.; De Muzio, F.; Cutolo, C.; Setola, S.V.; Grassi, R.; Grassi, F.; Ottaiano, A.; Nasti, G.; Tatangelo, F.; et al. Radiomics textural features by MR imaging to assess clinical outcomes following liver resection in colorectal liver metastases. *Radiol. Med.* **2022**, *127*, 461–470. [CrossRef]
58. Fusco, R.; Setola, S.V.; Raiano, N.; Granata, V.; Cerciello, V.; Pecori, B.; Petrillo, A. Analysis of a monocentric computed tomography dosimetric database using a radiation dose index monitoring software: Dose levels and alerts before and after the implementation of the adaptive statistical iterative reconstruction on CT images. *Radiol. Med.* **2022**, *127*, 733–742. [CrossRef]
59. Robert, C.; Long, G.V.; Brady, B.; Dutriaux, C.; Maio, M.; Mortier, L.; Hassel, J.C.; Rutkowski, P.; McNeil, C.; Kalinka-Warzocha, E.; et al. Nivolumab in previously untreated melanoma without BRAF mutation. *New Engl. J. Med.* **2015**, *372*, 320–330. [CrossRef]
60. Seth, R.; Messersmith, H.; Kaur, V.; Kirkwood, J.M.; Kudchadkar, R.; McQuade, J.L.; Provenzano, A.; Swami, U.; Weber, J.; Alluri, K.C.; et al. Systemic Therapy for Melanoma: ASCO Guideline. *J. Clin. Oncol.* **2020**, *38*, 3947–3970. [CrossRef]
61. Weber, J.; Mandala, M.; Del Vecchio, M.; Gogas, H.J.; Arance, A.M.; Cowey, C.L.; Dalle, S.; Schenker, M.; Chiarion-Sileni, V.; Marquez-Rodas, I.; et al. Adjuvant Nivolumab versus Ipilimumab in Resected Stage III or IV Melanoma. *New Engl. J. Med.* **2017**, *377*, 1824–1835. [CrossRef] [PubMed]
62. Wolchok, J.D.; Chiarion-Sileni, V.; Gonzalez, R.; Rutkowski, P.; Grob, J.J.; Cowey, C.L.; Lao, C.D.; Wagstaff, J.; Schadendorf, D.; Ferrucci, P.F.; et al. Overall Survival with Combined Nivolumab and Ipilimumab in Advanced Melanoma. *New Engl. J. Med.* **2017**, *377*, 1345–1356. [CrossRef]

63. Ascierto, P.A.; Del Vecchio, M.; Mandalá, M.; Gogas, H.; Arance, A.M.; Dalle, S.; Cowey, C.L.; Schenker, M.; Grob, J.J.; Chiarion-Sileni, V.; et al. Adjuvant nivolumab versus ipilimumab in resected stage IIIB-C and stage IV melanoma (CheckMate 238): 4-year results from a multicentre, double-blind, randomised, controlled, phase 3 trial. *Lancet Oncol.* **2020**, *21*, 1465–1477. [CrossRef] [PubMed]
64. Amaria, R.N.; Menzies, A.M.; Burton, E.M.; Scolyer, R.A.; Tetzlaff, M.T.; Antdbacka, R.; Ariyan, C.; Bassett, R.; Carter, B.; Daud, A.; et al. Neoadjuvant systemic therapy in melanoma: Recommendations of the International Neoadjuvant Melanoma Consortium. *Lancet Oncol.* **2019**, *20*, e378–e389. [CrossRef] [PubMed]
65. Gutzmer, R.; Stroyakovskiy, D.; Gogas, H.; Robert, C.; Lewis, K.; Protsenko, S.; Pereira, R.P.; Eigentler, T.; Rutkowski, P.; Demidov, L.; et al. Atezolizumab, vemurafenib, and cobimetinib as first-line treatment for unresectable advanced BRAF^{V600} mutation-positive melanoma (IMspire150): Primary analysis of the randomised, double-blind, placebo-controlled, phase 3 trial. *Lancet* **2020**, *395*, 1835–1844. [CrossRef]
66. Barretta, M.L.; Catalano, O.; Setola, S.V.; Granata, V.; Marone, U.; D'Errico Gallipoli, A. Gallbladder metastasis: Spectrum of imaging findings. *Abdom. Imaging* **2011**, *36*, 729–734. [CrossRef]
67. Chapman, P.B.; Hauschild, A.; Robert, C.; Haanen, J.B.; Ascierto, P.; Larkin, J.; Dummer, R.; Garbe, C.; Testori, A.; Maio, M.; et al. Improved survival with vemurafenib in melanoma with BRAF V600E mutation. *New Engl. J. Med.* **2011**, *364*, 2507–2516. [CrossRef]
68. Fusco, R.; Granata, V.; Sansone, M.; Rega, D.; Delrio, P.; Tatangelo, F.; Romano, C.; Avallone, A.; Pupo, D.; Giordano, M.; et al. Validation of the standardized index of shape tool to analyze DCE-MRI data in the assessment of neo-adjuvant therapy in locally advanced rectal cancer. *Radiol. Med.* **2021**, *126*, 1044–1054. [CrossRef] [PubMed]
69. Ascierto, P.A.; Kirkwood, J.M.; Grob, J.J.; Simeone, E.; Grimaldi, A.M.; Maio, M.; Palmieri, G.; Testori, A.; Marincola, F.M.; Mozzillo, N. The role of BRAF V600 mutation in melanoma. *J. Transl. Med.* **2012**, *10*, 85. [CrossRef] [PubMed]
70. Fusco, R.; Sansone, M.; Granata, V.; Setola, S.V.; Petrillo, A. A systematic review on multiparametric MR imaging in prostate cancer detection. *Infect. Agents Cancer* **2017**, *312*, 57. [CrossRef]
71. Granier, C.; De Guillebon, E.; Blanc, C.; Roussel, H.; Badoual, C.; Colin, E.; Saldmann, A.; Gey, A.; Oudard, S.; Tartour, E. Mechanisms of action and rationale for the use of checkpoint inhibitors in cancer. *ESMO Open* **2017**, *2*, e000213. [CrossRef] [PubMed]
72. Martínez-Lostao, L.; Anel, A.; Pardo, J. How Do Cyto-toxic Lymphocytes Kill Cancer Cells? *Clin. Cancer Res.* **2015**, *21*, 5047–5056. [CrossRef]
73. Hegde, P.S.; Chen, D.S. Top 10 Challenges in Cancer Immunotherapy. *Immunity* **2020**, *52*, 17–35. [CrossRef]
74. Zimmermannova, O.; Caiado, I.; Ferreira, A.G.; Pereira, C.F. Cell Fate Reprogramming in the Era of Cancer Immunotherapy. *Front. Immunol.* **2021**, *12*, 714822. [CrossRef]
75. Schoenfeld, A.J.; Hellmann, M.D. Acquired Resistance to Immune Checkpoint Inhibitors. *Cancer Cell* **2020**, *37*, 443–455. [CrossRef] [PubMed]
76. Stefanini, M.; Simonetti, G. Interventional Magnetic Resonance Imaging Suite (IMRIS): How to build and how to use. *Radiol. Med.* **2022**, *127*, 1063–1067. [CrossRef] [PubMed]
77. Renzulli, M.; Brandi, N.; Argalia, G.; Brocchi, S.; Farolfi, A.; Fanti, S.; Golfieri, R. Morphological, dynamic and functional characteristics of liver pseudolesions and benign lesions. *Radiol. Med.* **2022**, *127*, 129–144. [CrossRef] [PubMed]
78. Palatresi, D.; Fedeli, F.; Danti, G.; Pasqualini, E.; Castiglione, F.; Messerini, L.; Massi, D.; Bettarini, S.; Tortoli, P.; Busoni, S.; et al. Correlation of CT radiomic features for GISTs with pathological classification and molecular subtypes: Preliminary and monocentric experience. *Radiol. Med.* **2022**, *127*, 117–128. [CrossRef] [PubMed]
79. Ledda, R.E.; Silva, M.; McMichael, N.; Sartorio, C.; Branchi, C.; Milanese, G.; Nayak, S.M.; Sverzellati, N. The diagnostic value of grey-scale inversion technique in chest radiography. *Radiol. Med.* **2022**, *127*, 294–304. [CrossRef] [PubMed]
80. Ierardi, A.M.; Stellato, E.; Pellegrino, G.; Bonelli, C.; Cellina, M.; Renzulli, M.; Biondetti, P.; Carrafiello, G. Fluid-dynamic control microcatheter used with glue: Preliminary experience on its feasibility and safety. *Radiol. Med.* **2022**, *127*, 272–276. [CrossRef] [PubMed]
81. Sansone, M.; Marrone, S.; Di Salvio, G.; Belfiore, M.P.; Gatta, G.; Fusco, R.; Vanore, L.; Zuiani, C.; Grassi, F.; Vietri, M.T.; et al. Comparison between two packages for pectoral muscle removal on mammographic images. *Radiol. Med.* **2022**, *127*, 848–856. [CrossRef] [PubMed]
82. Granata, V.; Fusco, R.; Belli, A.; Danti, G.; Bicci, E.; Cutolo, C.; Petrillo, A.; Izzo, F. Diffusion weighted imaging and diffusion kurtosis imaging in abdominal oncological setting: Why and when. *Infect. Agents Cancer* **2022**, *17*, 25. [CrossRef] [PubMed]
83. Petrillo, A.; Fusco, R.; Di Bernardo, E.; Petrosino, T.; Barretta, M.L.; Porto, A.; Granata, V.; Di Bonito, M.; Fanizzi, A.; Massafra, R.; et al. Prediction of Breast Cancer Histological Outcome by Radiomics and Artificial Intelligence Analysis in Contrast-Enhanced Mammography. *Cancers* **2022**, *14*, 2132. [CrossRef] [PubMed]
84. Granata, V.; Fusco, R.; De Muzio, F.; Cutolo, C.; Setola, S.V.; Dell'Aversana, F.; Belli, A.; Romano, C.; Ottaiano, A.; Nasti, G.; et al. Magnetic Resonance Features of Liver Mucinous Colorectal Metastases: What the Radiologist Should Know. *J. Clin. Med.* **2022**, *11*, 2221. [CrossRef] [PubMed]
85. Cutolo, C.; Dell'Aversana, F.; Fusco, R.; Grazzini, G.; Chiti, G.; Simonetti, I.; Bruno, F.; Palumbo, P.; Pierpaoli, L.; Valeri, T.; et al. Combined Hepatocellular-Cholangiocarcinoma: What the Multidisciplinary Team Should Know. *Diagnostics* **2022**, *12*, 890. [CrossRef]

86. Committeri, U.; Fusco, R.; Di Bernardo, E.; Abbate, V.; Salzano, G.; Maglitto, F.; Dell'Aversana Orabona, G.; Piombino, P.; Bonavolontà, P.; Arena, A.; et al. Radiomics Metrics Combined with Clinical Data in the Surgical Management of Early-Stage (cT1-T2 N0) Tongue Squamous Cell Carcinomas: A Preliminary Study. *Biology* **2022**, *11*, 468. [CrossRef]
87. Reck, M.; Rodríguez-Abreu, D.; Robinson, A.G.; Hui, R.; Csőszi, T.; Fülöp, A.; Gottfried, M.; Peled, N.; Tafreshi, A.; Cuffe, S.; et al. Pembrolizumab versus chemotherapy for PD-L1-positive non- small-cell lung cancer. *N. Engl. J. Med.* **2016**, *375*, 1823–1833. [CrossRef]
88. Hamid, O.; Molinero, L.; Bolen, C.R.; Sosman, J.A.; Muñoz-Couselo, E.; Kluger, H.M.; McDermott, D.F.; Powderly, J.D.; Sarkar, I.; Ballinger, M.; et al. Safety, Clinical Activity, and Biological Correlates of Response in Patients with Metastatic Melanoma: Results from a Phase I Trial of Atezolizumab. *Clin. Cancer Res.* **2019**, *25*, 6061–6072. [CrossRef]
89. Kim, J.M.; Chen, D.S. Immune escape to PD-L1/PD-1 blockade: Seven steps to success (or failure). *Ann. Oncol.* **2016**, *8*, 1492–1504. [CrossRef]
90. Anagnostou, V.; Smith, K.N.; Forde, P.M.; Niknafs, N.; Bhattacharya, R.; White, J.; Zhang, T.; Adleff, V.; Phallen, J.; Wali, N.; et al. Evolution of Neoantigen Landscape during Immune Checkpoint Blockade in Non-Small Cell Lung Cancer. *Cancer Discov.* **2017**, *7*, 264–276. [CrossRef]
91. Wang, D.Y.; Eroglu, Z.; Ozgun, A.; Leger, P.D.; Zhao, S.; Ye, F.; Luke, J.J.; Joseph, R.W.; Haq, R.; Ott, P.A.; et al. Clinical Features of Acquired Resistance to Anti-PD-1 Therapy in Advanced Melanoma. *Cancer Immunol. Res.* **2017**, *5*, 357–362. [CrossRef]
92. McGranahan, N.; Rosenthal, R.; Hiley, C.T.; Rowan, A.J.; Watkins, T.B.K.; Wilson, G.A.; Birkbak, N.J.; Veeriah, S.; Van Loo, P.; Herrero, J.; et al. Allele-Specific HLA Loss and Immune Escape in Lung Cancer Evolution. *Cell* **2017**, *171*, 1259–1271.e11. [CrossRef]
93. Darnell, E.P.; Mooradian, M.J.; Baruch, E.N.; Yilmaz, M.; Reynolds, K.L. Immune-Related Adverse Events (irAEs): Diagnosis, Management, and Clinical Pearls. *Curr. Oncol. Rep.* **2020**, *22*, 39. [CrossRef]
94. Common Terminology Criteria for Adverse Events (CTCAE) V5. Available online: https://ctep.cancer.gov/protocolDevelopment/electronic_applications/ctc.htm (accessed on 25 October 2022).
95. Arnaud-Coffin, P.; Maillet, D.; Gan, H.K.; Stelmes, J.-J.; You, B.; Dalle, S.; Péron, J. A systematic review of adverse events in randomized trials assessing immune checkpoint inhibitors. *Int. J. Cancer* **2019**, *145*, 639–648. [CrossRef]
96. Simeone, E.; Grimaldi, A.M.; Festino, L.; Trojaniello, C.; Vitale, M.G.; Vanella, V.; Palla, M.; Ascierto, P.A. Immunotherapy in metastatic melanoma: A novel scenario of new toxicities and their management. *Melanoma Manag.* **2019**, *6*, MMT30. [CrossRef]
97. Nishino, M.; Hatabu, H.; Hodi, F.S. Imaging of Cancer Immunotherapy: Current Approaches and Future Directions. *Radiology* **2019**, *290*, 9–22. [CrossRef]
98. Brahmer, J.R.; Abu-Sbeih, H.; Ascierto, P.A.; Brufsky, J.; Cappelli, L.C.; Cortazar, F.B.; Gerber, D.E.; Hamad, L.; Hansen, E.; Johnson, D.B.; et al. Society for Immunotherapy of Cancer (SITC) clinical practice guideline on immune checkpoint inhibitor-related adverse events. *J. Immunother. Cancer* **2021**, *9*, e002435. [CrossRef]
99. Comstock, D.E.; Nishino, M.; Giardino, A.A. Headache in the setting of immunotherapy treatment for metastatic melanoma. *JAMA Oncol.* **2017**, *3*, 703–704. [CrossRef]
100. Faje, A.T.; Sullivan, R.; Lawrence, D.; Tritos, N.A.; Fadden, R.; Klibanski, A.; Nachtigall, L. Ipilimumab-induced hypophysitis: A detailed longitudinal analysis in a large cohort of patients with metastatic melanoma. *J. Clin. Endocrinol. Metab.* **2014**, *99*, 4078–4085. [CrossRef]
101. Min, L.; Hodi, F.S.; Giobbie-Hurder, A.; Ott, P.A.; Luke, J.J.; Donahue, H.; Davis, M.; Carroll, R.S.; Kaiser, U.B. Systemic high-dose corticosteroid treatment does not improve the outcome of ipilimumab-related hypophysitis: A retrospective cohort study. *Clin. Cancer Res.* **2015**, *21*, 749–755. [CrossRef]
102. Khunger, M.; Rakshit, S.; Pasupuleti, V.; Hernandez, A.V.; Mazzone, P.; Stevenson, J.; Pennell, N.A.; Velcheti, V. Incidence of Pneumonitis with Use of Programmed Death 1 and Programmed Death-Ligand 1 Inhibitors in Non-Small Cell Lung Cancer: A Systematic Review and Meta-Analysis of Trials. *Chest* **2017**, *152*, 271–281. [CrossRef] [PubMed]
103. Kalisz, K.R.; Ramaiya, N.H.; Laukamp, K.R.; Gupta, A. Immune Checkpoint Inhibitor Therapy-related Pneumonitis: Patterns and Management. *Radiographics* **2019**, *39*, 1923–1937. [CrossRef] [PubMed]
104. Bianchi, A.; Mazzoni, L.N.; Busoni, S.; Pinna, N.; Albanesi, M.; Cavigli, E.; Cozzi, D.; Poggesi, A.; Miele, V.; Fainardi, E.; et al. Assessment of cerebrovascular disease with computed tomography in COVID-19 patients: Correlation of a novel specific visual score with increased mortality risk. *Radiol. Med.* **2021**, *126*, 570–576. [CrossRef] [PubMed]
105. Cartocci, G.; Colaiacomo, M.C.; Lanciotti, S.; Andreoli, C.; De Cicco, M.L.; Brachetti, G.; Pugliese, S.; Capoccia, L.; Tortora, A.; Scala, A.; et al. Correction to: Chest CT for early detection and management of coronavirus disease (COVID-19): A report of 314 patients admitted to Emergency Department with suspected pneumonia. *Radiol. Med.* **2021**, *126*, 642. [CrossRef] [PubMed]
106. Masci, G.M.; Iafrate, F.; Ciccarelli, F.; Pambianchi, G.; Panebianco, V.; Pasculli, P.; Ciardi, M.R.; Mastroianni, C.M.; Ricci, P.; Catalano, C.; et al. Tocilizumab effects in COVID-19 pneumonia: Role of CT texture analysis in quantitative assessment of response to therapy. *Radiol. Med.* **2021**, *126*, 1170–1180. [CrossRef] [PubMed]
107. Francolini, G.; Desideri, I.; Stocchi, G.; Ciccone, L.P.; Salvestrini, V.; Garlatti, P.; Aquilano, M.; Greto, D.; Bonomo, P.; Meattini, I.; et al. Impact of COVID-19 on workload burden of a complex radiotherapy facility. *Radiol. Med.* **2021**, *126*, 717–721. [CrossRef]
108. McKay, M.J.; Foster, R. Radiation recall reactions: An oncologic enigma. *Crit. Rev. Oncol.* **2021**, *168*, 103527. [CrossRef] [PubMed]

109. Granata, V.; Fusco, R.; Catalano, O.; Avallone, A.; Palaia, R.; Botti, G.; Tatangelo, F.; Granata, F.; Cascella, M.; Izzo, F.; et al. Diagnostic accuracy of magnetic resonance, computed tomography and contrast enhanced ultrasound in radiological multimodality assessment of peribiliary liver metastases. *PLoS ONE* 2017, *12*, e0179951. [CrossRef]
110. Granata, V.; Fusco, R.; Catalano, O.; Avallone, A.; Leongito, M.; Izzo, F.; Petrillo, A. Peribiliary liver metastases MR findings. *Med. Oncol.* 2017, *34*, 124. [CrossRef]
111. Li, N.; Wakim, J.; Koethe, Y.; Huber, T.; Schenning, R.; Gade, T.P.; Hunt, S.J.; Park, B.J. Multicenter assessment of augmented reality registration methods for image-guided interventions. *Radiol. Med.* 2022, *127*, 857–865. [CrossRef]
112. Caruso, D.; Polici, M.; Rinzivillo, M.; Zerunian, M.; Nacci, I.; Marasco, M.; Magi, L.; Tarallo, M.; Gargiulo, S.; Iannicelli, E.; et al. CT-based radiomics for prediction of therapeutic response to Everolimus in metastatic neuroendocrine tumors. *Radiol. Med.* 2022, *127*, 691–701. [CrossRef]
113. Han, D.; Yu, N.; Yu, Y.; He, T.; Duan, X. Performance of CT radiomics in predicting the overall survival of patients with stage III clear cell renal carcinoma after radical nephrectomy. *Radiol. Med.* 2022, *127*, 837–847. [CrossRef]
114. Granata, V.; Fusco, R.; de Lutio di Castelguidone, E.; Avallone, A.; Palaia, R.; Delrio, P.; Tatangelo, F.; Botti, G.; Grassi, R.; Izzo, F.; et al. Diagnostic performance of gadoxetic acid-enhanced liver MRI versus multidetector CT in the assessment of colorectal liver metastases compared to hepatic resection. *BMC Gastroenterol.* 2019, *19*, 129. [CrossRef] [PubMed]
115. Masci, G.M.; Ciccarelli, F.; Mattei, F.I.; Grasso, D.; Accarpio, F.; Catalano, C.; Laghi, A.; Sammartino, P.; Iafrate, F. Role of CT texture analysis for predicting peritoneal metastases in patients with gastric cancer. *Radiol. Med.* 2022, *127*, 251–258. [CrossRef]
116. Tafuto, S.; von Arx, C.; De Divitiis, C.; Maura, C.T.; Palaia, R.; Albino, V.; Fusco, R.; Membrini, M.; Petrillo, A.; Granata, V.; et al. Electrochemotherapy as a new approach on pancreatic cancer and on liver metastases. *Int. J. Surg.* 2015, *21* (Suppl. S1), S78–S82. [CrossRef] [PubMed]
117. Zerunian, M.; Pucciarelli, F.; Caruso, D.; Polici, M.; Masci, B.; Guido, G.; De Santis, D.; Polverari, D.; Principessa, D.; Benvenga, A.; et al. Artificial intelligence based image quality enhancement in liver MRI: A quantitative and qualitative evaluation. *Radiol. Med.* 2022, *127*, 1098–1105. [CrossRef] [PubMed]
118. Kang, Y.J.; Cho, J.H.; Hwang, S.H. Diagnostic value of various criteria for deep lobe involvement in radiologic studies with parotid mass: A systematic review and meta-analysis. *Radiol. Med.* 2022, *127*, 1124–1133. [CrossRef]
119. Borgheresi, A.; De Muzio, F.; Agostini, A.; Ottaviani, L.; Bruno, A.; Granata, V.; Fusco, R.; Danti, G.; Flammia, F.; Grassi, R.; et al. Lymph Nodes Evaluation in Rectal Cancer: Where Do We Stand and Future Perspective. *J. Clin. Med.* 2022, *11*, 2599. [CrossRef]
120. Granata, V.; de Lutio di Castelguidone, E.; Fusco, R.; Catalano, O.; Piccirillo, M.; Palaia, R.; Izzo, F.; Gallipoli, A.D.; Petrillo, A. Irreversible electroporation of hepatocellular carcinoma: Preliminary report on the diagnostic accuracy of magnetic resonance, computer tomography, and contrast-enhanced ultrasound in evaluation of the ablated area. *Radiol. Med.* 2016, *121*, 122–131. [CrossRef]
121. Granata, V.; Grassi, R.; Fusco, R.; Belli, A.; Cutolo, C.; Pradella, S.; Grazzini, G.; La Porta, M.; Brunese, M.C.; De Muzio, F.; et al. Diagnostic evaluation and ablation treatments assessment in hepatocellular carcinoma. *Infect. Agents Cancer* 2021, *16*, 53. [CrossRef]
122. Granata, V.; Grassi, R.; Fusco, R.; Setola, S.V.; Belli, A.; Piccirillo, M.; Pradella, S.; Giordano, M.; Cappabianca, S.; Brunese, L.; et al. Abbreviated MRI Protocol for the Assessment of Ablated Area in HCC Patients. *Int. J. Environ. Res. Public Health* 2021, *18*, 3598. [CrossRef] [PubMed]
123. Petrillo, A.; Fusco, R.; Granata, V.; Filice, S.; Sansone, M.; Rega, D.; Delrio, P.; Bianco, F.; Romano, G.M.; Tatangelo, F.; et al. Assessing response to neo-adjuvant therapy in locally advanced rectal cancer using Intra-voxel Incoherent Motion modelling by DWI data and Standardized Index of Shape from DCE-MRI. *Ther. Adv. Med. Oncol.* 2018, *10*, 1758835918809875. [CrossRef] [PubMed]
124. Fusco, R.; Sansone, M.; Granata, V.; Grimm, R.; Pace, U.; Delrio, P.; Tatangelo, F.; Botti, G.; Avallone, A.; Pecori, B.; et al. Diffusion and perfusion MR parameters to assess preoperative short-course radiotherapy response in locally advanced rectal cancer: A comparative explorative study among Standardized Index of Shape by DCE-MRI, intravoxel incoherent motion- and diffusion kurtosis imaging-derived parameters. *Abdom. Radiol.* 2019, *44*, 3683–3700. [CrossRef]
125. Scola, E.; Desideri, I.; Bianchi, A.; Gadda, D.; Busto, G.; Fiorenza, A.; Amadori, T.; Mancini, S.; Miele, V.; Fainardi, E. Assessment of brain tumors by magnetic resonance dynamic susceptibility contrast perfusion-weighted imaging and computed tomography perfusion: A comparison study. *Radiol. Med.* 2022, *127*, 664–672. [CrossRef]
126. Vicini, S.; Bortolotto, C.; Rengo, M.; Ballerini, D.; Bellini, D.; Carbone, I.; Preda, L.; Laghi, A.; Coppola, F.; Faggioni, L. A narrative review on current imaging applications of artificial intelligence and radiomics in oncology: Focus on the three most common cancers. *Radiol. Med.* 2022, *127*, 819–836. [CrossRef]
127. Petrillo, A.; Fusco, R.; Petrillo, M.; Granata, V.; Delrio, P.; Bianco, F.; Pecori, B.; Botti, G.; Tatangelo, F.; Caracò, C.; et al. Standardized Index of Shape (DCE-MRI) and Standardized Uptake Value (PET/CT): Two quantitative approaches to discriminate chemo-radiotherapy locally advanced rectal cancer responders under a functional profile. *Oncotarget* 2017, *8*, 8143–8153. [CrossRef]
128. Wang, G.X.; Kurra, V.; Gainor, J.F.; Sullivan, R.J.; Flaherty, K.T.; Lee, S.I.; Fintelmann, F.J. Immune Checkpoint Inhibitor Cancer Therapy: Spectrum of Imaging Findings. *Radiographics* 2017, *37*, 2132–2144. [CrossRef]
129. De Cecco, C.N.; Buffa, V.; Fedeli, S.; Vallone, A.; Ruopoli, R.; Luzietti, M.; Miele, V.; Rengo, M.; Maurizi Enrici, M.; Fina, P.; et al. Preliminary experience with abdominal dual-energy CT (DECT): True versus virtual nonenhanced images of the liver. *Radiol. Med.* 2010, *115*, 1258–1266. [CrossRef]

130. Tirkes, T.; Hollar, M.A.; Tann, M.; Kohli, M.D.; Akisik, F.; Sandrasegaran, K. Response criteria in oncologic imaging: Review of traditional and new criteria. *Radiographics* **2013**, *33*, 1323–1341. [CrossRef]
131. Granata, V.; Fusco, R.; Setola, S.V.; Piccirillo, M.; Leongito, M.; Palaia, R.; Granata, F.; Lastoria, S.; Izzo, F.; Petrillo, A. Early radiological assessment of locally advanced pancreatic cancer treated with electrochemotherapy. *World J. Gastroenterol.* **2017**, *23*, 4767–4778. [CrossRef]
132. di Giacomo, V.; Trinci, M.; van der Byl, G.; Catania, V.D.; Calisti, A.; Miele, V. Ultrasound in newborns and children suffering from non-traumatic acute abdominal pain: Imaging with clinical and surgical correlation. *J. Ultrasound* **2014**, *18*, 385–393. [CrossRef] [PubMed]
133. Eisenhauer, E.; Therasse, P.; Bogaerts, J.; Schwartz, L.H.; Sargent, D.; Ford, R.; Dancey, J.; Arbuck, S.; Gwyther, S.; Mooney, M.; et al. New response evaluation criteria in solid tumours: Revised RECIST guideline (version 1.1). *Eur. J. Cancer* **2009**, *45*, 228–247. [CrossRef] [PubMed]
134. Granata, V.; Grassi, R.; Fusco, R.; Setola, S.V.; Palaia, R.; Belli, A.; Miele, V.; Brunese, L.; Grassi, R.; Petrillo, A.; et al. Assessment of Ablation Therapy in Pancreatic Cancer: The Radiologist's Challenge. *Front. Oncol.* **2020**, *10*, 560952. [CrossRef] [PubMed]
135. Chiti, G.; Grazzini, G.; Cozzi, D.; Danti, G.; Matteuzzi, B.; Granata, V.; Pradella, S.; Recchia, L.; Brunese, L.; Miele, V. Imaging of Pancreatic Neuroendocrine Neoplasms. *Int. J. Environ. Res. Public Health* **2021**, *18*, 8895. [CrossRef] [PubMed]
136. Wolchok, J.D.; Hoos, A.; O'Day, S.; Weber, J.S.; Hamid, O.; Lebbé, C.; Maio, M.; Binder, M.; Bohnsack, O.; Nichol, G.; et al. Guidelines for the evaluation of immune therapy activity in solid tumors: Immune-related response criteria. *Clin. Cancer Res.* **2009**, *15*, 7412–7420. [CrossRef]
137. Borcoman, E.; Kanjanapan, Y.; Champiat, S.; Kato, S.; Servois, V.; Kurzrock, R.; Goel, S.; Bedard, P.; Le Tourneau, C. Novel patterns of response under immunotherapy. *Ann. Oncol.* **2019**, *30*, 385–396. [CrossRef]
138. Nishino, M.; Giobbie-Hurder, A.; Gargano, M.; Suda, M.; Ramaiya, N.H.; Hodi, F.S. Developing a common language for tumor response to immunotherapy: Immune-related response criteria using unidimensional measurements. *Clin. Cancer Res.* **2013**, *19*, 3936–3943. [CrossRef]
139. Seymour, L.; Bogaerts, J.; Perrone, A.; Ford, R.; Schwartz, L.; Mandrekar, S.; Lin, N.; Litière, S.; Dancey, J.; Chen, A.; et al. iRECIST: Guidelines for response criteria for use in trials testing immunotherapeutics. *Lancet Oncol.* **2017**, *18*, e143–e152. [CrossRef]
140. Regine, G.; Stasolla, A.; Miele, V. Multidetector computed tomography of the renal arteries in vascular emergencies. *Eur. J. Radiol.* **2007**, *64*, 83–91. [CrossRef]
141. Choi, J.H.; Ahn, M.J.; Rhim, H.C.; Kim, J.W.; Lee, G.H.; Lee, Y.Y.; Kim, I.S. Comparison of WHO and RECIST criteria for response in metastatic colorectal carcinoma. *Cancer Res. Treat.* **2005**, *37*, 290–293. [CrossRef]
142. Regine, G.; Atzori, M.; Miele, V.; Buffa, V.; Galluzzo, M.; Luzietti, M.; Adami, L. Second-generation sonographic contrast agents in the evaluation of renal trauma. *Radiol. Med.* **2007**, *112*, 581–587, (In English and Italian). [CrossRef]
143. Choi, H.; Charnsangavej, C.; Faria, S.C.; Macapinlac, H.A.; Burgess, M.A.; Patel, S.R.; Chen, L.L.; Podoloff, D.A.; Benjamin, R.S. Correlation of computed tomography and positron emission tomography in patients with metastatic gastrointestinal stromal tumor treated at a single institution with imatinib mesylate: Proposal of new computed tomography response criteria. *J. Clin. Oncol.* **2007**, *25*, 1753–1759. [CrossRef]
144. Park, S.H.; Kim, Y.S.; Choi, J. Dosimetric analysis of the effects of a temporary tissue expander on the radiotherapy technique. *Radiol. Med.* **2021**, *126*, 437–444. [CrossRef]
145. Bozkurt, M.; Eldem, G.; Bozbulut, U.B.; Bozkurt, M.F.; Kılıçkap, S.; Peynircioğlu, B.; Çil, B.; Lay Ergün, E.; Volkan-Salanci, B. Factors affecting the response to Y-90 microsphere therapy in the cholangiocarcinoma patients. *Radiol. Med.* **2021**, *126*, 323–333. [CrossRef] [PubMed]
146. Gregory, J.; Dioguardi Burgio, M.; Corrias, G.; Vilgrain, V.; Ronot, M. Evaluation of liver tumour response by imaging. *JHEP Rep.* **2020**, *2*, 100100. [CrossRef] [PubMed]
147. Wahl, R.L.; Jacene, H.; Kasamon, Y.; Lodge, M.A. From RECIST to PERCIST: Evolving Considerations for PET response criteria in solid tumors. *J. Nucl. Med.* **2009**, *50* (Suppl. S1), 122S–150S. [CrossRef]
148. Skougaard, K.; Nielsen, D.; Jensen, B.V.; Hendel, H.W. Comparison of EORTC criteria and PERCIST for PET/CT response evaluation of patients with metastatic colorectal cancer treated with irinotecan and cetuximab. *J. Nucl. Med.* **2013**, *54*, 1026–1031. [CrossRef]
149. Kim, N.; Lee, E.S.; Won, S.E.; Yang, M.; Lee, A.J.; Shin, Y.; Ko, Y.; Pyo, J.; Park, H.J.; Kim, K.W. Evolution of Radiological Treatment Response Assessments for Cancer Immunotherapy: From iRECIST to Radiomics and Artificial Intelligence. *Korean J. Radiol.* **2022**, *23*, 1089. [CrossRef]
150. Ter Maat, L.S.; van Duin, I.A.J.; Elias, S.G.; van Diest, P.J.; Pluim, J.P.W.; Verhoeff, J.J.C.; de Jong, P.A.; Leiner, T.; Veta, M.; Suijkerbuijk, K.P.M. Imaging to predict checkpoint inhibitor outcomes in cancer. A systematic review. *Eur. J. Cancer* **2022**, *175*, 60–76. [CrossRef] [PubMed]
151. Bracco, S.; Zanoni, M.; Casseri, T.; Castellano, D.; Cioni, S.; Vallone, I.M.; Gennari, P.; Mazzei, M.A.; Romano, D.G.; Piano, M.; et al. Endovascular treatment of acute ischemic stroke due to tandem lesions of the anterior cerebral circulation: A multicentric Italian observational study. *Radiol. Med.* **2021**, *126*, 804–817. [CrossRef]
152. Nardone, V.; Boldrini, L.; Salvestrini, V.; Greco, C.; Petrianni, G.M.; Desideri, I.; De Felice, F. Are you planning to be a radiation oncologist? A survey by the young group of the Italian Association of Radiotherapy and Clinical Oncology (yAIRO). *Radiol. Med.* **2022**; Epub ahead of print. [CrossRef]

153. Giurazza, F.; Contegiacomo, A.; Calandri, M.; Mosconi, C.; Modestino, F.; Corvino, F.; Scrofani, A.R.; Marra, P.; Coniglio, G.; Failla, G.; et al. IVC filter retrieval: A multicenter proposal of two score systems to predict application of complex technique and procedural outcome. *Radiol. Med.* **2021**, *126*, 1007–1016. [CrossRef] [PubMed]
154. Barile, A. Some thoughts and greetings from the new Editor-in-Chief. *Radiol. Med.* **2021**, *126*, 3–4. [CrossRef]
155. Cappabianca, S.; Granata, V.; Di Grezia, G.; Mandato, Y.; Reginelli, A.; Di Mizio, V.; Grassi, R.; Rotondo, A. The role of nasoenteric intubation in the MR study of patients with Crohn's disease: Our experience and literature review. *Radiol. Med.* **2011**, *116*, 389–406. [CrossRef]
156. De Filippo, M.; Puglisi, S.; D'Amuri, F.; Gentili, F.; Paladini, I.; Carrafiello, G.; Maestroni, U.; Del Rio, P.; Ziglioli, F.; Pagnini, F. CT-guided percutaneous drainage of abdominopelvic collections: A pictorial essay. *Radiol. Med.* **2021**, *126*, 1561–1570. [CrossRef] [PubMed]
157. De Felice, F.; Boldrini, L.; Greco, C.; Nardone, V.; Salvestrini, V.; Desideri, I. ESTRO vision 2030: The young Italian Association of Radiotherapy and Clinical Oncology (yAIRO) commitment statement. *Radiol. Med.* **2021**, *126*, 1374–1376. [CrossRef]
158. Pecoraro, M.; Cipollari, S.; Marchitelli, L.; Messina, E.; Del Monte, M.; Galea, N.; Ciardi, M.R.; Francone, M.; Catalano, C.; Panebianco, V. Cross-sectional analysis of follow-up chest MRI and chest CT scans in patients previously affected by COVID-19. *Radiol. Med.* **2021**, *126*, 1273–1281. [CrossRef]
159. Delaunay, M.; Cadranel, J.; Lusque, A.; Meyer, N.; Gounant, V.; Moro-Sibilot, D.; Michot, J.M.; Raimbourg, J.; Girard, N.; Guisier, F.; et al. Immune-checkpoint inhibitors associated with interstitial lung disease in cancer patients. *Eur. Respir. J.* **2017**, *50*, 1700050. [CrossRef]
160. Piccolo, C.L.; Galluzzo, M.; Ianniello, S.; Trinci, M.; Russo, A.; Rossi, E.; Zeccolini, M.; Laporta, A.; Guglielmi, G.; Miele, V. Pediatric musculoskeletal injuries: Role of ultrasound and magnetic resonance imaging. *Musculoskelet. Surg.* **2017**, *101* (Suppl. S1), 85–102. [CrossRef]
161. Conte, P.; Ascierto, P.A.; Patelli, G.; Danesi, R.; Vanzulli, A.; Sandomenico, F.; Tarsia, P.; Cattelan, A.; Comes, A.; De Laurentiis, M.; et al. Drug-induced interstitial lung disease during cancer therapies: Expert opinion on diagnosis and treatment. *ESMO Open* **2022**, *7*, 100404. [CrossRef]
162. Luke, J.J.; Rutkowski, P.; Queirolo, P.; Del Vecchio, M.; Mackiewicz, J.; Chiarion-Sileni, V.; de la Cruz Merino, L.; Khattak, M.A.; Schadendorf, D.; Long, G.V.; et al. Pembrolizumab versus placebo as adjuvant therapy in completely resected stage IIB or IIC melanoma (KEYNOTE-716): A randomised, double-blind, phase 3 trial. *Lancet* **2022**, *399*, 1718–1729. [CrossRef]
163. Goldman, J.D.; Ascierto, P.A. Perspectives on COVID-19 and cancer immunotherapy: A review series. *J. Immunother. Cancer* **2021**, *9*, e002489. [CrossRef]
164. Kwak, J.J.; Tirumani, S.H.; Van den Abbeele, A.D.; Koo, P.J.; Jacene, H.A. Cancer immunotherapy: Imaging assessment of novel treatment response patterns and immune-related adverse events. *Radiographics* **2015**, *35*, 424–437. [CrossRef]
165. Assadsangabi, R.; Babaei, R.; Songco, C.; Ivanovic, V.; Bobinski, M.; Chen, Y.J.; Nabavizadeh, S.A. Multimodality oncologic evaluation of superficial neck and facial lymph nodes. *Radiol. Med.* **2021**, *126*, 1074–1084. [CrossRef]
166. Petralia, G.; Zugni, F.; Summers, P.E.; Colombo, A.; Pricolo, P.; Grazioli, L.; Colagrande, S.; Giovagnoni, A.; Padhani, A.R.; Italian Working Group on Magnetic Resonance. Whole-body magnetic resonance imaging (WB-MRI) for cancer screening: Recommendations for use. *Radiol. Med.* **2021**, *126*, 1434–1450. [CrossRef]
167. Tirumani, S.H.; Ramaiya, N.H.; Keraliya, A.; Bailey, N.D.; Ott, P.A.; Hodi, F.S.; Nishino, M. Radiographic profiling of immune-related adverse events in advanced melanoma patients treated with ipilimumab. *Cancer Immunol. Res.* **2015**, *3*, 1185–1192. [CrossRef]
168. Palmucci, S.; Roccasalva, F.; Puglisi, S.; Torrisi, S.E.; Vindigni, V.; Mauro, L.A.; Ettorre, G.C.; Piccoli, M.; Vancheri, C. Clinical and radiological features of idiopathic interstitial pneumonias (IIPs): A pictorial review. *Insights Imaging* **2014**, *5*, 347–364. [CrossRef]
169. Khoja, L.; Day, D.; Chen, T.W.-W.; Siu, L.L.; Hansen, A.R. Tumour-and class specific patterns of immune-related adverse events of immune checkpoint inhibitors: A systematic review. *Ann. Oncol.* **2017**, *28*, 2377–2385. [CrossRef]
170. Suresh, K.; Voong, K.R.; Shankar, B.; Forde, P.M.; Ettinger, D.S.; Marrone, K.A.; Kelly, R.J.; Hann, C.L.; Levy, B.; Feliciano, J.L.; et al. Pneumonitis in Non–Small Cell Lung Cancer Patients Receiving Immune Checkpoint Immunotherapy: Incidence and Risk Factors. *J. Thorac. Oncol.* **2018**, *13*, 1930–1939. [CrossRef]
171. Tay, R.Y.; Califano, R. Checkpoint Inhibitor Pneumonitis Real World Incidence and Risk. *J. Thorac. Oncol.* **2018**, *13*, 1812–1814. [CrossRef]
172. Larkin, J.; Chiarion-Sileni, V.; Gonzalez, R.; Grob, J.J.; Cowey, L.; Lao, C.D.; Schadendorf, D.; Dummer, R.; Smylie, M.; Rutkowwski, P.; et al. Combined nivolumab and ipilimumab or monotherapy in untreated melanoma. *N. Engl. J. Med.* **2015**, *373*, 23–34. [CrossRef]
173. D'Agostino, V.; Caranci, F.; Negro, A.; Piscitelli, V.; Tuccillo, B.; Fasano, F.; Sirabella, G.; Marano, I.; Granata, V.; Grassi, R.; et al. A Rare Case of Cerebral Venous Thrombosis and Disseminated Intravascular Coagulation Temporally Associated to the COVID-19 Vaccine Administration. *J. Pers. Med.* **2021**, *11*, 285. [CrossRef]
174. Agostini, A.; Borghesi, A.; Carotti, M.; Ottaviani, L.; Badaloni, M.; Floridi, C.; Giovagnoni, A. Third-generation iterative reconstruction on a dual-source, high-pitch, low-dose chest CT protocol with tin filter for spectral shaping at 100 kV: A study on a small series of COVID-19 patients. *Radiol. Med.* **2021**, *126*, 388–398. [CrossRef]

175. Palmisano, A.; Scotti, G.M.; Ippolito, D.; Morelli, M.J.; Vignale, D.; Gandola, D.; Sironi, S.; De Cobelli, F.; Ferrante, L.; Spessot, M.; et al. Chest CT in the emergency department for suspected COVID-19 pneumonia. *Radiol. Med.* **2021**, *126*, 498–502. [CrossRef]
176. Lombardi, A.F.; Afsahi, A.M.; Gupta, A.; Gholamrezanezhad, A. Severe acute respiratory syndrome (SARS), Middle East respiratory syndrome (MERS), influenza, and COVID-19, beyond the lungs: A review article. *Radiol. Med.* **2021**, *126*, 561–569. [CrossRef]
177. Gabelloni, M.; Faggioni, L.; Cioni, D.; Mendola, V.; Falaschi, Z.; Coppola, S.; Corradi, F.; Isirdi, A.; Brandi, N.; Coppola, F.; et al. Extracorporeal membrane oxygenation (ECMO) in COVID-19 patients: A pocket guide for radiologists. *Radiol. Med.* **2022**, *13*, 369–382. [CrossRef]
178. Grassi, R.; Cappabianca, S.; Urraro, F.; Feragalli, B.; Montanelli, A.; Patelli, G.; Granata, V.; Giacobbe, G.; Russo, G.M.; Grillo, A.; et al. Chest CT Computerized Aided Quantification of PNEUMONIA Lesions in COVID-19 Infection: A Comparison among Three Commercial Software. *Int. J. Environ. Res. Public Health* **2020**, *17*, 6914. [CrossRef]
179. Fusco, R.; Grassi, R.; Granata, V.; Setola, S.V.; Grassi, F.; Cozzi, D.; Pecori, B.; Izzo, F.; Petrillo, A. Artificial Intelligence and COVID-19 Using Chest CT Scan and Chest X-ray Images: Machine Learning and Deep Learning Approaches for Diagnosis and Treatment. *J. Pers. Med.* **2021**, *11*, 993. [CrossRef]
180. Özel, M.; Aslan, A.; Araç, S. Use of the COVID-19 Reporting and Data System (CO-RADS) classification and chest computed tomography involvement score (CT-IS) in COVID-19 pneumonia. *Radiol. Med.* **2021**, *126*, 679–687. [CrossRef]
181. Ippolito, D.; Giandola, T.; Maino, C.; Pecorelli, A.; Capodaglio, C.; Ragusi, M.; Porta, M.; Gandola, D.; Masetto, A.; Drago, S.; et al. Acute pulmonary embolism in hospitalized patients with SARS-CoV-2-related pneumonia: Multicentric experience from Italian endemic area. *Radiol. Med.* **2021**, *126*, 669–678. [CrossRef]
182. Moroni, C.; Cozzi, D.; Albanesi, M.; Cavigli, E.; Bindi, A.; Luvarà, S.; Busoni, S.; Mazzoni, L.N.; Grifoni, S.; Nazerian, P.; et al. Chest X-ray in the emergency department during COVID-19 pandemic descending phase in Italy: Correlation with patients' outcome. *Radiol. Med.* **2021**, *126*, 661–668. [CrossRef]
183. Cereser, L.; Girometti, R.; Da Re, J.; Marchesini, F.; Como, G.; Zuiani, C. Inter-reader agreement of high-resolution computed tomography findings in patients with COVID-19 pneumonia: A multi-reader study. *Radiol. Med.* **2021**, *126*, 577–584. [CrossRef] [PubMed]
184. Rawashdeh, M.A.; Saade, C. Radiation dose reduction considerations and imaging patterns of ground glass opacities in coronavirus: Risk of over exposure in computed tomography. *Radiol. Med.* **2021**, *126*, 380–387. [CrossRef] [PubMed]
185. Granata, V.; Ianniello, S.; Fusco, R.; Urraro, F.; Pupo, D.; Magliocchetti, S.; Albarello, F.; Campioni, P.; Cristofaro, M.; Di Stefano, F.; et al. Quantitative Analysis of Residual COVID-19 Lung CT Features: Consistency among Two Commercial Software. *J. Pers. Med.* **2021**, *11*, 1103. [CrossRef]
186. Granata, V.; Fusco, R.; Bicchierai, G.; Cozzi, D.; Grazzini, G.; Danti, G.; De Muzio, F.; Maggialetti, N.; Smorchkova, O.; D'Elia, M.; et al. Diagnostic protocols in oncology: Workup and treatment planning: Part 1: The optimization of CT protocol. *Eur. Rev. Med. Pharmacol. Sci.* **2021**, *25*, 6972–6994.
187. Fusco, R.; Granata, V.; Petrillo, A. Introduction to Special Issue of Radiology and Imaging of Cancer. *Cancers* **2020**, *12*, 2665. [CrossRef] [PubMed]
188. Scapicchio, C.; Gabelloni, M.; Barucci, A.; Cioni, D.; Saba, L.; Neri, E. A deep look into radiomics. *Radiol. Med.* **2021**, *126*, 1296–1311. [CrossRef]
189. Neri, E.; Coppola, F.; Larici, A.R.; Sverzellati, N.; Mazzei, M.A.; Sacco, P.; Dalpiaz, G.; Feragalli, B.; Miele, V.; Grassi, R. Structured reporting of chest CT in COVID-19 pneumonia: A consensus proposal. *Insights Imaging* **2020**, *11*, 92. [CrossRef]
190. Cellina, M.; Pirovano, M.; Ciocca, M.; Gibelli, D.; Floridi, C.; Oliva, G. Radiomic analysis of the optic nerve at the first episode of acute optic neuritis: An indicator of optic nerve pathology and a predictor of visual recovery? *Radiol. Med.* **2021**, *126*, 698–706. [CrossRef]
191. Santone, A.; Brunese, M.C.; Donnarumma, F.; Guerriero, P.; Mercaldo, F.; Reginelli, A.; Miele, V.; Giovagnoni, A.; Brunese, L. Radiomic features for prostate cancer grade detection through formal verification. *Radiol. Med.* **2021**, *126*, 688–697. [CrossRef]
192. Granata, V.; Fusco, R.; Barretta, M.L.; Picone, C.; Avallone, A.; Belli, A.; Patrone, R.; Ferrante, M.; Cozzi, D.; Grassi, R.; et al. Radiomics in hepatic metastasis by colorectal cancer. *Infect. Agents Cancer* **2021**, *16*, 39. [CrossRef]
193. Granata, V.; Grassi, R.; Fusco, R.; Galdiero, R.; Setola, S.V.; Palaia, R.; Belli, A.; Silvestro, L.; Cozzi, D.; Brunese, L.; et al. Pancreatic cancer detection and characterization: State of the art and radiomics. *Eur. Rev. Med. Pharmacol. Sci.* **2021**, *25*, 3684–3699. [CrossRef] [PubMed]
194. Agazzi, G.M.; Ravanelli, M.; Roca, E.; Medicina, D.; Balzarini, P.; Pessina, C.; Vermi, W.; Berruti, A.; Maroldi, R.; Farina, D. CT texture analysis for prediction of EGFR mutational status and ALK rearrangement in patients with non-small cell lung cancer. *Radiol. Med.* **2021**, *126*, 786–794. [CrossRef] [PubMed]
195. Agüloğlu, N.; Aksu, A.; Akyol, M.; Katgı, N.; Doksöz, T.Ç. Importance of Pretreatment 18F-FDG PET/CT Texture Analysis in Predicting EGFR and ALK Mutation in Patients with Non-Small Cell Lung Cancer. *Nuklearmedizin* **2022**, *61*, 433–439. [CrossRef] [PubMed]
196. Mayerhoefer, M.E.; Materka, A.; Langs, G.; Häggström, I.; Szczypiński, P.; Gibbs, P.; Cook, G. Introduction to Radiomics. *J. Nucl. Med.* **2020**, *61*, 488–495. [CrossRef]
197. Yip, S.S.; Aerts, H.J. Applications and limitations of radiomics. *Phys. Med. Biol.* **2016**, *61*, R150–R166. [CrossRef]

198. Granata, V.; Bicchierai, G.; Fusco, R.; Cozzi, D.; Grazzini, G.; Danti, G.; De Muzio, F.; Maggialetti, N.; Smorchkova, O.; D'Elia, M.; et al. Diagnostic protocols in oncology: Workup and treatment planning. Part 2: Abbreviated MR protocol. *Eur. Rev. Med. Pharmacol. Sci.* **2021**, *25*, 6499–6528. [CrossRef]
199. Granata, V.; Fusco, R.; Catalano, O.; Setola, S.V.; de Lutio di Castelguidone, E.; Piccirillo, M.; Palaia, R.; Grassi, R.; Granata, F.; Izzo, F.; et al. Multidetector computer tomography in the pancreatic adenocarcinoma assessment: An update. *Infect. Agents Cancer* **2016**, *11*, 57. [CrossRef]
200. Granata, V.; Fusco, R.; Setola, S.V.; Galdiero, R.; Picone, C.; Izzo, F.; D'Aniello, R.; Miele, V.; Grassi, R.; Grassi, R.; et al. Lymphadenopathy after BNT162b2 Covid-19 Vaccine: Preliminary Ultrasound Findings. *Biology* **2021**, *10*, 214. [CrossRef]
201. Binczyk, F.; Prazuch, W.; Bozek, P.; Polanska, J. Radiomics and artificial intelligence in lung cancer screening. *Transl. Lung Cancer Res.* **2021**, *10*, 1186–1199. [CrossRef]
202. Fiz, F.; Viganò, L.; Gennaro, N.; Costa, G.; La Bella, L.; Boichuk, A.; Cavinato, L.; Sollini, M.; Politi, L.S.; Chiti, A.; et al. Radiomics of Liver Metastases: A Systematic Review. *Cancers* **2020**, *12*, 2881. [CrossRef]
203. Granata, V.; Fusco, R.; Avallone, A.; Catalano, O.; Piccirillo, M.; Palaia, R.; Nasti, G.; Petrillo, A.; Izzo, F. A radiologist's point of view in the presurgical and intraoperative setting of colorectal liver metastases. *Future Oncol.* **2018**, *14*, 2189–2206. [CrossRef] [PubMed]
204. Benedetti, G.; Mori, M.; Panzeri, M.M.; Barbera, M.; Palumbo, D.; Sini, C.; Muffatti, F.; Andreasi, V.; Steidler, S.; Doglioni, C.; et al. CT-derived radiomic features to discriminate histologic characteristics of pancreatic neuroendocrine tumors. *Radiol. Med.* **2021**, *126*, 745–760. [CrossRef] [PubMed]
205. Gurgitano, M.; Angileri, S.A.; Rodà, G.M.; Liguori, A.; Pandolfi, M.; Ierardi, A.M.; Wood, B.J.; Carrafiello, G. Interventional Radiology ex-machina: Impact of Artificial Intelligence on practice. *Radiol. Med.* **2021**, *126*, 998–1006. [CrossRef] [PubMed]
206. Granata, V.; Fusco, R.; Avallone, A.; De Stefano, A.; Ottaiano, A.; Sbordone, C.; Brunese, L.; Izzo, F.; Petrillo, A. Radiomics-Derived Data by Contrast Enhanced Magnetic Resonance in RAS Mutations Detection in Colorectal Liver Metastases. *Cancers* **2021**, *13*, 453. [CrossRef] [PubMed]
207. Granata, V.; Fusco, R.; Costa, M.; Picone, C.; Cozzi, D.; Moroni, C.; La Casella, G.V.; Montanino, A.; Monti, R.; Mazzoni, F.; et al. Preliminary Report on Computed Tomography Radiomics Features as Biomarkers to Immunotherapy Selection in Lung Adenocarcinoma Patients. *Cancers* **2021**, *13*, 3992. [CrossRef]
208. Taha, B.; Boley, D.; Sun, J.; Chen, C.C. State of Radiomics in Glioblastoma. *Neurosurgery* **2021**, *89*, 177–184. [CrossRef]
209. Yu, Y.; He, Z.; Ouyang, J.; Tan, Y.; Chen, Y.; Gu, Y.; Mao, L.; Ren, W.; Wang, J.; Lin, L.; et al. Magnetic resonance imaging radiomics predicts preoperative axillary lymph node metastasis to support surgical decisions and is associated with tumor microenvironment in invasive breast cancer: A machine learning, multicenter study. *eBioMedicine* **2021**, *69*, 103460. [CrossRef]
210. Taha, B.; Boley, D.; Sun, J.; Chen, C. Potential and limitations of radiomics in neuro-oncology. *J. Clin. Neurosci.* **2021**, *90*, 206–211. [CrossRef]
211. Frix, A.N.; Cousin, F.; Refaee, T.; Bottari, F.; Vaidyanathan, A.; Desir, C.; Vos, W.; Walsh, S.; Occhipinti, M.; Lovinfosse, P.; et al. Radiomics in Lung Diseases Imaging: State-of-the-Art for Clinicians. *J. Pers. Med.* **2021**, *11*, 602. [CrossRef]
212. Fusco, R.; Sansone, M.; Filice, S.; Granata, V.; Catalano, O.; Amato, D.M.; Di Bonito, M.; D'Aiuto, M.; Capasso, I.; Rinaldo, M.; et al. Integration of DCE-MRI and DW-MRI Quantitative Parameters for Breast Lesion Classification. *Biomed. Res. Int.* **2015**, *2015*, 237863. [CrossRef]
213. Fusco, R.; Granata, V.; Grazzini, G.; Pradella, S.; Borgheresi, A.; Bruno, A.; Palumbo, P.; Bruno, F.; Grassi, R.; Giovagnoni, A.; et al. Radiomics in medical imaging: Pitfalls and challenges in clinical management. *Jpn. J. Radiol.* **2022**, *40*, 919–929. [CrossRef]
214. Nakamura, Y.; Higaki, T.; Honda, Y.; Tatsugami, F.; Tani, C.; Fukumoto, W.; Narita, K.; Kondo, S.; Akagi, M.; Awai, K. Advanced CT techniques for assessing hepatocellular carcinoma. *Radiol. Med.* **2021**, *126*, 925–935. [CrossRef]
215. Chianca, V.; Albano, D.; Messina, C.; Vincenzo, G.; Rizzo, S.; Del Grande, F.; Sconfienza, L.M. An update in musculoskeletal tumors: From quantitative imaging to radiomics. *Radiol. Med.* **2021**, *126*, 1095–1105. [CrossRef] [PubMed]
216. Halefoglu, A.M.; Ozagari, A.A. Tumor grade estimation of clear cell and papillary renal cell carcinoma using contrast-enhanced MDCT and FSE T2 weighted MR imaging: Radiology-pathology correlation. *Radiol. Med.* **2021**, *126*, 1139–1148. [CrossRef] [PubMed]
217. Granata, V.; Fusco, R.; Risi, C.; Ottaiano, A.; Avallone, A.; De Stefano, A.; Grimm, R.; Grassi, R.; Brunese, L.; Izzo, F.; et al. Diffusion-Weighted MRI and Diffusion Kurtosis Imaging to Detect RAS Mutation in Colorectal Liver Metastasis. *Cancers* **2020**, *12*, 2420. [CrossRef]
218. Granata, V.; Fusco, R.; Setola, S.V.; Simonetti, I.; Cozzi, D.; Grazzini, G.; Grassi, F.; Belli, A.; Miele, V.; Izzo, F.; et al. An update on radiomics techniques in primary liver cancers. *Infect. Agents Cancer* **2022**, *17*, 6. [CrossRef] [PubMed]
219. Avanzo, M.; Stancanello, J.; El Naqa, I. Beyond imaging: The promise of radiomics. *Phys. Med.* **2017**, *38*, 122–139. [CrossRef] [PubMed]
220. Fornacon-Wood, I.; Faivre-Finn, C.; O'Connor, J.P.B.; Price, G.J. Radiomics as a personalized medicine tool in lung cancer: Separating the hope from the hype. *Lung Cancer* **2020**, *146*, 197–208. [CrossRef]
221. Bogowicz, M.; Vuong, D.; Huellner, M.W.; Pavic, M.; Andratschke, N.; Gabrys, H.S.; Guckenberger, M.; Tanadini-Lang, S. CT radiomics and PET radiomics: Ready for clinical implementation? *Q. J. Nucl. Med. Mol. Imaging* **2019**, *63*, 355–370. [CrossRef]

222. Granata, V.; Fusco, R.; Sansone, M.; Grassi, R.; Maio, F.; Palaia, R.; Tatangelo, F.; Botti, G.; Grimm, R.; Curley, S.; et al. Magnetic resonance imaging in the assessment of pancreatic cancer with quantitative parameter extraction by means of dynamic contrast-enhanced magnetic resonance imaging, diffusion kurtosis imaging and intravoxel incoherent motion diffusion-weighted imaging. *Ther. Adv. Gastroenterol.* **2020**, *13*, 1756284819885052. [CrossRef]
223. Granata, V.; Fusco, R.; Setola, S.V.; Picone, C.; Vallone, P.; Belli, A.; Incollingo, P.; Albino, V.; Tatangelo, F.; Izzo, F.; et al. Microvascular invasion and grading in hepatocellular carcinoma: Correlation with major and ancillary features according to LIRADS. *Abdom. Radiol.* **2019**, *44*, 2788–2800. [CrossRef]
224. Granata, V.; Fusco, R.; Setola, S.V.; De Muzio, F.; Dell' Aversana, F.; Cutolo, C.; Faggioni, L.; Miele, V.; Izzo, F.; Petrillo, A. CT-Based Radiomics Analysis to Predict Histopathological Outcomes Following Liver Resection in Colorectal Liver Metastases. *Cancers* **2022**, *14*, 1648. [CrossRef]
225. Sun, J.; Li, H.; Gao, J.; Li, J.; Li, M.; Zhou, Z.; Peng, Y. Performance evaluation of a deep learning image reconstruction (DLIR) algorithm in "double low" chest CTA in children: A feasibility study. *Radiol. Med.* **2021**, *126*, 1181–1188. [CrossRef]
226. Granata, V.; Faggioni, L.; Grassi, R.; Fusco, R.; Reginelli, A.; Rega, D.; Maggialetti, N.; Buccicardi, D.; Frittoli, B.; Rengo, M.; et al. Structured reporting of computed tomography in the staging of colon cancer: A Delphi consensus proposal. *Radiol. Med.* **2022**, *127*, 21–29. [CrossRef] [PubMed]
227. Granata, V.; Fusco, R.; De Muzio, F.; Cutolo, C.; Setola, S.V.; Dell'Aversana, F.; Ottaiano, A.; Nasti, G.; Grassi, R.; Pilone, V.; et al. EOB-MR Based Radiomics Analysis to Assess Clinical Outcomes following Liver Resection in Colorectal Liver Metastases. *Cancers* **2022**, *14*, 1239. [CrossRef]
228. Arimura, H.; Soufi, M.; Kamezawa, H.; Ninomiya, K.; Yamada, M. Radiomics with artificial intelligence for precision medicine in radiation therapy. *J. Radiat. Res.* **2019**, *60*, 150–157. [CrossRef] [PubMed]
229. Fusco, R.; Granata, V.; Mazzei, M.A.; Meglio, N.D.; Roscio, D.D.; Moroni, C.; Monti, R.; Cappabianca, C.; Picone, C.; Neri, E.; et al. Quantitative imaging decision support (QIDS^{TM}) tool consistency evaluation and radiomic analysis by means of 594 metrics in lung carcinoma on chest CT scan. *Cancer Control* **2021**, *28*, 1073274820985786. [CrossRef] [PubMed]
230. Zanfardino, M.; Franzese, M.; Pane, K.; Cavaliere, C.; Monti, S.; Esposito, G.; Salvatore, M.; Aiello, M. Bringing radiomics into a multi-omics framework for a comprehensive genotype-phenotype characterization of oncological diseases. *J. Transl. Med.* **2019**, *17*, 337. [CrossRef] [PubMed]
231. Izzo, F.; Piccirillo, M.; Albino, V.; Palaia, R.; Belli, A.; Granata, V.; Setola, S.; Fusco, R.; Petrillo, A.; Orlando, R.; et al. Prospective screening increases the detection of potentially curable hepatocellular carcinoma: Results in 8,900 high-risk patients. *HPB* **2013**, *15*, 985–990. [CrossRef] [PubMed]
232. Granata, V.; Fusco, R.; De Muzio, F.; Cutolo, C.; Setola, S.V.; Dell' Aversana, F.; Ottaiano, A.; Avallone, A.; Nasti, G.; Grassi, F.; et al. Contrast MR-Based Radiomics and Machine Learning Analysis to Assess Clinical Outcomes following Liver Resection in Colorectal Liver Metastases: A Preliminary Study. *Cancers* **2022**, *14*, 1110. [CrossRef]
233. Liu, J.; Wang, C.; Guo, W.; Zeng, P.; Liu, Y.; Lang, N.; Yuan, H. A preliminary study using spinal MRI-based radiomics to predict high-risk cytogenetic abnormalities in multiple myeloma. *Radiol. Med.* **2021**, *126*, 1226–1235. [CrossRef]
234. Qin, H.; Que, Q.; Lin, P.; Li, X.; Wang, X.R.; He, Y.; Chen, J.Q.; Yang, H. Magnetic resonance imaging (MRI) radiomics of papillary thyroid cancer (PTC): A comparison of predictive performance of multiple classifiers modeling to identify cervical lymph node metastases before surgery. *Radiol. Med.* **2021**, *126*, 1312–1327. [CrossRef]
235. Fusco, R.; Di Bernardo, E.; Piccirillo, A.; Rubulotta, M.R.; Petrosino, T.; Barretta, M.L.; Mattace Raso, M.; Vallone, P.; Raiano, C.; Di Giacomo, R.; et al. Radiomic and Artificial Intelligence Analysis with Textural Metrics Extracted by Contrast-Enhanced Mammography and Dynamic Contrast Magnetic Resonance Imaging to Detect Breast Malignant Lesions. *Curr. Oncol.* **2022**, *29*, 159. [CrossRef]
236. Neri, E.; Granata, V.; Montemezzi, S.; Belli, P.; Bernardi, D.; Brancato, B.; Caumo, F.; Calabrese, M.; Coppola, F.; Cossu, E.; et al. Structured reporting of x-ray mammography in the first diagnosis of breast cancer: A Delphi consensus proposal. *Radiol. Med.* **2022**, *127*, 471–483. [CrossRef] [PubMed]
237. Granata, V.; Fusco, R.; De Muzio, F.; Cutolo, C.; Mattace Raso, M.; Gabelloni, M.; Avallone, A.; Ottaiano, A.; Tatangelo, F.; Brunese, M.C.; et al. Radiomics and Machine Learning Analysis Based on Magnetic Resonance Imaging in the Assessment of Colorectal Liver Metastases Growth Pattern. *Diagnostics* **2022**, *12*, 1115. [CrossRef] [PubMed]
238. Brunese, L.; Brunese, M.C.; Carbone, M.; Ciccone, V.; Mercaldo, F.; Santone, A. Automatic PI-RADS assignment by means of formal methods. *Radiol. Med.* **2022**, *127*, 83–89. [CrossRef] [PubMed]
239. Bellardita, L.; Colciago, R.R.; Frasca, S.; De Santis, M.C.; Gay, S.; Palorini, F.; La Rocca, E.; Valdagni, R.; Rancati, T.; Lozza, L. Breast cancer patient perspective on opportunities and challenges of a genetic test aimed to predict radio-induced side effects before treatment: Analysis of the Italian branch of the REQUITE project. *Radiol. Med.* **2021**, *126*, 1366–1373. [CrossRef]
240. Caruso, D.; Pucciarelli, F.; Zerunian, M.; Ganeshan, B.; De Santis, D.; Polici, M.; Rucci, C.; Polidori, T.; Guido, G.; Bracci, B.; et al. Chest CT texture-based radiomics analysis in differentiating COVID-19 from other interstitial pneumonia. *Radiol. Med.* **2021**, *126*, 1415–1424. [CrossRef]
241. Karmazanovsky, G.; Gruzdev, I.; Tikhonova, V.; Kondratyev, E.; Revishvili, A. Computed tomography-based radiomics approach in pancreatic tumors characterization. *Radiol. Med.* **2021**, *126*, 1388–1395. [CrossRef]

242. Danti, G.; Flammia, F.; Matteuzzi, B.; Cozzi, D.; Berti, V.; Grazzini, G.; Pradella, S.; Recchia, L.; Brunese, L.; Miele, V. Gastrointestinal neuroendocrine neoplasms (GI-NENs): Hot topics in morphological, functional, and prognostic imaging. *Radiol. Med.* **2021**, *126*, 1497–1507. [CrossRef]
243. Satake, H.; Ishigaki, S.; Ito, R.; Naganawa, S. Radiomics in breast MRI: Current progress toward clinical application in the era of artificial intelligence. *Radiol. Med.* **2022**, *127*, 39–56. [CrossRef]
244. Chiloiro, G.; Cusumano, D.; de Franco, P.; Lenkowicz, J.; Boldrini, L.; Carano, D.; Barbaro, B.; Corvari, B.; Dinapoli, N.; Giraffa, M.; et al. Does restaging MRI radiomics analysis improve pathological complete response prediction in rectal cancer patients? A prognostic model development. *Radiol. Med.* **2022**, *127*, 11–20. [CrossRef] [PubMed]
245. Gregucci, F.; Fiorentino, A.; Mazzola, R.; Ricchetti, F.; Bonaparte, I.; Surgo, A.; Figlia, V.; Carbonara, R.; Caliandro, M.; Ciliberti, M.P.; et al. Radiomic analysis to predict local response in locally advanced pancreatic cancer treated with stereotactic body radiation therapy. *Radiol. Med.* **2022**, *127*, 100–107. [CrossRef] [PubMed]
246. Herbst, R.S.; Soria, J.C.; Kowanetz, M.; Fine, G.D.; Hamid, O.; Gordon, M.S.; Sosman, J.A.; McDermott, D.F.; Powderly, J.D.; Gettinger, S.N.; et al. Predictive correlates of response to the anti-PD-L1 antibody MPDL3280A in cancer patients. *Nature* **2014**, *515*, 563–567. [CrossRef] [PubMed]
247. Fusco, R.; Petrillo, M.; Granata, V.; Filice, S.; Sansone, M.; Catalano, O.; Petrillo, A. Magnetic Resonance Imaging Evaluation in Neoadjuvant Therapy of Locally Advanced Rectal Cancer: A Systematic Review. *Radiol. Oncol.* **2017**, *51*, 252–262. [CrossRef]
248. Sun, R.; Limkin, E.J.; Vakalopoulou, M.; Dercle, L.; Champiat, S.; Han, S.R.; Verlingue, L.; Brandao, D.; Lancia, A.; Ammari, S.; et al. A radiomics approach to assess tumour-infiltrating CD8 cells and response to anti-PD-1 or anti-PD-L1 immunotherapy: An imaging biomarker, retrospective multicohort study. *Lancet Oncol.* **2018**, *19*, 1180–1191. [CrossRef]
249. Tang, C.; Hobbs, B.; Amer, A.; Li, X.; Behrens, C.; Canales, J.R.; Cuentas, E.P.; Villalobos, P.; Fried, D.; Chang, J.Y.; et al. Development of an Immune-Pathology Informed Radiomics Model for Non-Small Cell Lung Cancer. *Sci. Rep.* **2018**, *8*, 1922. [CrossRef]
250. Tunali, I.; Tan, Y.; Gray, J.E.; Katsoulakis, E.; Eschrich, S.A.; Saller, J.; Aerts, H.J.W.L.; Boyle, T.; Qi, J.; Guvenis, A.; et al. Hypoxia-Related Radiomics and Immunotherapy Response: A Multicohort Study of Non-Small Cell Lung Cancer. *JNCI Cancer Spectr.* **2021**, *5*, pkab048. [CrossRef]
251. Tunali, I.; Tan, Y.; Gray, J.E.; Eschrich, S.; Guvenis, A.; Gillies, R.; Schabath, M. Clinical-radiomic models predict overall survival among non-small cell lung cancer patients treated with immunotherapy. *J. Thorac. Oncol.* **2019**, *14*, S1129. [CrossRef]
252. Granata, V.; Cascella, M.; Fusco, R.; dell'Aprovitola, N.; Catalano, O.; Filice, S.; Schiavone, V.; Izzo, F.; Cuomo, A.; Petrillo, A. Immediate Adverse Reactions to Gadolinium-Based MR Contrast Media: A Retrospective Analysis on 10,608 Examinations. *Biomed. Res. Int.* **2016**, *2016*, 3918292. [CrossRef]
253. Thomas, H.M.T.; Hippe, D.S.; Forouzannezhad, P.; Sasidharan, B.K.; Kinahan, P.E.; Miyaoka, R.S.; Vesselle, H.J.; Rengan, R.; Zeng, J.; Bowen, S.R. Radiation and immune checkpoint inhibitor-mediated pneumonitis risk stratification in patients with locally advanced non-small cell lung cancer: Role of functional lung radiomics? *Discov. Oncol.* **2022**, *13*, 85. [CrossRef]
254. Granata, V.; Fusco, R.; Avallone, A.; Catalano, O.; Filice, F.; Leongito, M.; Palaia, R.; Izzo, F.; Petrillo, A. Major and ancillary magnetic resonance features of LI-RADS to assess HCC: An overview and update. *Infect. Agents Cancer* **2017**, *12*, 23. [CrossRef]
255. Matsoukas, S.; Scaggiante, J.; Schuldt, B.R.; Smith, C.J.; Chennareddy, S.; Kalagara, R.; Majidi, S.; Bederson, J.B.; Fifi, J.T.; Mocco, J.; et al. Accuracy of artificial intelligence for the detection of intracranial hemorrhage and chronic cerebral microbleeds: A systematic review and pooled analysis. *Radiol. Med.* **2022**, *127*, 1106–1123. [CrossRef]
256. De Robertis, R.; Geraci, L.; Tomaiuolo, L.; Bortoli, L.; Beleù, A.; Malleo, G.; D'Onofrio, M. Liver metastases in pancreatic ductal adenocarcinoma: A predictive model based on CT texture analysis. *Radiol. Med.* **2022**, *127*, 1079–1084. [CrossRef]
257. Park, J.E.; Kim, D.; Kim, H.S.; Park, S.Y.; Kim, J.Y.; Cho, S.J.; Shin, J.H.; Kim, J.H. Quality of science and reporting of radiomics in oncologic studies: Room for improvement according to radiomics quality score and TRIPOD statement. *Eur. Radiol.* **2020**, *30*, 523–536. [CrossRef]
258. Zwanenburg, A.; Vallières, M.; Abdalah, M.A.; Aerts, H.J.W.L.; Andrearczyk, V.; Apte, A.; Ashrafinia, S.; Bakas, S.; Beukinga, R.J.; Boellaard, R.; et al. The Image Biomarker Standardization Initiative: Standardized Quantitative Radiomics for High-Throughput Image-based Phenotyping. *Radiology* **2020**, *295*, 328–338. [CrossRef]

Disclaimer/Publisher's Note: The statements, opinions and data contained in all publications are solely those of the individual author(s) and contributor(s) and not of MDPI and/or the editor(s). MDPI and/or the editor(s) disclaim responsibility for any injury to people or property resulting from any ideas, methods, instructions or products referred to in the content.

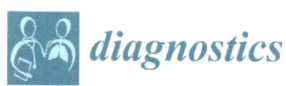 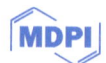

Interesting Images

The Many Hidden Faces of Gallbladder Carcinoma on CT and MRI Imaging—From A to Z

Damaris Neculoiu [1], Lavinia Claudia Neculoiu [1,*], Ramona Mihaela Popa [1] and Rosana Mihaela Manea [1,2]

[1] Department of Radiology and Medical Imaging, Clinical Emergency County Hospital of Brașov, 500326 Brașov, Romania
[2] Faculty of Medicine, "Transilvania" University of Brașov, Nicolae Bălcescu 56, 500019 Brașov, Romania
* Correspondence: neculoiulavinia@gmail.com

Abstract: Gallbladder carcinoma represents the most aggressive biliary tract cancer and the sixth most common gastrointestinal malignancy. The diagnosis is a challenging clinical task due to its clinical presentation, which is often non-specific, mimicking a heterogeneous group of diseases, as well as benign processes such as complicated cholecystitis, xanthogranulomatous cholecystitis, adenomyomatosis, porcelain gallbladder or metastasis to the gallbladder (most frequently derived from melanoma, renal cell carcinoma). Risk factors include gallstones, carcinogen exposure, porcelain gallbladder, typhoid carrier state, gallbladder polyps and abnormal pancreaticobiliary ductal junction. Typical imaging features on CT or MRI reveal three major patterns: asymmetric focal or diffuse wall-thickening of the gallbladder, a solid mass that replaces the gallbladder and invades the adjacent organs or as an intraluminal enhancement mass arising predominantly from the gallbladder fundus. The tumor can spread to the liver, the adjacent internal organs and lymph nodes. Depending on the disease stage, surgical resection is the curative treatment option in early stages and adjuvant combination chemotherapy at advanced stages. The purpose of this scientific paper is to fully illustrate and evaluate, through multimodality imaging findings (CT and MRI), different presentations and imaging scenarios of gallbladder cancer in six patients and thoroughly analyze the risk factors, patterns of spread and differential diagnosis regarding each particular case.

Keywords: gallbladder; gallbladder cancer; biliary tract cancer; CT; MRI; oncology; surgery; metastases

Citation: Neculoiu, D.; Neculoiu, L.C.; Popa, R.M.; Manea, R.M. The Many Hidden Faces of Gallbladder Carcinoma on CT and MRI Imaging—From A to Z. *Diagnostics* 2024, 14, 475. https://doi.org/10.3390/diagnostics14050475

Academic Editors: Kazushi Numata, Francescamaria Donati and Piero Boraschi

Received: 2 December 2023
Revised: 11 February 2024
Accepted: 19 February 2024
Published: 22 February 2024

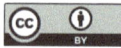

Copyright: © 2024 by the authors. Licensee MDPI, Basel, Switzerland. This article is an open access article distributed under the terms and conditions of the Creative Commons Attribution (CC BY) license (https://creativecommons.org/licenses/by/4.0/).

Gallbladder cancer is the most common malignancy of the biliary tract and the sixth most common cancer of the gastrointestinal system [1]. According to GLOBOCAN estimates, gallbladder cancer is relatively rare and stands in 24th place among the most frequent type of cancers worldwide with more than 115,949 new cases in 2020 [2,3]. In the majority of cases, gallbladder carcinoma is asymptomatic or the clinical presentation is often vague, non-specific and discovered at an advanced stage [4,5]. Imaging plays a crucial and decisive role in the diagnosis, staging and subsequent management planning [6]. Occasionally, gallbladder cancer might be discovered following a cholecystectomy. Moreover, gallbladder cancer is thought to be favored by chronic cholelithiasis, cholecystolithiasis, gallbladder polyps and porcelain gallbladder [7]. The prevalence of the disease is primarily among elderly women over 60 years-old. The highest incidence occurs in South American countries, Chile, Ecuador, India, Pakistan, Japan and South Korea. Incidence of gallbladder cancer is 1–2 cases per 100,000 people [3,8,9]. However, gallbladder carcinoma still remains a relatively rare pathology with a poor prognosis and it usually presents at a very advanced stage [1]. Late-stage illness frequently manifests with anorexia, weight loss, abdominal pain and jaundice [3].

Diagnostic imaging modalities for the gallbladder cancer include ultrasound, computerized tomography (CT) and magnetic resonance imaging (MRI). CT and MRI are both effective imaging modalities, but MRI provides superior soft-tissue characterization of the gallbladder and biliary tree. The use of hepatobiliary contrast agents (gadolinium chelates) with increased hepatobiliary excretion in abdominal MRI imaging may offer valuable information by providing enhanced images of the biliary tree [10].

We hereby fully illustrate the case of a 67-year-old female patient, who was admitted to the Emergency Department with intense pain localized in the right renal fossa, radiating to the right abdominal flank, accompanied by nausea with an onset of approximately two weeks. During the physical examination, a reduced abdominal wall mobility with respiratory movements was observed, along with pain in the right hypochondrium and muscular defense. Her medical history included hypertension grade 3 and congestive heart failure. Laboratory tests showed elevated inflammatory markers (leukocytosis, procalcitonin, CRP) and hypochromic microcytic anemia.

Biphasic (arterial phase followed by venous phase) contrast-enhanced emergency CT was performed (Figure 1), which clearly highlighted a gallbladder hydrops, with asymmetric, irregular gallbladder mural thickening, associated with multiple intraluminal mixed stones (Panel A). The tumoral mass extends directly into the adjacent liver parenchyma in segments IV and V and is in contact with the ascending colon (Panel C). Hepatomegaly can be observed (right hepatic lobe measures = 190 mm), with nodular lesions, disseminated in both hepatic lobes, hypodense, with rim peripheral contrast enhancement, more numerous in the right lobe, presenting various sizes (up to 35 mm in segment V) highly suggestive of liver metastases (Panel B and Panel C). Lymphatic metastases are common in gallbladder cancer. In this particular case, CT showed multiple lymph nodes enlargements in the hilar, mesenteric, celiac and precaval regions, up to 26/25 mm (measured in the hepatic hilum), with associated central necrosis (Panel D).

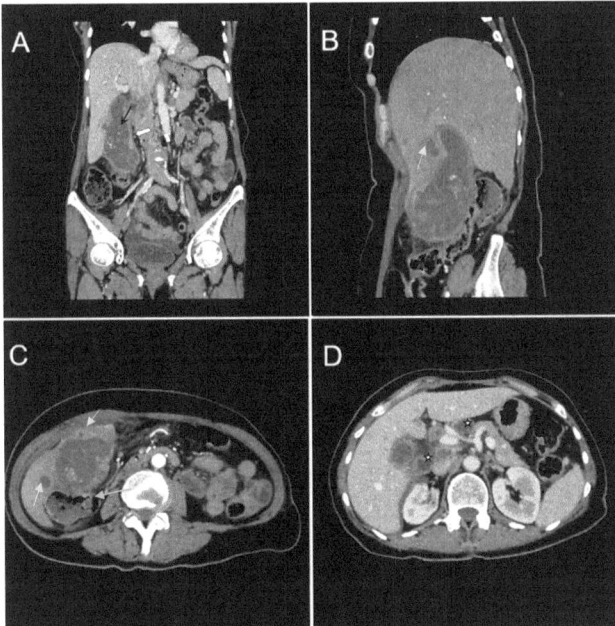

Figure 1. Multiplanar sections of contrast-enhanced CT acquisitions richly illustrating a low differentiated gallbladder adenocarcinoma. (**A**) Gallbladder hydrops (>40 mm transverse measurement, 142 mm longitudinal measurement) with asymmetric gallbladder mural thickening, 7 mm (white arrow), and multiple intraluminal mixed stones, 5–8 mm (black arrow). (**B,C**) Liver metastases—hypodense nodular hepatic lesions with rim contrast enhancement (yellow arrow). (**C**) Tumoral extension into IV, V segments of the right hepatic lobe and contact with the ascending colon (green arrow). (**D**) Lymphatic metastases (white stars).

The patient was transferred to the General Surgery Department for specialized treatment (intravenous antibiotics, intravenous hydration and correction of electrolyte abnormalities). After laparoscopy and laparotomy, a subhepatic perforated tumor with duodenum and transvers colon invasion was revealed. A partial cholecystectomy was performed with cholecystostomy and intraperitoneal drain. The postoperative evolution progressed without incident.

Formalin-fixed paraffin-embedded tissue sections from gallbladder and liver were examined histologically. The microscopic description was suggestive of poorly differentiated gallbladder adenocarcinoma (G3); pT3NxMx. The liver metastatic site was pathologically confirmed. TNM according to the AJCC (American Joint Committee on Cancer) 8th edition gallbladder cancer staging system was in this case T3N2M1. Oncology follow-up and adjuvant chemotherapy were recommended.

A 55-year-old female patient was admitted to the Emergency Department with right hypochondrium pain and weight loss for 2 weeks, which had worsened over the last two days accompanied by nausea and vomiting. No medical history was noted. Physical examination revealed normal abdominal wall mobility with respiratory movements and a sensitive right hypochondrium. Blood sample demonstrated normal levels of leukocytes and inflammatory markers.

Contrast-enhanced emergency CT (Figure 2) revealed mucosal hyperenhancement of the gallbladder, with irregular, mural thickening (16 mm), a gallstone (15 mm) and pericholecystic fluid and loco-regional inflammatory reactive lymph nodes (Panel A, Panel B and Panel C).

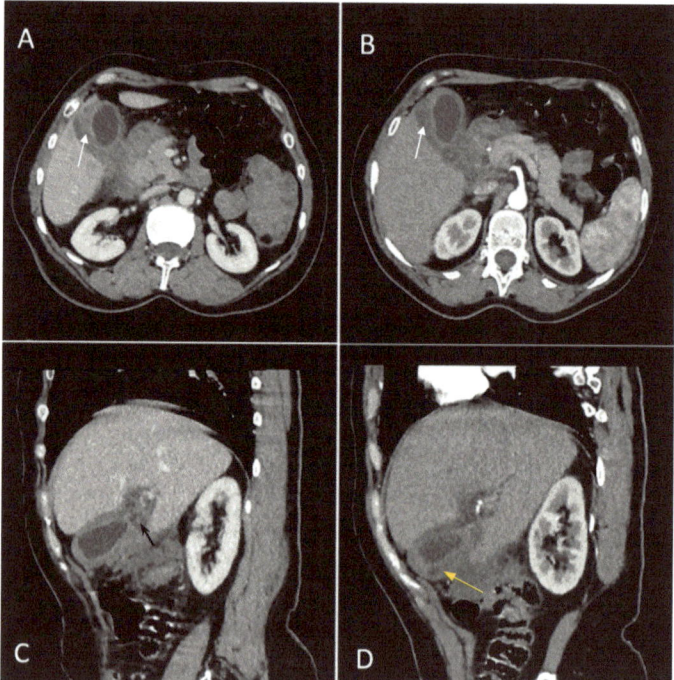

Figure 2. Multiplanar sections of contrast-enhanced CT acquisitions richly illustrating gallbladder carcinoma. (**A,B**) Gallbladder with irregular mural thickening, 16 mm (white arrow), pericholecystic fluid and loco-regional inflammatory lymph nodes. (**C**) Gallbladder with an intraluminal gallstone, 15 mm (black arrow). (**D**) Abscess adjacent to the gallbladder with subtle peripheral contrast enhancement (yellow arrow).

The CT scan depicted an abscess adjacent to the gallbladder with subtle peripheral contrast enhancement, measuring up to 12 mm in size along with inflammatory alterations in the adjacent hepatic parenchyma (Panel D). Inflammatory fat stranding can be observed at the omentum, periduodenum and pericolonic areas, as well as free intraperitoneal fluid.

An acute cholecystitis complicated by pericholecystic abscess was diagnosed. The patient refused hospitalization and specialized treatment. The following day the patient returned to the Emergency Department with severe pain and was admitted directly to the General Surgery Department. Nevertheless, blood sample demonstrated increased levels of CEA (67.83 ng/mL) and CA 19-9 (110.20 U/mL), markers which brought to question the CT imaging diagnosis of an acute cholecystitis complicated by pericholecystic abscess.

Therefore, clinical suspicion of gallbladder carcinoma was raised and an MRI cholangiography was performed (Figure 3). A laparoscopic cholecystectomy was performed and a subhepatic tumoral block with transvers colon invasion was identified. The patient was referred to the Oncology Department for further specialized treatment and follow-up.

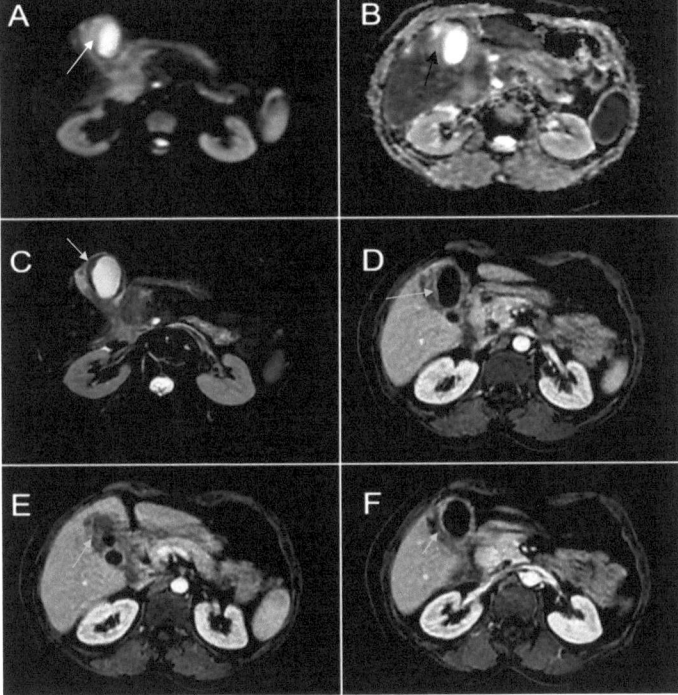

Figure 3. Abdominal MRI sequences highlighting imaging features suggestive of gallbladder carcinoma. (**A**) Diffusion-weighted imaging (DWI B800) showing bright high signal intensity of the wall thickening of the gallbladder (white arrow). (**B**) On apparent diffusion coefficient (ADC) map, the wall thickening is dark (black arrow)—illustrating markedly diffusion restriction—which in correlation with increased levels of CEA and CA 19-9 is highly suggestive of gallbladder carcinoma. (**C**) Axial T2-weighted FIESTA showing asymmetric strongly inhomogeneous wall thickening involving the gallbladder (yellow arrow). (**D–F**). Axial contrast-enhanced T1-weighted images showing heterogeneous enhancement of the wall thickening (green arrows).

A 49-year-old woman with no relevant medical history presented with a 1-week his-tory of abdominal pain, jaundice, dark-colored urine and clay-colored stool. Physical examinations revealed normal abdominal wall mobility with respiratory movements, pain and abdominal tenderness in the epigastric region. Laboratory results upon admission revealed elevated transaminases (ASAT 314 U/L, ALAT 484 U/L) and icteric cholestasis (GGT 311 U/L, bilirubin 8.59 mg/dL). The complete blood count was normal.

Contrast-enhanced emergency CT was performed (Figure 4), which richly highlighted a large heterogeneous intraluminal gallbladder mass, localized in the gallbladder fundus, measuring 58/34 mm, irregular, peripheral contrast enhancement on arterial and venous phase and with central hypodensity suggestive of areas of necrosis, extending to the surrounding liver (segment V) (Panel A and Panel C). CT showed a gallstone (17 mm) wedged in the gallbladder neck and intrahepatic biliary dilatation (Panel C and D). The common bile duct was dilated due to the presence of a possible tumoral extension to biliary tract or by the compressive effect of the multiple hilar lymphadenopathies; mesenteric, celiac and retroperitoneal lymphadenopathies with areas of necrosis, measuring up to 25/15 mm were also noted (Panel B). Abdominal contrast-enhanced MRI was performed (Figure 5).

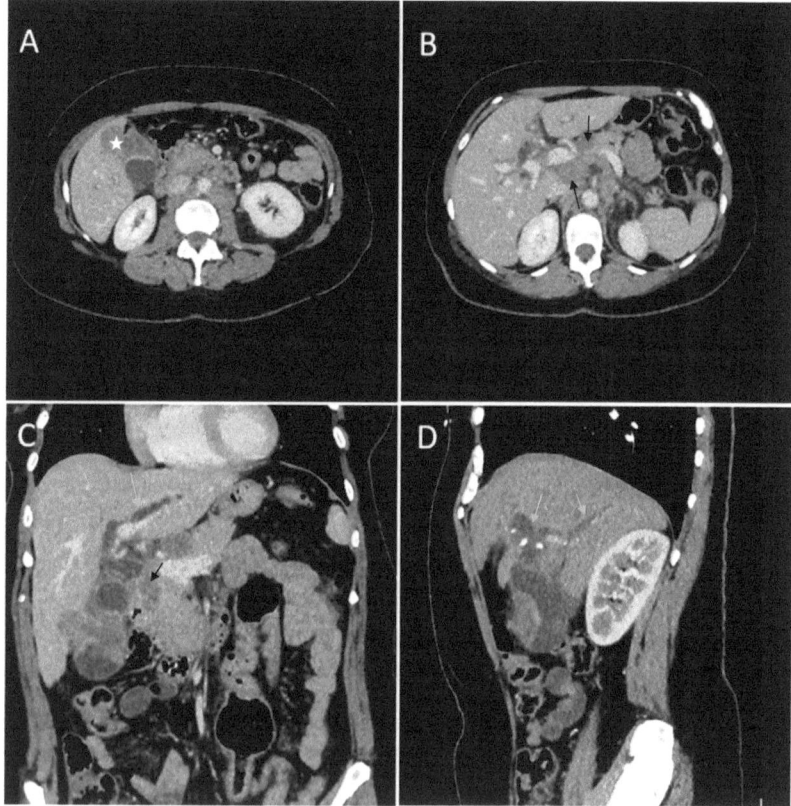

Figure 4. Multiplanar sections of contrast-enhanced CT acquisitions richly illustrating gallbladder carcinoma. (**A**) Heterogeneous ill-defined intraluminal irregular mass located predominantly in the gallbladder fundus (white star). (**B**) Multiple lymphadenopathies with areas of necrosis included (black arrows). (**C**) Gallbladder mass presents extension in the surrounding liver (segment V). (**D**) Intrahepatic biliary dilatation in both hepatic lobes, predominantly perihilar (green arrows).

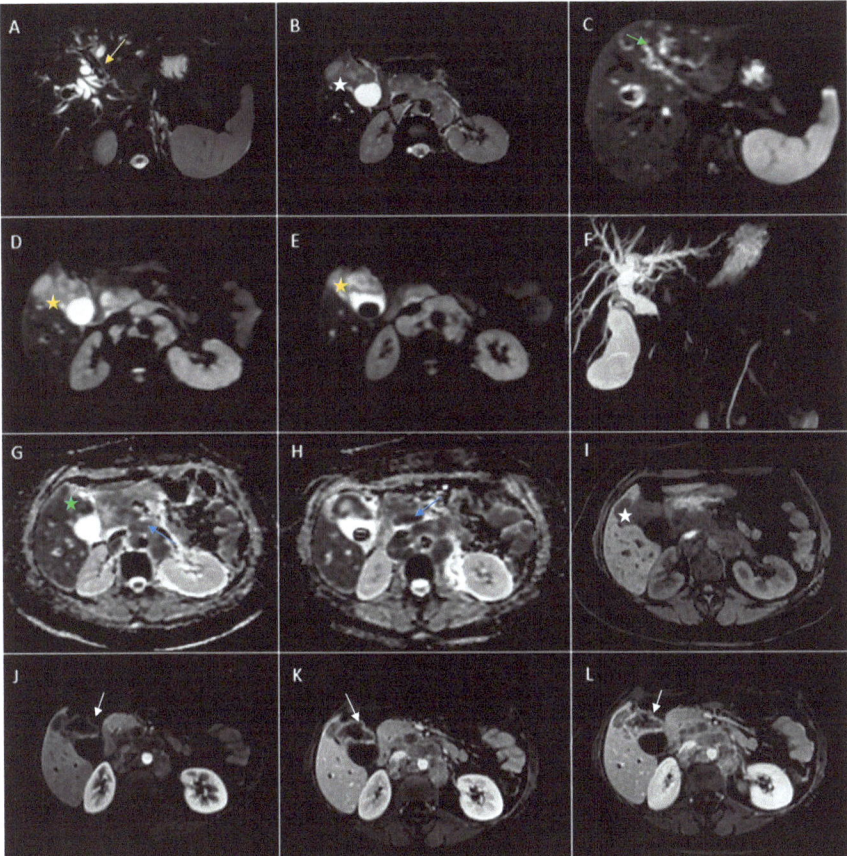

Figure 5. Abdominal MRI vividly illustrating synchronous gallbladder and biliary tract carcinoma with multiple large lymphadenopathies localized in the hepatic hilum, surrounding the cephalic region of the pancreas and in the celiac region. (**A**) Axial T2-weighted FS showed significant intrahepatic biliary dilatation in both hepatic lobes (yellow arrow). (**B**) Axial T2-weighted FS showed hypointense intraluminal gallbladder mass (white star) and multiple large lymphadenopathies. (**C**) Axial diffusion-weighted imaging (DWI B800) showed irregular, asymmetrical thickening of the walls of the intrahepatic bile ducts with high signal intensity suggestive of cholangitis (green arrow). (**D,E**). DWI B800 highlighted the gallbladder mass; inhomogeneous areas of high signal (yellow stars). (**F**) Coronal 3D MRCP showed enlarged gallbladder with an intraluminal gallstone and dilated intrahepatic and extrahepatic biliary tree. (**G,H**). On apparent diffusion coefficient (ADC) map, the gallbladder mass is dark, illustrating markedly diffusion restriction (green star). Multiple large lymphadenopathies are also observed mainly in the lombo-aortic region, in the cephalic pancreatic region and in the hepatic hilum (blue arrow). (**I**) Axial T1-weighted image showing hypointense irregular tumoral gallbladder mass (white star). (**J–L**). Axial contrast-enhanced (arterial phase followed by venous phase) T1-weighted image showing rim-enhancing of the tumoral gallbladder mass (white arrow).

Furthermore, endoscopic retrograde cholangiopancreatography showed a stenosis (with the length of 14–15 mm) at the middle third of the major biliary tract, therefore a stent was placed.

In this case, the probable diagnosis was of synchronous gallbladder and biliary tract carcinoma with multiple large lymphadenopathies localized in the hepatic hilum, surrounding the cephalic region of the pancreas and in the celiac region.

Endoscopic ultrasound-guided fine-needle aspiration (EUS-FNA) for gallbladder tissue was performed. Histopathology showed small cell neuroendocrine carcinoma of the gallbladder. Immunohistochemical stains were positive for CK7, synaptophysin (Syn) and chromogranin A (CgA), and the Ki-67 indexes were over 97% cells.

A 69-year-old female patient with a past medical history of diabetes type II presented to the Emergency Department with a 2-day upper abdominal pain, accompanied by hypotension and oligoanuria. Routine laboratory evaluation showed elevated inflammatory markers (leukocytosis, procalcitonin 100 ng/mL, CRP 126 mg/L), elevated transaminases and ferritin. The patient underwent contrast-enhanced computed tomography (Figure 6). CT images depicted a distended gallbladder (99 mm in longitudinal measurement), with asymmetrical thick-walled gallbladder (16 mm), heterogeneous contrast enhancement (Panel A), with a gallbladder neck stone (10 mm), extended to the duodenum (Panel B and Panel C). CT showed multiple low-attenuation hepatic masses with peripheral enhancement, adjacent to the gallbladder fossa (segment V) and intrahepatic biliary tract dilatation. Below the liver and adjacent to the gallbladder fundus, fat standing and free fluid were observed. These imaging findings were suggestive of acute cholecystitis complicated by an intrahepatic abscess or gallbladder carcinoma with wall perforation into the adjacent liver.

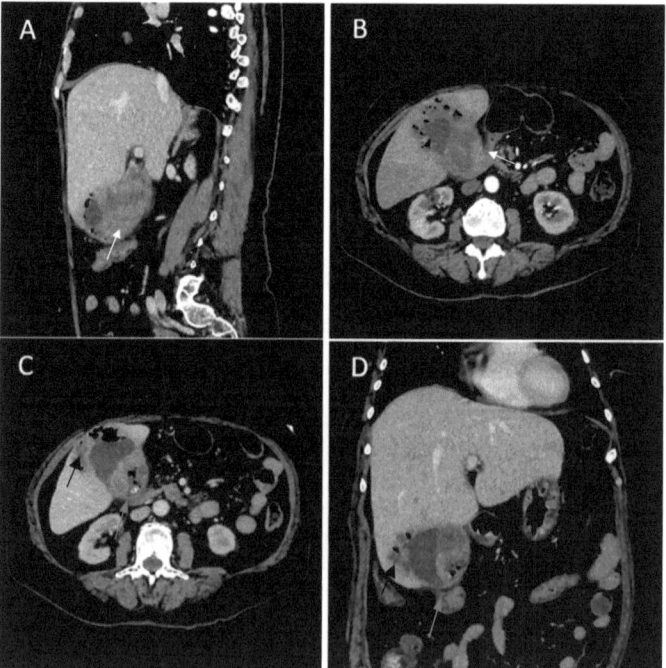

Figure 6. Multiplanar sections of contrast-enhanced CT acquisitions richly illustrating gallbladder carcinoma with an associated necrotizing infectious component. (**A,B**). Distended gallbladder with asymmetrical thick-walled gallbladder (16 mm) (white arrow). (**C,D**). Abscess adjacent to the gallbladder (black arrow); extension to the duodenum (blue arrow).

Antibiotic therapy and percutaneous US-guided drainage for liver abscess represented the first-line treatment, without response. After that, surgical drainage and cholecystostomy was performed.

Histopathological analysis revealed gallbladder carcinoma and palliative chemotherapy was proposed.

A 63-year-old man with a history of severe hyponatremia, known prostate adenocarcinoma and gastroduodenal ulcer with Billroth I gastric resection presented with nausea, vomiting, dizziness and weight loss for one month. On physical examination, abdominal tenderness was noted. Routine laboratory evaluation demonstrated normal leukocytes and inflammatory markers, moderate anemia and severe hyponatremia (serum sodium was 108 mmol/L). Contrast-enhanced CT (Figure 7) showed a heterogeneous intraluminal gallbladder mass, measuring 25/24/35 mm, localized in gallbladder fundus (Panel A, Panel B, Panel C and Panel D). The mass had no invasion of the adjacent structures and no associated imaging findings. An abdominal MRI was performed (Figure 8).

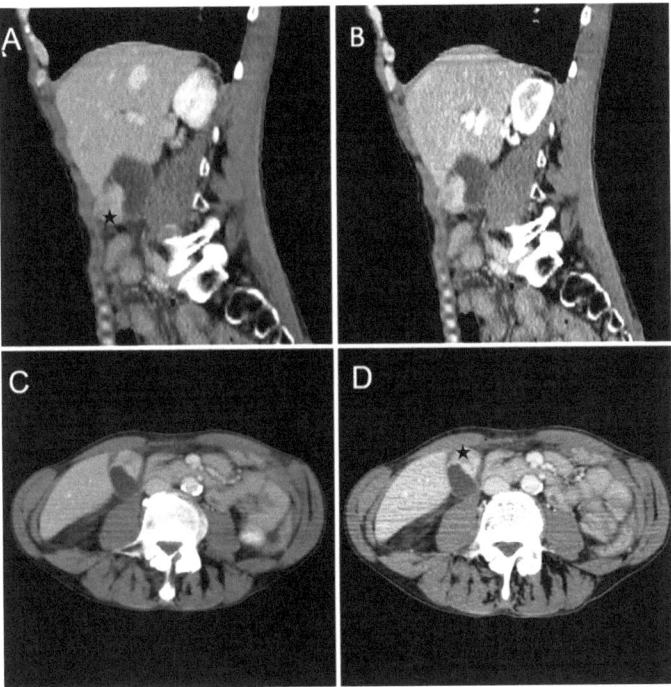

Figure 7. Multiplanar sections of contrast-enhanced CT acquisitions richly illustrating gallbladder carcinoma. (**A–D**). Heterogeneous, contrast-enhancing intraluminal gallbladder mass located in the gallbladder fundus region (black star).

Furthermore, a laparoscopic cholecystectomy was performed. The histopathological exam revealed gallbladder carcinoma.

The particularity of this case report is amply illustrated by severe hyponatremia presented as paraneoplastic SIADH syndrome (syndrome of inappropriate antidiuretic hormone secretion) in a patient with gallbladder carcinoma.

A 67-year-old female patient with a past medical history of hypertension and autoimmune thyroiditis presented to the Emergency Department with abdominal pain accompanied by nausea and weight loss. Physical examinations revealed abdominal tenderness with a palpable mass in the right hypochondrium. Blood sample demonstrated elevated inflammatory markers, hypochromic microcytic anemia, hepatic cytolysis and increased levels of CEA (12.5 ng/mL) and CA 19-9 (51 U/mL). Contrast-enhanced emergency CT (Figure 9) showed a large mass with heterogeneous enhancement, measuring 94/57 mm, that partially replaced the gallbladder and invaded the liver (segment IVb), pyloric antrum and duodenum II. Bulky celiac and mesenteric lymphadenopathies with areas of necrosis, measuring up to 27/25 mm were present.

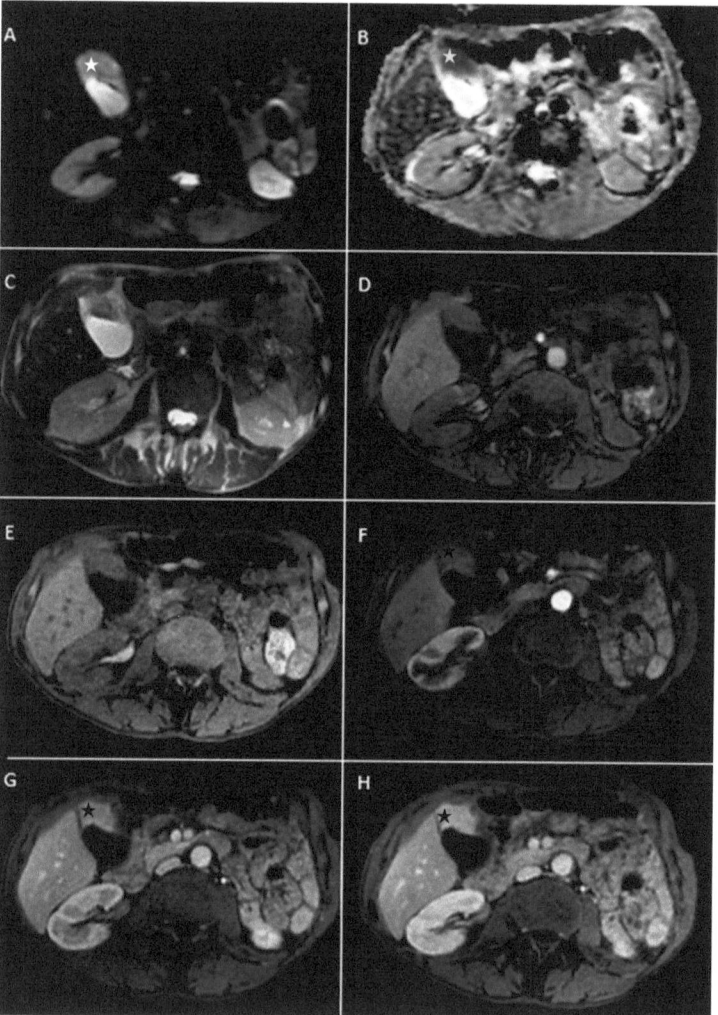

Figure 8. Abdominal MRI sequences highlighting gallbladder carcinoma. (**A**) Diffusion-weighted imaging (DWI B800) showing areas of moderate-high signal of the intraluminal gallbladder mass located in the fundus area (white star). (**B**) On ADC map, the intraluminal gallbladder mass is dark—diffusion restriction (yellow star). (**C**,**D**). Axial T2-weighted showing distended gallbladder with a heterogeneous hypointense intraluminal mass and axial T1 dual ECHO showing isointense gallbladder mass. (**E**) Axial T1-weighted image showing isointense gallbladder mass. (**F**–**H**). Axial contrast-enhanced T1-weighted image (arterial phase followed by venous phase) showing strong contrast-enhancement of the intraluminal gallbladder mass (black star).

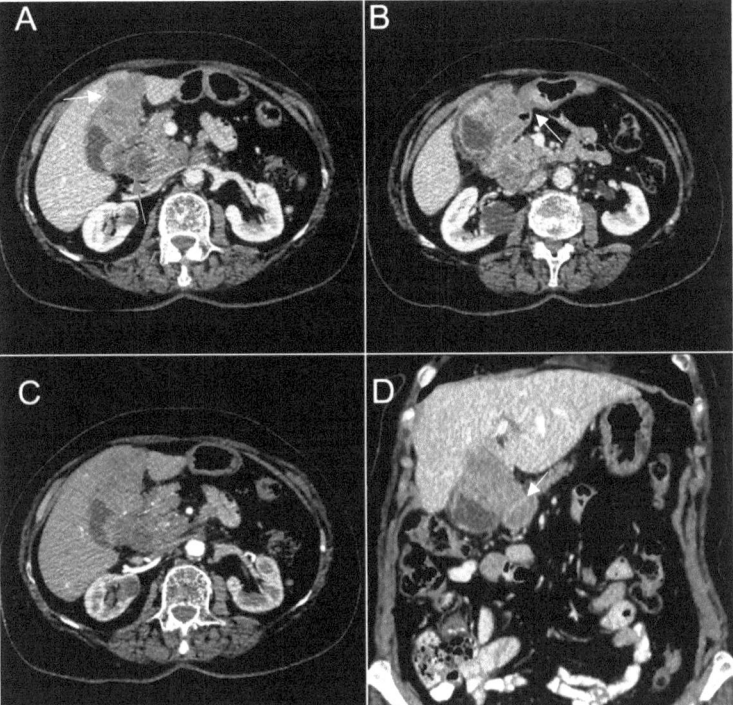

Figure 9. Multiplanar sections of contrast-enhanced CT acquisitions richly illustrating gallbladder carcinoma. (**A–D**). A large, inhomogeneous pseudonodular mass with heterogeneous contrast enhancement, with invasion in the adjacent liver, pyloric antrum and duodenum II (white arrows). (**A**) Lymphatic metastases; with compressive effect on the inferior vena cava and right renal artery and vein (blue arrow).

Abdominal MRI was performed (Figure 10).

Endoscopic ultrasound-guided fine-needle aspiration (EUS-FNA) for gallbladder tissue was performed and revealed epithelial gallbladder carcinoma. The biopsy specimens were processed for frozen sectioning. Formalin-fixed paraffin-embedded tissue sections from the gallbladder were examined histologically. The microscopic description revealed proliferation of polygonal cells, abundant clear cytoplasm, large nuclei with irregular membranes and atypical mitotic divisions.

The clinical symptoms of gallbladder cancer are often vague and non-specific and include pain in the right hypochondriac region, nausea and vomiting. In the late stages of the disease weight loss, anorexia and jaundice are often seen [11,12]. In contrast, some patients present with symptoms of acute cholecystitis and malignancy may be incidentally found following a cholecystectomy [13]. Detection of gallbladder at an early stage is difficult because the symptoms often mimic benign conditions.

The major risk factors include being an elderly woman (over 60 years old, F:M ratio 3:1), cholelithiasis and gallstones (in 60–90% cases) [10]. Regarding our cases, five of them were female and one was male. Other risk factors include:

- √ chronic inflammation due to typhoid carrier state;
- √ gallbladder polyps (more than 10 mm);
- √ porcelain gallbladder;
- √ smoking and obesity [3,11];
- √ anomalous pancreaticobiliary ductal junction, which is a rare congenital anomaly [12].

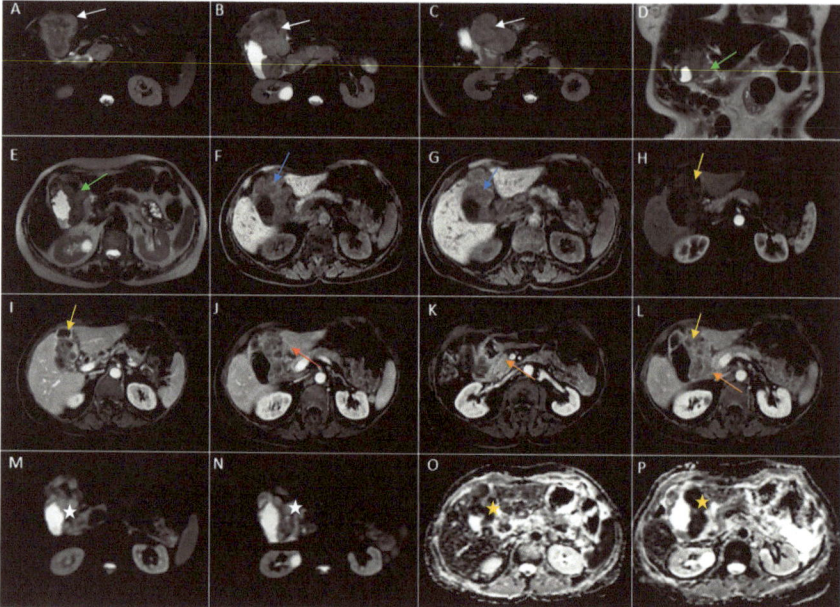

Figure 10. Abdominal MRI images vividly illustrating epithelial gallbladder carcinoma. (**A–C**). Axial T2-weighted FS showing inhomogeneous moderate hypointense heterogeneous tumoral parietal mass surrounding the gallbladder (white arrow). (**D,E**). Coronal and axial T2-weighted images showing hypointense heterogeneous tumoral gallbladder mass (green arrow). (**F,G**). Axial T1-weighted illustrating iso-hypointense tumoral mass (blue arrow). (**H–L**). Axial contrast-enhanced T1-weighted image (arterial phase followed by venous phase) showing a heterogeneous enhancement of the gallbladder mass with areas of necrosis (yellow arrows). The mass invades the adjacent liver ((**J**), red arrow) and duodenum II ((**K,L**), orange arrows). (**M,N**). Diffusion-weighted imaging (DWI B800) showing bright signal of the large gallbladder mass (white stars). (**O,P**). On ADC map, the large gallbladder mass is dark, illustrating diffusion restriction (yellow stars).

Gallbladder carcinoma might be found incidentally in 1–3% following a cholecystectomy [14]. Because of advanced disease at diagnosis, the typical 5-year survival is only 5% [15].

Imaging has a key role in the diagnosis, staging, characterization and planning management of gallbladder cancer.

Diagnostic imaging modalities for the gallbladder cancer include ultrasound, computerized tomography (CT) and magnetic resonance imaging (MRI). Ultrasound is frequently the initial imaging modality for evaluating gallbladder disease. In locally advanced gallbladder cancer, ultrasound has a sensitivity of 85% and a specificity of 80% in diagnosis. Moreover, ultrasound is limited to evaluate locoregional extension, nodal and metastatic disease. CT and MRI are commonly indicated for the comprehensive assessment of disease extension. Biphasic arterial phase (at 20 to 30 s) followed by venous phase (50 to 60 s) contrast-enhanced CT is useful to evaluate gallbladder cancer. CT demonstrates a sensitivity of 99% and a specificity of 76% in determining resectability. MRI is a noninvasive imaging method and demonstrates superior sensitivity compared to CT, providing superior soft-tissue characterization of the gallbladder and biliary tree [10].

Computed tomography (CT) and magnetic resonance imaging (MRI) reveal three major patterns of disease. Gallbladder carcinoma could present as a mass that completely replaces the gallbladder and invades the adjacent liver or as an intraluminal enhancement mass (in 25% of cases) arising from the fundus (60%) or body (30%) [15–18]. Regarding our six patients, two of them presented with a mass that replaced a part of gallbladder and invaded the adjacent liver (Case 3 and 6) and one of them as a suspicious intraluminal gallbladder lesion localized in gallbladder fundus on CT and MRI (Case 5).

A third presentation of gallbladder carcinoma is either irregular focal or diffuse wall-thickening of the gallbladder [15,19]. Regarding our cases, three of them had presented with this imaging scenario (Cases 1, 2 and 4).

Tumor can spread to the liver (65%), colon (15%), duodenum (15%) and pancreas (6%) [12,15]. Regarding our cases, in Case 1 the tumor spread to the liver and duodenum and transvers colon and in Cases 4 and 6 metastatic spread to the liver and duodenum can be noted.

Tumor extending to biliary tract is associated with poor prognosis. This aspect was presented in Case 3. Also, in Cases 1, 3 and 6, local lymphatic tumoral spread was presented [15,20].

Associated findings include a checklist of:

- √ gallstones (Cases 1, 2);
- √ biliary dilatation (Case 3);
- √ metastases in the liver parenchyma (segments IV, V) (Cases 1, 3);
- √ peritoneum;
- √ bulky porta hepatis, adenopathy (Cases 1, 3, 5);
- √ invasion of the liver and bowel (Cases 1, 3, 4, 5, 6) [15,18].

Adenocarcinoma is the most common morphologic subtype of gallbladder cancer (over 90% of cases), followed by adenosquamous and squamous cell type (10–15%). Small cell carcinoma, neuroendocrine cell tumors and metastases are the rare types [10]. In our six cases, different subtypes of gallbladder cancer were observed, three of which were adenocarcinoma (Cases 1, 4 and 6). In two cases (Cases 3 and 5), the histopathology showed small cell neuroendocrine carcinoma. Neuroendocrine carcinoma of gallbladder is a rare entity and it tends to be more aggressive compared with gallbladder adenocarcinoma [21].

In our Case 5 report (Figure 7), the patient presented gallbladder carcinoma with endocrine manifestation. Gallbladder cancer associated with SIADH syndrome represents a very rare entity with few cases reported in the current literature. Hyponatremia (<135 mmol/L) is correlated with a negative prognosis and in some case is a predictive factor for cancer patients. Paraneoplastic syndrome of inappropriate antidiuretic hormone secretion (SIADH) is induced by the abnormal secretion of antidiuretic hormone by tumoral cells [21]. In our case, the final diagnosis was gallbladder carcinoma associated with SIADH as a paraneoplastic syndrome.

Moreover, the American Joint Committee on Cancer 8th edition gallbladder cancer staging system is staged by the depth of tumor invasion (T), presence of lymph node metastases (N) and presence of distant metastases (M) [1]. The T component describes the depth that the tumor has grown from the inside through the outer layers. The N component indicates invasion in lymph nodes. The M component describes distant metastases, the most common sites of metastases being represented by the peritoneum and liver parenchyma [10,22].

Furthermore, for the most important imaging part regarding differential diagnostic, imaging represents a helpful modality for distinguishing between benign and malign gallbladder diseases, in most cases [15,23]. Differential diagnosis includes a group of diseases, such as complicated or chronic cholecystitis, xanthogranulomatous cholecystitis, adenomyomatosis, adenoma, porcelain and metastases [15].

A gallbladder tumor is usually represented on imaging as focal or diffuse asymmetric mural thickening [10,24].

The presence of symmetric wall thickening often indicates a benign origin, such as acute or chronic cholecystitis or adenomyomatosis [24].

Acute cholecystitis complicated by pericholecystic abscess are frequently differentiated from gallbladder cancer due to their typically rapid and severe acute clinical presentation.

Also, acute cholecystitis on contrast-enhanced CT shows increased gallbladder wall enhancement associated with hyperemia, frequently associated with gallstones (Figure 11) [10].

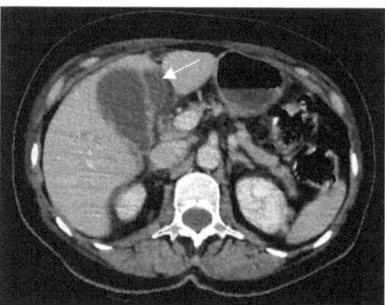

Figure 11. A 67-year-old woman undergoing contrast-enhanced CT for suspected abdominal acute appendicitis. CT images show pericholecystic abscess (white arrow) and symmetric wall thickening suggestive of acalculous cholecystitis.

Moreover, the differential diagnosis between xanthogranulomatous cholecystitis (Figure 12) and gallbladder tumor, can be challenging, particularly in patients with proliferative fibrosis. Xanthogranulomatous cholecystitis is an uncommon form of chronic cholecystitis characterized by aggressive inflammatory changes, by intramural hypoattenuating nodules and by fat detection on MRI in thickened wall (Figure 13) [25–29].

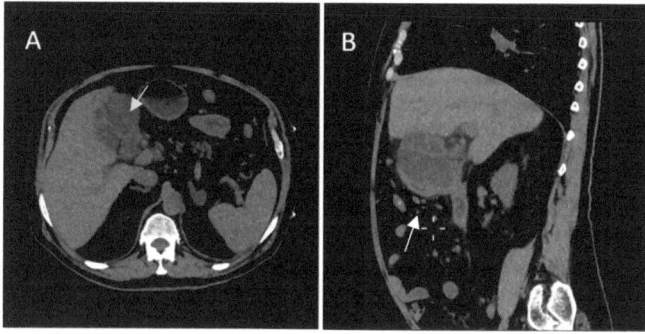

Figure 12. A 70-year-old male with a history of hypertension, type 2 diabetes, peripheral venous thrombosis, presented at our Emergency Department with abdominal pain accompanied by diarrhea, night sweats and fever. His laboratory findings showed elevated inflammatory markers. Computerized tomography (CT) revealed (**B**)—diffuse wall thickening with intramural low-density nodules and bands in thickened walls (white arrow) associated with (**A**) pericholecystic inflammatory change (yellow arrow).

Furthermore, gallbladder adenomyomatosis is a benign gallbladder lesion. Imaging shows a focal or diffuse gallbladder mural thickening, which can mimic cancer. The invaginations or diverticula are frequently called Rokitansky–Aschoff sinuses, which can be easily visualized on MRI imaging [19,20,30]. The differential diagnosis for intraluminal polypoid tumors includes both benign and malignant lesions: adenomatous polyp, cholesterol polyp, carcinoid tumor and metastasis from melanoma or renal cell carcinoma [31].

Metastases to the gallbladder are rare, usually with a late diagnosis and represent an end-stage of malignancy, being commonly associated with metastases to other tissues (patients with an established diagnosis of disseminated cancer) and usually presenting poor and unfavorable prognosis. The most common primary tumor metastasizing to the gallbladder is melanoma (55% of cases) (Figures 14–16), followed by breast cancer (13%), hepatocellular carcinoma (13%) and renal cell carcinoma (7%) [32,33].

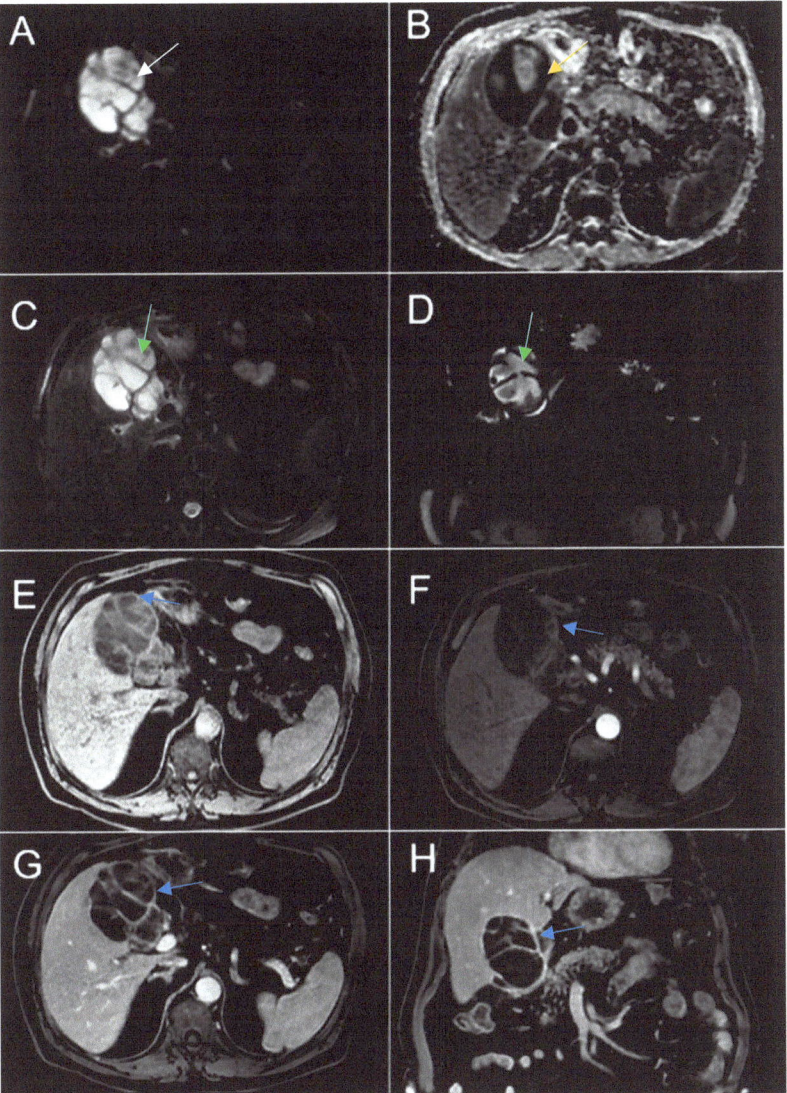

Figure 13. Abdominal MRI vividly illustrating Xanthogranulomatous Cholecystitis. (**A**) Diffusion-weighted imaging (DWI B800—bright high signal) demonstrated restricted diffusion (white arrow), but malignancy typically demonstrates lower ADC values. (**B**) On ADC map, the wall thickening is dark (yellow arrow). (**C**,**D**). Intramural areas of necrosis are high signal intensity on axial and coronal T2-weighted images (green arrows). (**E**–**H**). Axial unenhanced and contrast-enhanced T1-weighted images showing diffusely thickened wall, with multiple intramural nodules with peripheral contrast enhancement (blue arrows).

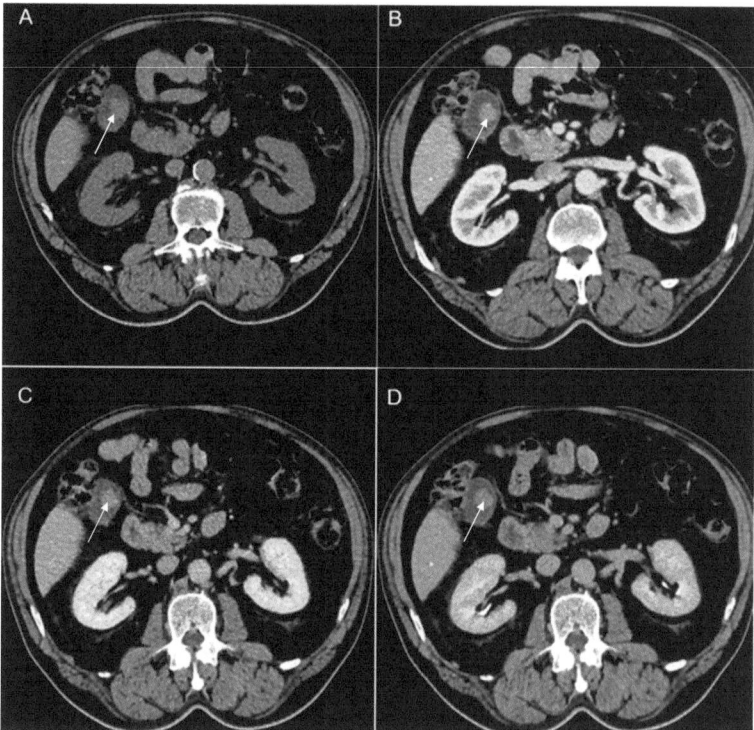

Figure 14. We present a rare and unusual case of a 67-year-old male with a medical history of cutaneous melanoma on right thorax stage IV. CT images fully illustrated a contrast-enhancing polypoid pseudonodular mass located in the gallbladder fundus measuring 21/20 mm (white arrows). (**A**) Native examination: 55–60 HU. (**B**) Arterial phase: 95–119 HU. (**C**) Venous phase: 80–100 HU. (**D**) Delayed phase (3 min): 75–80 HU. MRI was performed (Figure 15). Melanin is usually hyperdense on unenhanced CT images and hyperintense on T1-weighted MRI; this criterion plays an essential role in the differential diagnosis between primary or secondary gallbladder lesions. The patient followed immunotherapy.

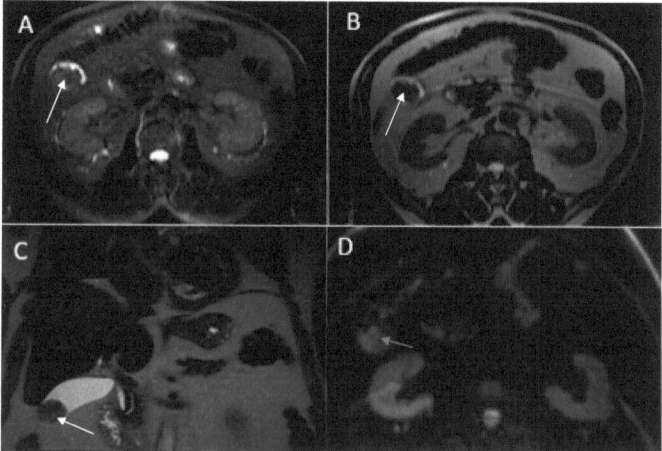

Figure 15. *Cont.*

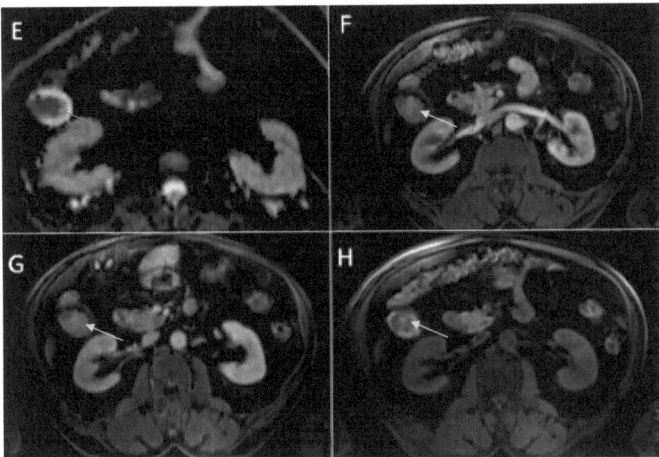

Figure 15. Abdominal MRI. (**A**) Axial T2-weighted FS showing markedly hypointense pseudonodular tumoral gallbladder lesion (white arrow). (**B**) Axial T2-weighted showing hypointense gallbladder lesion (white arrow). (**C**) Coronal T2-HASTE hypointense gallbladder lesion (white arrow). (**D**) Diffusion-weighted imaging (DWI B800) showing bright hypersignal of the lesion (blue arrow). (**E**) Restricted diffusion (blue arrow) on apparent diffusion coefficient (ADC) map. (**F**,**G**) Axial contrast-enhanced T1-weighted image showing a strongly enhancing polypoid pseudonodular mass in the gallbladder fundus. (**H**) Axial T1-weighted image FS showing hyperintense nodular lesion component (yellow arrows), highly suggestive of melanin.

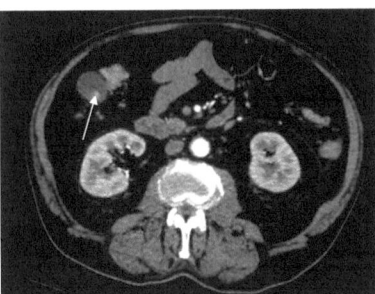

Figure 16. Remarkable treatment response to immunotherapy; intracholecystic metastatic lesion from cutaneous melanoma after immunotherapy appears in remission (white arrow).

Author Contributions: All authors have worked on conception and design of the scientific paper, on the data collection and analysis and interpretation of data and images and on the revised article. All authors gave final approval of the version to be submitted. All authors have read and agreed to the published version of the manuscript.

Funding: This research received no external funding.

Institutional Review Board Statement: Ethical review and approval were waived for this study, due to being a retrospective case report series, which did not impact the management of the patients.

Informed Consent Statement: Informed written consent has been obtained from the patients.

Data Availability Statement: The data presented in this study are available on request from the corresponding author (N, L.C.).

Conflicts of Interest: The authors declare no conflicts of interest.

References

1. Ramachandran, A.; Srivastava, D.N.; Madhusudhan, K.S. Gallbladder cancer revisited: The evolving role of a radiologist. *Br. J. Radiol.* **2021**, *94*, 20200726. [CrossRef]
2. Rawla, P.; Sunkara, T.; Thandra, K.C.; Barsouk, A. Epidemiology of gallbladder cancer. *Clin. Exp. Hepatol.* **2019**, *5*, 93–102. [CrossRef]
3. Halaseh, S.A.; Halaseh, S.A.; Halaseh, S.; Halaseh, S.; Shakman, R.; Shakman, R. A Review of the Etiology and Epidemiology of Gallbladder Cancer: What You Need to Know. *Cureus* **2022**, *14*, e28260. [CrossRef]
4. Liu, Z.; Zhu, G.; Jiang, X.; Zhao, Y.; Zeng, H.; Jing, J.; Ma, X. Survival Prediction in Gallbladder Cancer Using CT Based Machine Learning. *Front. Oncol.* **2020**, *10*, 604288. [CrossRef]
5. Hundal, R.; Shaffer, E.A. Gallbladder cancer: Epidemiology and outcome. *Clin. Epidemiol.* **2014**, *6*, 99–109. [CrossRef]
6. Kalra, N.; Gupta, P.; Singhal, M.; Gupta, R.; Gupta, V.; Srinivasan, R.; Mittal, B.R.; Dhiman, R.K.; Khandelwal, N. Cross-sectional Imaging of Gallbladder Carcinoma: An Update. *J. Clin. Exp. Hepatol.* **2018**, *9*, 334–344. [CrossRef] [PubMed]
7. John, S.; Moyana, T.; Shabana, W.; Walsh, C.; McInnes, M.D.F. Gallbladder Cancer: Imaging Appearance and Pitfalls in Diagnosis. *Can. Assoc. Radiol. J.* **2020**, *71*, 448–458. [CrossRef] [PubMed]
8. Furlan, A.; Ferris, J.V.; Hosseinzadeh, K.; Borhani, A.A. Gallbladder carcinoma update: Multimodality imaging evaluation, staging, and treatment options. *Am. J. Roentgenol.* **2008**, *191*, 1440–1447. [CrossRef] [PubMed]
9. Randi, G.; Malvezzi, M.; Levi, F.; Ferlay, J.; Negri, E.; Franceschi, S.; La Vecchia, C. Epidemiology of biliary tract cancers: An update. *Ann. Oncol.* **2009**, *20*, 146–159. [CrossRef] [PubMed]
10. Lopes Vendrami, C.; Magnetta, M.J.; Mittal, P.K.; Moreno, C.C.; Miller, F.H. Gallbladder carcinoma and its differential diagnosis at MRI: What radiologists should know. *RadioGraphics* **2021**, *41*, 78–95. [CrossRef] [PubMed]
11. Adam, K.M.; Abdelrahim, E.Y.; Doush, W.M.; Abdelaziz, M.S. Clinical presentation and management modalities of gallbladder cancer in Sudan: A single-center study. *JGH Open* **2023**, *7*, 365–371. [CrossRef]
12. Gupta, P.; Meghashyam, K.; Marodia, Y.; Gupta, V.; Basher, R.; Das, C.K.; Yadav, T.D.; Irrinki, S.; Nada, R.; Dutta, U. Locally advanced gallbladder cancer: A review of the criteria and role of imaging. *Abdom. Imaging* **2020**, *46*, 998–1007. [CrossRef]
13. Franco, N. Outcomes of Patients with Gallbladder Cancer Presenting with Acute Cholecystitis. *Researchsquare* **2023**. [CrossRef]
14. Alkhayyat, M.; Saleh, M.A.; Qapaja, T.; Abureesh, M.; Almomani, A.; Mansoor, E.; Chahal, P. Epidemiology of gallbladder cancer in the Unites States: A population-based study. *Chin. Clin. Oncol.* **2021**, *10*, 25. [CrossRef] [PubMed]
15. Zaheer, A.; Raman, S.P. *Diagnostic Imaging: Gastrointestinal*; Elsevier: Amsterdam, The Netherlands, 2015.
16. Ganeshan, D.; Kambadakone, A.; Nikolaidis, P.; Subbiah, V.; Subbiah, I.M.; Devine, C. Current update on gallbladder carcinoma. *Abdom. Imaging* **2021**, *46*, 2474–2489. [CrossRef] [PubMed]
17. Levy, A.D.; Murakata, L.A.; Rohrmann, C.A. Gallbladder carcinoma: Radiologic-pathologic correlation. *RadioGraphics* **2001**, *21*, 295–314. [CrossRef] [PubMed]
18. George, R.; Godara, S.; Dhagat, P.; Som, P. Computed tomographic findings in 50 cases of gall bladder carcinoma. *Med. J. Armed Forces India* **2007**, *63*, 215–219. [CrossRef]
19. Ratanaprasatporn, L.; Uyeda, J.W.; Wortman, J.R.; Richardson, I.; Sodickson, A.D. Multimodality imaging, including dual-energy CT, in the evaluation of gallbladder disease. *RadioGraphics* **2018**, *38*, 75–89. [CrossRef]
20. Gourgiotis, S.; Kocher, H.M.; Solaini, L.; Yarollahi, A.; Tsiambas, E.; Salemis, N.S. Gallbladder cancer. *Am. J. Surg.* **2008**, *196*, 252–264. [CrossRef]
21. Ng, E.S.; Venkateswaran, K.; Ganpathi, S.I.; Chuah, B.Y. Small cell gallbladder carcinoma complicated by paraneoplastic hyponatremia: A case report and literature review. *J. Gastrointest. Cancer* **2010**, *41*, 264–268. [CrossRef]
22. Amin, M.B.; Greene, F.L.; Edge, S.B.; Compton, C.C.; Gershenwald, J.E.; Brookland, R.K.; Meyer, L.; Gress, D.M.; Byrd, D.R.; Winchester, D.P. The Eighth Edition AJCC Cancer Staging Manual: Continuing to build a bridge from a population-based to a more "personalized" approach to cancer staging. *CA Cancer J. Clin.* **2017**, *67*, 93–99. [CrossRef] [PubMed]
23. Kitazume, Y.; Taura, S.-I.; Nakaminato, S.; Noguchi, O.; Masaki, Y.; Kasahara, I.; Kishino, M.; Tateishi, U. Diffusion-weighted magnetic resonance imaging to differentiate malignant from benign gallbladder disorders. *Eur. J. Radiol.* **2016**, *85*, 864–873. [CrossRef] [PubMed]
24. Soundararajan, R.; Marodia, Y.; Gupta, P.; Rana, P.; Chhabra, M.; Kalage, D.; Dutta, U.; Sandhu, M. Imaging patterns of wall thickening type of gallbladder cancer. *Clin. Exp. Hepatol.* **2022**, *8*, 255–266. [CrossRef] [PubMed]
25. Gri, J.; Hatahet, M.A.; Chopra, S. Xanthogranulomatous pyelonephritis: A rare case report of a 54 year old female (a potentially fatal infection). *Int. J. Surg. Case Rep.* **2021**, *85*, 106287. [CrossRef] [PubMed]
26. Suzuki, H.; Wada, S.; Araki, K.; Kubo, N.; Watanabe, A.; Tsukagoshi, M.; Kuwano, H. Xanthogranulomatous cholecystitis: Difficulty in differentiating from gallbladder cancer. *World J. Gastroenterol.* **2015**, *21*, 10166–10173. [CrossRef]
27. Kang, T.; Kim, S.; Park, H.; Lim, S.; Jang, K.; Choi, D.; Lee, S. Differentiating xanthogranulomatous cholecystitis from wall-thickening type of gallbladder cancer: Added value of diffusion-weighted MRI. *Clin. Radiol.* **2013**, *68*, 992–1001. [CrossRef]
28. Xu, Z.; Cai, T.; Zhang, X.; Wu, J.; Liu, C. Xanthogranulomatous pyelonephritis infected with the *Providencia stuartii*: A case report and literature review. *BMC Nephrol.* **2021**, *22*, 356. [CrossRef]
29. Chang, B.J.; Kim, S.H.; Park, H.Y.; Lim, S.W.; Kim, J.; Lee, K.H.; Lee, K.T.; Rhee, J.C.; Lim, J.H.; Lee, J.K. Distinguishing xanthogranulomatous cholecystitis from the wall-thickening type of early-stage gallbladder cancer. *Gut Liver* **2010**, *4*, 518–523. [CrossRef]

30. Bonatti, M.; Vezzali, N.; Lombardo, F.; Ferro, F.; Zamboni, G.; Tauber, M.; Bonatti, G. Gallbladder adenomyomatosis: Imaging findings, tricks and pitfalls. *Insights Imaging* **2017**, *8*, 243–253. [CrossRef]
31. Zemour, J.; Marty, M.; Lapuyade, B.; Collet, D.; Chiche, L. Gallbladder tumor and pseudotumor: Diagnosis and management. *J. Visc. Surg.* **2014**, *151*, 289–300. [CrossRef]
32. Cocco, G.; Pizzi, A.D.; Basilico, R.; Fabiani, S.; Taraschi, A.L.; Pascucci, L.; Boccatonda, A.; Catalano, O.; Schiavone, C. Imaging of gallbladder metastasis. *Insights Imaging* **2021**, *12*, 100. [CrossRef] [PubMed]
33. Christou, D.; Katodritis, N.; Decatris, M.P.; Katodritou, A.; Michaelides, I.; Nicolaou, N.; Kounoushis, M.; Hadjicostas, P. Melanoma of the gallbladder: Appropriate surgical management and review of the literature. *Clin. Case Rep.* **2014**, *2*, 313–318. [CrossRef] [PubMed]

Disclaimer/Publisher's Note: The statements, opinions and data contained in all publications are solely those of the individual author(s) and contributor(s) and not of MDPI and/or the editor(s). MDPI and/or the editor(s) disclaim responsibility for any injury to people or property resulting from any ideas, methods, instructions or products referred to in the content.

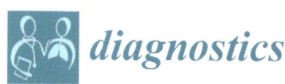
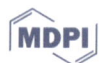

Interesting Images

An Isolated Intestinal Juvenile Polyp Diagnosed by Abdominal Ultrasonography and Resected by Double-Balloon Endoscopy: A Case Report and Literature Review

Masumi Nagata, Keisuke Jimbo *, Nobuyasu Arai, Kosuke Kashiwagi, Kaori Tokushima, Mitsuyoshi Suzuki, Takahiro Kudo and Toshiaki Shimizu

Department of Pediatrics, Faculty of Medicine, Juntendo University, Tokyo 113-8421, Japan
* Correspondence: kjinbo@juntendo.ac.jp; Tel.: +81-(0)3-3813-3111

Abstract: Juvenile polyps, typically localized in the rectum and sigmoid colon, are a common cause of pediatric bloody stool. An isolated small intestinal juvenile polyp is uncommon and generally difficult to diagnose. The first case of an isolated juvenile polyp diagnosed by abdominal ultrasonography before acute abdomen had developed and resected by double-balloon endoscopy is presented along with a review of previous reports including this case. A two-year-old Japanese boy was referred to our institute for further evaluation of anemia persisting from one year of age. Laboratory findings showed mild iron deficiency anemia and elevated fecal human hemoglobin (Hb) and fecal calprotectin values. Upper and lower endoscopic findings showed no abnormalities. Because the abdominal ultrasonography performed one year later demonstrated a 15 mm jejunal polyp, combined with a similar finding on small intestinal capsule endoscopy, this was diagnosed as an isolated lesion. The lesion was resected by cautery with double-balloon endoscopy and diagnosed as a juvenile polyp pathologically. All clinical symptoms disappeared, and all laboratory data improved after treatment, without recurrence for more than one year after the procedure. Abdominal ultrasonographic screening and the fecal calprotectin value led to the diagnosis and non-surgical invasive treatment of an isolated small intestinal juvenile polyp.

Keywords: anemia; double-balloon endoscopy; fecal calprotectin; intestinal juvenile polyp; ultrasonography

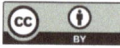

A two-year-old Japanese boy was referred to our institute for further evaluation and treatment of protracted iron deficiency anemia. The anemia improved with iron supplements, but relapsed following cessation of the medication. Similar episodes were repeated frequently, and fecal human Hb level was also elevated. The patient had no significant personal or family history. At the first visit to our institute, the patient had no growth retardation and no significant abnormalities in vital signs. During the period of iron administration, no physical abnormalities were observed. Moreover, he had no significant external deformities and normal psychomotor development.

The patient's initial laboratory tests showed Hb 11.2 g/dL, mean corpuscular volume 80.5 fL, mean corpuscular Hb concentration 26.4%, total protein 6.1 g/dL, albumin 4.1 g/dL, immunoglobulin G 461 mg/dL, and ferritin 19 ng/mL. Fecal examinations showed fecal human Hb 215 ng/mL and fecal calprotectin 134 µg/g. Both upper gastrointestinal endoscopy and colonoscopy performed at two years of age showed normal mucosal findings. At three years of age, the patient was re-evaluated by abdominal ultrasonography (AUS) concurrent with capsule endoscopy (CE). Abdominal ultrasonography showed a movable mass lesion in the mid-abdomen, and color Doppler flow showed a blood flow signal toward the mass, leading to the diagnosis of a pedunculated polyp. The polyp was localized in the upper jejunum, with a diameter of approximately 15 mm, and multiple anechoic cysts in the parenchyma, suggesting a juvenile polyp (Figure 1a,b). A same mass lesion was also identified in the upper jejunum by CE, with no abnormalities in the remaining small intestine (Figure 2a).

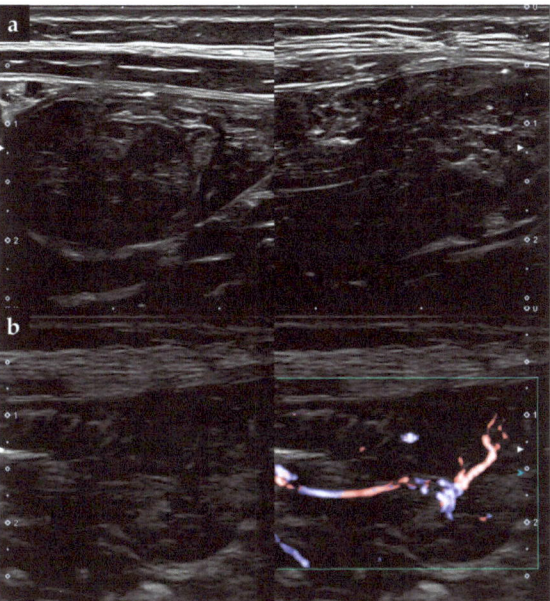

Figure 1. The ultrasonographic findings of the isolated small intestinal polyp. (**a**) Multiple anechoic cysts are identified within the parenchyma of the polyp. (**b**) The pedunculated polyp has a diameter of 15 mm and shows increased internal vascularity.

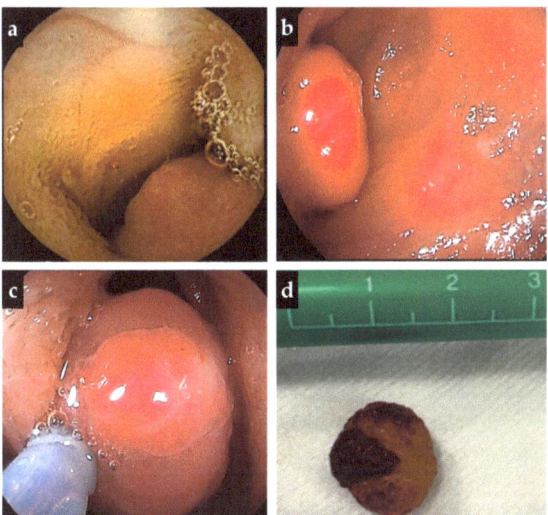

Figure 2. The findings of capsule endoscopy and double-balloon endoscopy. (**a**) Capsule endoscopy shows a polyp-like lesion at the upper jejunum, but no similar lesions are observed in other small intestinal segments. (**b,c**) A pedunculated polyp is found 75 cm anorectally from the pylorus and resected by cautery using a high-frequency snare. (**d**) The diameter of the resected polyp is 15 mm.

One month after CE, oral DBE was performed, and an isolated pedunculated polyp, identified 75 cm anorectally from the pylorus, was resected by cautery with a high-frequency snare (Figure 2b–d). The histopathology of the polyp suggesting a hamartomatous polyp, which was consistent with a juvenile polyp (Figure 3). The polyp was removed by DBE with no complications. The patient was discharged a day after polypectomy, following the disappearance of gastrointestinal symptoms and fecal human Hb and calprotectin elevation. Iron supplements were stopped, and the anemia disappeared. At one-year post-treatment, there were no abnormal laboratory data, and no new polyps were identified on abdominal ultrasonographic screening.

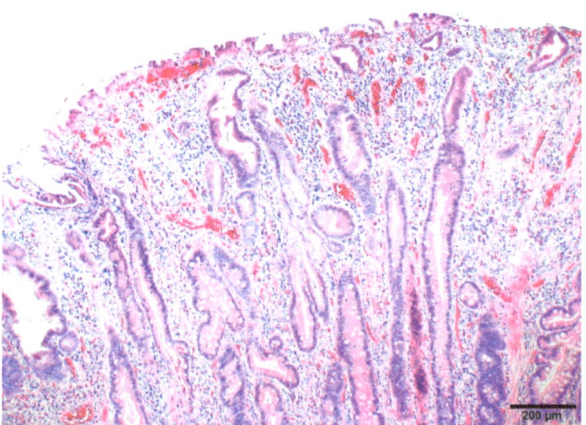

Figure 3. The histopathological findings of the resected polyp (hematoxylin and eosin staining). The histology shows mixed findings of dilated and serrated glandular ducts with partial granulation, consistent with a hamartomatous polyp.

Juvenile polyps tend to be localized to the rectum and sigmoid colon and are also associated with iron deficiency anemia due to protracted bloody stool and intussusception involving polyps as the pathologic advanced lesions [1,2]. The pathology is applicable to the small intestine, as well as the colon, particularly in Peutz–Jeghers syndrome, suggesting that small intestinal polyps larger than 15 mm in diameter should be resected to prevent intussusception [3]. Knowledge regarding the diagnostic difficulty and rate of small intestinal polyps is extremely limited because of the insufficient spread of small intestinal endoscopy [4]. In the present case, it was an isolated jejunal juvenile polyp, and occurrence in the small intestine except in juvenile polyposis syndrome is extremely rare and has been reported infrequently [5].

Therefore, a review of this disorder, including the present case, was conducted, examining clinical features, onset age, sex differences, treatments, and examination procedures. Searching in the PubMed database, seven cases were reported between 1981 and 2022, including the present case [5–10]. Intussusception and anemia were present in four and three of the seven cases, respectively. Two of the three cases of anemia had suffered for a long duration until diagnosis. The present case also required two years from identification of anemia to diagnosis, suggesting the diagnostic difficulty of an isolated small intestinal polyp [5,7]. No recurrent and malignant cases were found, and no cases of an isolated juvenile polyp were diagnosed as polyposis later. All isolated small intestinal polyps were located in the jejunum, and the diagnosis was established by ultrasonographic identification of jejunojejunal intussusception in three of seven cases, and surgical resection of the polyps was required in five of seven cases. Except for the present case, only one patient with chronic iron deficiency anemia diagnosed by small intestinal CE and who underwent polypectomy using single-balloon endoscopy was not treated surgically [5]. The findings suggest that isolated small intestinal juvenile polyps were diagnosed mainly with the onset of intestinal intussusception, leading to surgery in most patients.

The facts seem to suggest the diagnostic difficulty of this disorder preceding intussusception. Abdominal ultrasonographic screening is thus extremely valuable for patients with chronic iron deficiency anemia presenting at around one year of age and relapsing after withdrawal of iron supplements, because no standard criteria for the acceptable age to perform small intestinal CE have been established.

In addition, elevated fecal calprotectin values and their utility as a diagnostic aid have been reported in colonic juvenile polyps [11]. Hestvik et al. reported that the median fecal calprotectin value was 75 µg/g (95% CI: 53–119) in healthy children aged one to four years [12], and Roca et al. recommended the cut-off value of 285.9 µg/g for healthy children aged one to four years [13]. Fecal calprotectin values measured at four points prior to polypectomy in the present case were 103, 134, 205, and 327 µg/g (in chronological order), demonstrating a similar level of elevation to that reported previously. However, no data related to fecal calprotectin in small intestinal juvenile polyps were found, and fecal calprotectin may also be useful as a diagnostic aid for isolated small intestinal juvenile polyps, although this was derived from the data of the present case alone. The present case is particularly valuable because the diagnosis of an isolated small intestinal juvenile polyp could be made based on the patient's symptoms without surgical complications such as intussusception and is the first report of treatment by DBE.

Isolated small intestinal juvenile polyps may be treated non-surgically without intussusception developing with immediate diagnosis of the polyp using abdominal ultrasonographic screening and fecal calprotectin appropriately to make the differential diagnosis of protracted iron deficiency anemia.

Author Contributions: M.N. and K.J. contributed to manuscript writing and editing, and data collection; N.A., K.K. and K.T. contributed to data analysis; M.S., T.K. and T.S. contributed to conceptualization and supervision. All authors have read and agreed to the published version of the manuscript.

Funding: This work was supported by a Japan Society for the Promotion of Science KAKENHI Grant-in-Aid for Young Scientists (grant number 20K16905).

Informed Consent Statement: Written informed consent was obtained from the parents to publish this paper.

Data Availability Statement: Not applicable.

Acknowledgments: The authors would like to thank the family for their permission to publish this case report.

Conflicts of Interest: The authors declare that they have no conflict of interest to disclose.

References

1. Mandhan, P. Juvenile colorectal polyps in children: Experience in Pakistan. *Pediatr. Surg. Int.* **2004**, *20*, 339–342. [CrossRef] [PubMed]
2. Yan, J.; Shen, Q.; Peng, C.; Pang, W.; Chen, Y. Colocolic intussusception in children: A case series and review of the literature. *Front. Surg.* **2022**, *9*, 873624. [CrossRef] [PubMed]
3. Van Lier, M.G.F.; Mathus-Vliegen, E.M.H.; Wagner, A.; van Leerdam, M.E.; Kuipers, E.J. High cumulative risk of intussusception in patients with Peutz–Jeghers Syndrome: Time to update surveillance guidelines? *Am. J. Gastroenterol.* **2011**, *106*, 940–945. [CrossRef] [PubMed]
4. Honda, W.; Ohmiya, N.; Hirooka, Y.; Nakamura, M.; Miyahara, R.; Ohno, E.; Kawashima, H.; AkihiroItoh; Watanabe, O.; Ando, T.; et al. Enteroscopic and radiologic diagnoses, treatment, and prognoses of small-bowel tumors. *Gastrointest. Endosc.* **2012**, *76*, 344–354. [CrossRef] [PubMed]
5. Krasaelap, A.; Lerner, D.; Southern, J.; Noe, J.; Chugh, A. Endoscopic removal of a single, painless, juvenile polyp in the small intestine causing anemia. *J. Pediatr. Gastroenterol. Nutr.* **2020**, *71*, 491–493. [CrossRef] [PubMed]
6. Kang, S.I.; Kang, J.; Kim, M.J.; Kim, I.K.; Lee, J.; Lee, K.Y. Laparoscopic-assisted resection of jejunojejunal intussusception caused by a juvenile polyp in an adult. *Case Rep. Surg.* **2014**, *2014*, 856765. [CrossRef]

7. Ceccanti, S.; Frediani, S.; Manganaro, F.; Barbato, M.; Marcheggiano, A.; Cozzi, D.A. Laparoscopic-assisted resection of juvenile polyp of the jejunum in a 3-year-old girl. *J. Pediatr. Surg.* **2012**, *47*, 426–429. [CrossRef]
8. Sah, S.P.; Agrawal, C.S.; Jha, P.C.; Rani, S. Juvenile polyps in the small intestine presenting as jejunojejunal intussusception in a 10-year-old child: Report of a case. *Surg. Today* **2002**, *32*, 828–830. [CrossRef] [PubMed]
9. Garcia Crespo, J.M.; Martin Pinto, F.; Dominguez Vallejo, J. Intestinal polyp of infrequent localization: Presentation of 2 cases. *An. Esp. Pediatr.* **1984**, *21*, 855–857. [PubMed]
10. Zimmermann, H.; Stauch, G.; Kamran, D. Juvenile polyp in the small bowel (author's transl). *Z. Kinderchir.* **1981**, *33*, 89–93. [CrossRef] [PubMed]
11. Das, S.R.; Karim, A.; RukonUzzaman, M.; Mazumder, M.W.; Alam, R.; Benzamin, M.; Marjan, P.; Sarker, N.; Akther, H.; Mondal, M. Juvenile polyps in Bangladeshi children and their association with fecal calprotectin as a biomarker. *Pediatr. Gastroenterol. Hepatol. Nutr.* **2022**, *25*, 52–60. [CrossRef] [PubMed]
12. Hestvik, E.; Tumwine, J.K.; Tylleskar, T.; Grahnquist, L.; Ndeezi, G.; Kaddu-Mulindwa, D.H.; Aksnes, L.; Olafsdottir, E. Faecal calprotectin concentrations in apparently healthy children aged 0-12 years in urban Kampala, Uganda: A community-based survey. *BMC. Pediatr.* **2011**, *11*, 9. [CrossRef] [PubMed]
13. Roca, M.; Rodriguez Varela, A.; Donat, E.; Cano, F.; Hervas, D.; Armisen, A.; Ana, A.; Maria, J.V.; Ander, S.; Ribes-Koninckx, C. Fecal calprotectin and eosinophil-derived neurotoxin in healthy children between 0 and 12 years. *J. Pediatr. Gastroenterol. Nutr.* **2017**, *65*, 394–398. [CrossRef] [PubMed]

Disclaimer/Publisher's Note: The statements, opinions and data contained in all publications are solely those of the individual author(s) and contributor(s) and not of MDPI and/or the editor(s). MDPI and/or the editor(s) disclaim responsibility for any injury to people or property resulting from any ideas, methods, instructions or products referred to in the content.

MDPI AG
Grosspeteranlage 5
4052 Basel
Switzerland
Tel.: +41 61 683 77 34

Diagnostics Editorial Office
E-mail: diagnostics@mdpi.com
www.mdpi.com/journal/diagnostics

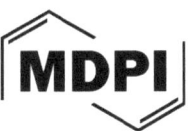

Disclaimer/Publisher's Note: The title and front matter of this reprint are at the discretion of the Guest Editors. The publisher is not responsible for their content or any associated concerns. The statements, opinions and data contained in all individual articles are solely those of the individual Editors and contributors and not of MDPI. MDPI disclaims responsibility for any injury to people or property resulting from any ideas, methods, instructions or products referred to in the content.

www.ingramcontent.com/pod-product-compliance
Lightning Source LLC
LaVergne TN
LVHW072329090526
838202LV00019B/2379